THE NEURAL BASIS
OF MOTOR CONTROL

THE NEURAL BASIS
OF MOTOR CONTROL

Vernon B. Brooks, Ph.D.

Professor of Physiology
The University of Western Ontario
London, Canada

New York   Oxford
OXFORD UNIVERSITY PRESS
1986

Oxford University Press

Oxford   New York   Toronto
Delhi   Bombay   Calcutta   Madras   Karachi
Petaling Jaya   Singapore   Hong Kong   Tokyo
Nairobi   Dar es Salaam   Cape Town
Melbourne   Auckland

and associated companies in
Beirut   Berlin   Ibadan   Nicosia

Published by Oxford University Press, Inc.,
200 Madison Avenue, New York, New York 10016

Oxford is a registered trademark of Oxford University Press

Library of Congress Cataloging-in-Publication Data
Brooks, Vernon B.
The neural basis of motor control.
Includes bibliographies and indexes.
1. Sensory-motor integration.   I. Title.
[DNLM: 1. Motor Activity.   2. Movement.
3.   Nervous System—physiology.   WE 103 B8733n]
QP369.B76   1986   612'.811   85-18780
ISBN 0-19-503683-2
ISBN 0-19-503684-0 (pbk.)

2   4   6   8   10   9   7   5   3   1

Printed in the United States of America
on acid free paper

Permission to reprint figures from the following sources is gratefully acknowledged:

Figs. 1.1, 1.3, 2.2, and 3.4 reprinted from Brooks, V. B., 1983. Motor control: how posture and movements are governed. *Physical Therapy*, 63:664-673. Figs. 1.4, 4.1, 4.2, 11.13, and 13.2 reprinted from Mountcastle, Vernon B., ed., *Medical physiology*, 14th ed., 1980, The C. V. Mosby Co., St. Louis, MO. Fig. 2.1 reprinted from Mc-Naught, A. B., and Callander, R., 1983. *Illustrated physiology*, 4th ed. Reprinted by permission of Churchill Livingstone, Edinburgh. Figs. 2.3B, 6.1, 8.3, and 11.12 reprinted by permission of the publisher from *Principles of neural science*, ed. E. R. Kandel and J. H. Schwartz. Copyright 1981 by Elsevier Science Publishing Co., Inc. Fig. 2.3C reprinted with permission from Mogenson, G. J., Jones, D. L., and Yim, C. Y., 1980. From motivation to action. *Prog. Neurobiol.* 14. Pergamon Press. Fig. 2.4 reprinted from M. M. Mesnlam, The functional anatomy and hemispheric specialization of directed attention, in *Trends in Neuroscience*, 6, p. 387. Copyright 1983 by Elsevier Publications (Cambridge). Fig. 2.5 reprinted by permission of the publisher from *Corticospinal neurons. Their role in movement*, by C. G. Phillips and R. Porter, p. 18. Copyright 1977 by Academic Press. Fig. 2.6 reprinted from Marsden, C. D., 1982. The mysterious motor function of the basal ganglia: The Robert Wartenberg Lecture. *Neurology* (NY) 32:514-39. Figs. 2.7, 5.4, 7.5D, 7.6, 7.7E, 7.8, 9.3, 9.4, 9.5D, 9.10, 9.14, 11.4, 12.8, 12.14, 12.15, 13.3, 13.7, 13.16, 14.3, 14.6, and 14.12 reprinted from *Exp. Brain Res.*, by permission of Springer-Verlag, Heidelberg. Fig. 3.3 reprinted from Houk, James, Feedback control of muscle: a synthesis of the peripheral mechanisms. In Mountcastle, Vernon B., ed. *Medical physiology*, 13th ed., 1974, The C. V. Mosby Co., St. Louis, MO. Figs. 3.5A,B, 4.3, 4.4B, 4.10, 12.3A, and 13.14 reprinted from *J. Physiol.* (London) with permission of the Physiological Society. Figs. 3.6, 4.5A, 4.6, 4.8B, 4.9A,B, 5.1, 5.5, 6.2A, 6.3B, 6.10A, 7.11, 7.12, 8.1, 8.2, 12.4, 12.6, 13.1, and 14.2 all from Motor control, 1981, Sect. I, vol. 2. *Handbook of physiology*, ed. V. B. Brooks. Reprinted with permission of the American Physiological Society, Bethesda, MD. Fig. 4.4A reprinted from McComas, A. J., 1977. Neuromuscular functions and disorders. Boston: Butterworths, p. 65. Figs. 4.4C, 4.5A, 5.13B, 7.5A-C, 10.9, 12.12A, and 13.10A,B, reprinted from *Brain Res.* or *Prog. Brain Res.*, with permission of Elsevier Biomedical Press B. V., Amsterdam. Figs. 4.5B, 6.3A, 7.7A-D, 9.5A,B,C, 9.10, 12.5, 12.12B, 12.13, and 13.4 reprinted from *J. Neurophysiol.* with the permission of the American Physiological Society, Bethesda, MD. Fig. 4.6A,B reprinted with permission from *Neuroscience*, 5, Fel'dman, A. G. Superposition of motor programs. 1980, Pergamon Press Ltd. Fig. 4.7 reprinted from Matthews, P. B. C., 1972, Mammalian muscle receptors and their central actions. London: Edward Arnold, p. 148. Previously unpublished record from experiments of Johnson and Matthews, 1962, The effects of fusimotor activity on the static responsiveness of primary and secondary ending of muscle spindles in the decerebrate cat, *Acta Physiol. Scand.* 44, 376–86. Fig. 4.9C reprinted from Houk, J. C., Crago, P. E., and Rymer, W. Z., 1981. Function of the spindle dynamic response in stiffness regulation. In *Muscle receptors and movement*, ed. A. Taylor and A. Prochazka, p. 307. London: Macmillan. Figs. 4.11 and 4.12 reprinted from *Exercise and Sports Science Reviews*, ed. R. L. Terjung, vol. 12, pp. 157–209. Copyright © 1984 by Macmillan Publishing Company. Reproduced by permission of the publisher. Fig. 5.2A, Fig. 5.6B, and 12.11 reprinted from Motor coordination, 1981, vol. 5. *Handbook of behavioral neurobiology*, ed. A. L. Towe and E. S. Luschei. Reprinted by permission of Plenum Publishing Co. Fig. 5.2B reprinted from Hultborn, H. M., Illert, M., and Santini, M., 1976. Convergence on interneurones mediating the reciprocal Ia inhibition of motoneurones. *Acta Physiol. Scand.* 96:193–201. Fig. 5.6A reprinted from Oscarsson, O., 1973. Functional organization of spinocerebellar paths. In Somatosensory system, vol. 2. *Handbook of sensory physiology*, ed. A. Iggo, p. 343. Berlin: Springer-Verlag. Figs. 5.7, 5.8, 5.11, 5.12, 9.1, and 11.1 reprinted from Barr, M. L., and Kiernan, J. A., 1983. *The human nervous system*, 4th ed. Philadelphia: Harper & Row. Figs. 5.9, 5.10, 11.2, 11.11, and 12.1 reprinted from Humphrey, D. R., 1983. Corticospinal systems and their control by premotor cortex, basal ganglia and cerebellum. In The clinical neurosciences, vol. 5. *Neurobiology*, ed. W. D. Willis, Jr. and R. N. Rosenberg. New York: Churchill Livingstone. Fig. 5.13A from Shinoda, Y. 1981. Divergent projection of individual corticospinal axons to motoneurons of multiple muscles in the monkey. *Neurosci. Lett.* 23: 7-12. Reprinted with permission of Elsevier Scientific Publishers. Fig. 6.5 from Chan, C. W. Y., Melvill Jones, G., and Catchglove, R. F. H., 1979. The "late" electromyographic response to limb displacement in man. *Clin. Neurophysiol.* 46: 182–88. Reprinted with permission of Elsevier Biomedical Press B. V., Amsterdam. Fig. 6.7 from Kwan, H. C., Murphy, J. T., and Repeck, M. W. 1979. Control of stiffness by the medium-latency electromyographic response to limb perturbation. *Can. J. Physiol. Pharmacol.* 57:277–85. Reprinted with permission of the National Research Council of Canada. Fig. 6.8 from Chan, C. W. Y., Melvill Jones, G., Kearney, R. E., and Watt, D. G. D., 1979. The "late" electromyographic response to limb displacement in man. *Electroencephalog. Clin. Neurophysiol.* 46:173–81. Reprinted by permission of Elsevier North-Holland Scientific Publishers, Shannon. Figs. 6.9, Fig. 6.10B, Fig. 8.4A,B, and 9.12 reprinted from Cerebral motor control in man, 1978, ed. J. E. Desmedt. *Prog. Clin. Neurophysiol.* 4. Reprinted with permission of S. Karger AG, Basel. Figs. 7.1 and 7.2 from Viviani, P., and Terzuolo, C., 1980. Spacetime invariance in learned motor skills. In Tutorials in motor behavior, ed. G. E. Stelmach and J. Requin. *Adv. Psychol.* 1:525–33. Reprinted with permission of Elsevier Biomedical Press B. V., Amsterdam. Figs. 7.3, 12.2, and 12.3B from Motor control mechanisms in health and disease, 1983, ed. J. E. Desmedt. *Adv. Neurol.* 39:12–29. Reprinted with permission of Raven Press, New York. Fig. 7.9 from Nelson, W. L., 1983. Physical principles for economics of skilled movements. *Biol. Cybern.* 46:135–47. Reprinted with permission of Springer-Verlag, Heidelberg. Fig. 8.5 from Lance, J. W., and McLeod, J. B., 1981. *A physiological approach to clinical neurology*. London: Butterworths. Figs. 9.9 and 9.13

Preface

Motor control is a rapidly growing field because of its basic interest and its practical implications. Postures and movements are our only physical means of interacting with the environment (besides external glandular secretions). Since we express our thoughts and emotions through postures and movements, they indicate our intentions, often revealingly so in our ubiquitous "body language"! The subject of motor control is of prime interest to physiologists and psychologists alike. How we perform motor tasks is relevant to all studies of work and sports, including kinesiology. How we can improve impaired performance is of central concern to the clinical neurological sciences and their associated specialties, to orthopedic surgery, to physical medicine and rehabilitation, and directly to the allied health professions, particularly occupational and physical therapy.

The field of motor control had its formal opening in the Western World with a symposium on "Muscular Afferents and Motor Control" led by Ragnar Granit in Stockholm in 1965, followed by his 1970 monograph on *The Basis of Motor Control*. That volume critically melded existing physiology and the newly declared "motor" theme, particularly in relation to the properties of alpha and gamma motoneurons (MNs). At the same time the first few, of many, North American conferences began to focus the views of a growing number of research workers. A meeting on "Neurophysiological Basis of Normal and Abnormal Motor Activities" was convened in 1966 by Yahr and Purpura, and a "Symposium on Cerebral and Cerebellar Motor Control" in 1968 by the author. That was a heady time, when common concerns became obvious for disciplines that were soon to merge into neuroscience.

The impetus of research in the fifties yielded a cornucopia of new understanding of brain systems, which in turn spawned new views of brain function. Two ingredients are needed for such productivity: a sense of direction for the research and an adequate level of financial support. Both had been in place since the early fifties, when Granit and Eccles led the way in studying the integrative action of the central nervous system by means of cellular analysis and McCulloch propounded theoretical means to show that the brain was a computing machine made of neurons. *Motor control* was born in the sixties amidst a flood of new facts and rules, for instance about sense organs in joints and muscles, for spinal interneurons and recruitment of motoneurons, for central transmitters, for cerebral and cerebellar circuits, and for many central input–output relations. New methods evolved in all aspects of neuroscience, including recording from single neurons in humans and in behaviorally trained monkeys. It was a Gold Rush of discovery, it was a roaring time!

New concepts flourished, particularly in the seventies, when recent knowledge about neural connections and functions was applied to how muscles hold and move joints. (Most of us were unaware of the Russian developments in biomechanics in the late fifties and early sixties and of Bernstein's fundamental theories of the interactions between brain, body and the environment, dating back to the thirties and forties. Alignment with parallel discoveries in the West had to await distribution of their translated works, some of which are listed at the end of Chapter 1). Terms such as "purpose," "volition" and "reflex" were redefined in the sixties and seventies. Engineering models began to enrich our views by assigning roles in control systems to modular assemblies of neurons in many parts of the brain, even to neurons within those parts. The comparison of intended and actual occurrences became recognized as a control device. Analogies to the logic flow of computer programs became commonplace. Feedback and feedforward controls, serial and parallel processing, and finally functions of distributed and adaptive systems, all found their neural counterparts. In little more than a decade motor control had come of age.

Today's exciting frontiers are revealing ever more subtle versatilities of the brain. Analyses of neural circuits and their codes continue but are now allied with the study of neuropsychology, biomechanics and plasticity in the nervous system. Circuit connections can now be altered temporarily by modulation of synaptic transmitters and permanently by induced growth of new connections. Practical pharmacology is advancing by leaps and bounds, and development of prosthetic devices is converging with neuroscience and robotics. We are witnessing the emergence of a new multidisciplinary movement science. Its applications offer the future health teams diverse, rational tools with tremendous therapeutic potential.

The Neural Basis of Motor Control provides a coherent text for students who have had courses in the neural sciences. The text presents a wide view of the integrative action of the nervous system in the control of posture and movement; its aim is to create basic understanding rather than to provide special professional instruction. Readers are expected to understand cellular processes like conduction, facilitation, inhibition, synaptic transmission, muscular contraction, as well as the structures and functions of the autonomic, limbic, sensory, motor and associative brain systems. Items of particular importance are reviewed in the text.

This text has been constructed on the basis of many years' experience in teaching undergraduate and graduate students in science and medicine. The book can be used at several levels, depending on the amount of time assigned for study of the text and background reading. Chapters are divided into units that can be covered mostly in one contact hour, some a little less and some a little more. Each chapter concludes with a brief summary of the most essential concepts presented in it. The depth of understanding students will reach by studying the text depends on the topics covered and on the required reading. To deal with all topics requires about 20 weekly sessions of 2 hours each in my experience. Furthermore, the teacher can grade the intensity of study by either requiring reading of the text only or selecting additional readings from the list of references at the end of each chapter. A number of reviews at different levels are usually provided about each topic (often at the end of the same chapter) to allow choices of course level. Some comments are made at the end of Chap. 1 about the levels of the major sources.

The text is written as if the workings of the brain were an orderly process that is well understood. This is of course not so for a field in a wild flux of rapid evolution. We need a simple map, however, to board this fast-moving train so that we may recognize the landscape as it flits by the windows. Reviews make up the bulk of the references, because it has been the author's experience that the majority of students seek to enlarge their view of the world through informed opinions rather than incidental detail. Original research papers usually contain too much about methods and results, and too little about the wider meaning of the work. This is especially pertinent in a changing field like motor control. Those who want to know more, should consult the reviews and their reference lists. That will also underscore the need for the innumerable (justified) qualifications that embroider even simple statements in the research literature. Such qualifications have mostly been omitted in this text in order to preserve a discernible story line. Learning how to read research reports is a separate matter. The illustrations are largely taken from reviews, and are referenced to the original material as citations in those reviews, to encourage students to increase their familiarity with some of the cited reviews. When investigators are referred to by name in the text, some of their writing is cited at the end of the chapter.

I hope that this book will be of value to all students who want to understand motor control, students in physiology, physiological psychology, the clinical neurological sciences, orthopedic surgery, the medical and surgical specialties, physical medicine and rehabilitation, physical education, kinesiology, and the health-allied professions, particularly occupational and physical therapy.

London, Ontario   V.B.B.
Canada
June 1985

References

Bernstein, N. 1967. *The coordination and regulation of movements*. Oxford: Pergamon Press.

Brooks, V. B. 1975. Opening remarks for the Symposium on Mechanisms in Motor Control. *Can. J. Neurol. Sci.* 2:221–222. (a listing of the early conferences on motor control)

Eccles, J. C. 1953. *The neurophysiological basis of mind*. Oxford: Clarendon Press.

Granit, R. 1981. Comments on history of motor control. In *Motor control*. Sect. 1, vol. 2. *Handbook of physiology*, ed. V. B. Brooks, pp. 1–16. Bethesda, Md.: American Physiological Society.

Jung, R. 1984. Sensory research in historical perspective: some philosophical foundations of perception. In *Sensory processes*. Sect. 1, vol. 3. *Handbook of physiology*, ed. I. Darian-Smith, pp. 1–74. Bethesda, Md.: American Physiological Society.

McCulloch, W. S. 1965. *Embodiments of mind*. Cambridge, Mass.: The M. I. T. Press.

Acknowledgments

This book grew out of the stimulation I received from teaching courses on motor control. I want to thank the students for the fun and joy that they have generated in the shared rediscovery of the subject every year. Two kinds of editorial assistance call for special thanks. First I must acknowledge the invaluable help given by Sherry Watts who composed many of the illustrations, largely taken from previous publications. Her help with this task has been a pleasure for many years. Second, I want to express my thanks for constructive comments to Christina Chan, Jon Hore, Keith Hayes, and Gordon Mogenson who read early drafts of some chapters, and to Pat Goldman-Rakic, Paul MacLean, and Victor Wilson, who read some later ones. Steve Spencer assisted in the editing of the introductory chapter. Finally, I wish to express my debt to Jeffrey House of the Oxford University Press for his support and editorial guidance from beginning to end.

Contents

THE NEURAL BASIS
OF MOTOR CONTROL

I
Motor Control

This part surveys the field of motor control with the aim of grasping the scope and the present state of the field. We recognize that control of posture and movements requires the cooperation of the nervous system, the muscles and the skeleton. Motor control is an interface between the neurosciences, kinesiology and biomechanics. In this survey we therefore raise many topics and point at their relations, but detailed discussion is reserved for later parts (beginning with Chap. 3.2). In line with the purpose of surveying the field, references at the end of the first chapter identify some general background reading and broad reviews.

1

What Is Motor Control?

The term motor control refers to the study of postures and movements and also to the functions of mind and body that govern posture and movement. In this context "posture" means the static position of any part of the body, rather than just the description of a standing or sitting position of the whole body, as its common usage suggests. Postures of the limbs, the trunk and the whole body are maintained by muscular effort. "Movements" are the transition from one posture to another. Postures and movements can be assumed consciously or as automatic adjustments, a distinction that formerly denoted "voluntary" as opposed to "reflex" actions. However, these words no longer adequately describe what is meant. Reflexes are best defined as responses evoked with great probability by particular stimuli. In fact, there is a continuum in the degree to which volition affects movements.

We are born with only rudimentary motor abilities; the rest have to be learned by active practice during infancy, childhood and thereafter. We have to learn to stand and to walk, to use our hands, to acquire practical skills, and to participate in sports. This learning is never directed at the control of single muscles but instead concerns the choice and timing of many. Control has to be acquired over their functional combinations that act on the joints on which they are inserted. In fact, control has to be acquired over related joints. Thus, motor learning is concerned with the *coordination* of joints, and as a matter of detail, the muscles that move and hold them. Motivation, alertness, concentration and other states of mind are critical in motor learning, because they determine how well we attend to the learning and execution of any motor task. These two processes of learning and doing are inevitably intertwined; we learn as we do and we do only as well as we have learned.

Once a particular movement has been learned, we use a plan of motor action to carry out that particular task when necessary. For example, hitting a ball with a golf club (Fig. 1.1) requires coordination of the trunk, legs and arms in relation to each other so that the right forces act at the right joints at just the right times. How is this achieved? It appears that we need to have memories of two items: how it felt to make a particular movement and the result that was achieved by it. Athletes are said to "visualize" their performance before beginning. We select the desired movement according to the remembered result (for instance, where the ball went the last time we hit it "like that"). The task is carried out and modified by adjustments, so that the sensations from the evolving movement match the memory of "how it felt."

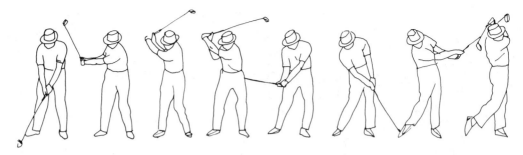

Fig. 1.1. Outline drawings of a golfer during a swing. Note how postures of the trunk accommodate shifts of the body's center of gravity, and how head, neck, trunk and all four limbs are coordinated by skeletomuscular linkages. (From Brooks, 1983)

Motor memory is twofold: how it felt to make the effort and what result was achieved by it.

Accurate perceptions of the force needed to make a movement or to maintain a posture are essential for their correct generation. Our "sense of effort" is based on messages that arise from sense organs in and near muscles (muscle spindles and Golgi tendon organs). The information contained in these messages is used in two ways: it regulates ongoing, present activity, and it guides, as part of the motor memory, the execution of such a task in the future. Thus our sense of effort and its memory are essential to both the execution and planning of motor action.

When a motor action is planned, the overall strategy is organized into smaller component parts or "programs" that are assembled in the brain. For example, as adults we have long since learned how to use our feet for standing and walking, but precise ways to move them, involving a new plan made up of new component programs, must be learned for any particular task, be it playing golf, working at a skilled craft or compensating for a physical disability. As an indication of the complexity involved, consider the requirements for a successful golf swing. The stance must be right to afford stability during the movement with the feet placed far enough apart and the legs and trunk braced to prevent sway when the center of gravity shifts as the club is brought for-

ward. Bracing involves two components of its own: setting the muscles at the proper steady tensions as well as setting the readiness to respond to stretch of any muscle with contraction of that same muscle (i.e., the gain of the stretch reflex, referred to as tone). The stance and tone of the lower limbs and trunk must be correct before a successful swing can be executed. The upper arms also must be placed and braced appropriately for the coming movement. The point is, not only do the muscles involved in the desired movement require programmed activity, but so do the muscles in the rest of the body that provide postural support for the moving parts—that ensure their correct static position. In a normal subject, these various muscle actions are generated in proper combinations to produce the desired action. This also applies to simpler motor tasks like the one illustrated in Fig. 1.2A, where the tips of the index fingers of each hand were brought together. In this case the number of programs necessary to complete the motor plan are fewer but the general requirement for coordination of postures and movements in a smooth sequence is the same.

The interdependence of movements and postures that we have described has important implications for physical and occupational therapy and for physical education. New postures of the trunk and limbs can often be learned to permit the performance of movements that could not be made before because of some disability. Fortunately, it is becoming possible to calculate new, usable combinations of postures and movements that can substitute for inefficient or disordered ones (Chap. 9.6). Therapists and coaches can then teach individuals these new combinations.

1. Planning and Programs

Learned tasks such as the action sequences depicted in Figs. 1.1 and 1.2A are produced by overall plans (also called complex motor programs) that create smooth, fast, skillful action. Motor programs are a set of muscle commands that are structured before the motor acts begin and that can be sent to the muscles with the correct timing so that the entire sequence can be carried out in the absence of peripheral feedback. In fact, feedback is normally used to adjust programmed movements. Looking at the brain as the machinery where programs are structured, we can think of motor plans and programs as communications within the central nervous system (the brain and spinal cord) that are based on past experience and can contribute to the generation of intended postures and movements. Feedback brings the program commands up to date with how their execution is coming along and corrects errors. Motor plans are made up of several programs that, in turn, consist of coordinated, smaller learned subroutines called subprograms. These subprograms not only encode actual muscle activity but also act as commands for the initiation of other subprograms that also produce motor action and command yet other subprograms. This hierarchy of plans, programs and subprograms finally exits into nonlearned automatic ("reflex") adjustments. Subprograms can have various levels of complexity. Some large subprograms can be discerned in Fig. 1.1: the golf swing and stroke are made up of sequences of movements and postures. Like all movements, they involve many joints because the skeleton is linked by many muscles. It

is the existence of the mechanical skeletomuscular linkages across the joints that demands muscular coordination. The neural bases for spinal subroutines and their interplay with supraspinal guidance are taken up in Chaps. 4 and 5 and continue to occupy us in Chaps. 6–10. Programs of the middle level intrude early, however, because their use is almost ubiquitous. We emerge into the realm of motor plans from the highest level as soon as we consider the structure and function of the middle level (in Chaps. 11–14).

Movements that involve a number of joints are difficult to learn in their entirety because multijoint (or "compound") movements, and the use of muscles acting across those joints, depend on complex motor programs. These movements may therefore be attempted first with the use of successive, less complex movements, each of which can be modified independently. When a successful combination has been achieved, the entire action sequence is learned and thereafter planned as a single unit. In practice, we reach skillful performance by successive approximations. The brain focuses on supporting or moving what is the most important part of the body for the action, for instance the hand or the head or the eyes. The "supporting players," the joints and muscles that support and transport the "star" of attention for the brain (be it hand, head or eyes), are coordinated in subsidiary fashion.

When an overall program fails, the brain reverts to composing multijoint movements once more from sequential simple movements. This decomposition from the complex into the simple has been shown to occur after (neo)cerebellar damage as in the poorly coordinated movements of arms and fingers of a patient with cerebellar disease (Fig. 1.2B). The fingers do not meet because individual movements become inaccurate (dysmetric) during cerebellar dysfunction, which is aggravated by their poor coordination. Simple movements are easier to think about in the abstract, but they do not ordinarily occur by themselves because various postural muscles always cooperate with intended movements to support the body and limbs. Simple movements, however, can be studied in isolation if support is provided for the body and the moving joint. A good demonstration that daily use of overall plans or programs for successive multijoint movements do, in fact, relate to posture, are the stereotyped adjustments made by normal subjects against postural sway caused by a disturbance (Chap. 9.6).

Although the simple single joint movements just described are easier to think about and examine, they do not normally occur alone because there is always cooperation from various postural muscles. Simple movements can be studied by providing support for the moving part and the rest of the body. For example, if the body is supported in a chair and the elbow is resting on a stable platform, simple movements at the elbow or wrist joint can be studied.

As mentioned earlier, even steady holding postures (like the arm positions in the first diagrams of Figs. 1.1 and 1.2A) are dependent on motor programs. In this case, the subprograms would code for the control of tensions (i.e., degree of muscle activity) at the various joints involved (shoulder, elbow, wrist and fingers). During movement, programs produce a controlled change in posture with planned speed and force toward another planned posture. In other words, both the end point of the movement and the path to be taken are programmed, but the chain of controlled events can be modified by sensory information when necessary to achieve the desired path and final goal.

2. Sensory Feedback

A critical element in any programmed posture or movement is the timing of the application of muscular force. For example, in fast movements this requires planning for both the onset and duration of the burst of activity in the mover, the agonist

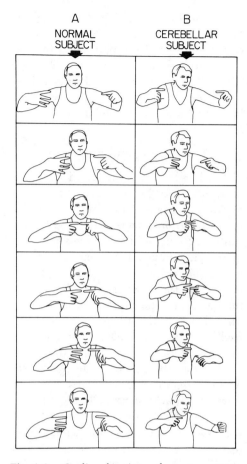

Fig. 1.2. Outline drawings of a movement sequence in which a normal subject (A) brings the tips of the index fingers together and then pulls them apart. (B) Equivalent sequence for a patient with cerebellar disease. Upper and lower arms are poorly coordinated, and the fingertips miss each other.

muscle. How detailed is the timed planning of such force by motor programs and subprograms? Do they contain *all* the necessary instructions that are fed forward from the brain to muscles via the spinal cord, or does a component of feedback regulation of timing exist? Complete feedforward of instructions, without any feedback, probably only occurs in all-out high-speed movements without much concern for skilled control. This is the type of programming that might be exhibited by an inexperienced baseball player who swings at the ball as hard as possible "with eyes closed" and only hopes that contact might be made. This type of fast movement is termed "ballistic" because the course the limb will follow is totally determined by the initial burst of activity in the agonist muscle, just as the ballistic flight of a bullet is determined by the initial charge in the cartridge. A more modern analogy would be a nonguided rocket whose ballistic flight path is determined by the brief, explosive burn of its engine. In skilled ballistic movements, the program for movement not only times the activity in the agonist but also in its opponent, the antagonist. An example of a skilled ballistic movement is given in Fig. 1.3, showing how agonist and antagonist actions are both *planned together* before the movement, which characteristically lasts less than 0.2 seconds because it is made with a sudden, steep increase of muscular force. Planned flight termination confers a measure of skill: soft rocket landings are made possible by programmed firing of the braking engine. In "skilled ballistic" movements (Fig. 1.1), programmed antagonist actions are part of the plan to temper the "initial impulse" and to protect the wrists of our golfer from being jarred on impact. A skilled ballistic movement is represented by the tracings on the left-hand side of Fig. 1.3.

Figure 1.3 illustrates how the early planning of timing and muscle activity translates into movement. Before and after movements, indicated by vertical broken lines, positions are maintained by tonic EMG levels. For example, a flexed posture at the elbow joint would require tonic activity in the biceps brachii muscle. The extension movement begins with relaxation of the antagonist muscle (biceps in our example), whose activity was necessary to maintain the premovement posture but would oppose the desired movement. The propelling (agonist) muscle, triceps brachii, also commonly relaxes just before its burst of activity that initiates the movement, but this is not illustrated in Fig. 1.3. The linked timing of activity onset in agonist and antagonist is indicated by arrows

in the figure and betrays early planning of not only the initiation of movement but also its termination. The brain therefore must calculate increases and decreases of force (which translate into acceleration and deceleration of the limb) even before the movement begins. Figure 1.3 indicates the relatively long time needed for coupling the electrical excitation of muscle fibers to the mechanical changes of the contractile elements. We see in the diagrams of EMG and kinematic variables for programmed movements that the antagonist has to be excited even while the mechanical action of the agonist is still being carried out. This is no more than an apparent paradox; it is in fact an outward sign of the inward advance planning of the brain. That the activity in the opposing muscles is programmed (and not therefore dependent on sensory feedback) becomes obvious when a nonyielding obstacle is unexpectedly placed in the path of the intended movement. The same patterns of muscle activity and resultant force are produced, whether they actually result in movement of the limb, or force is generated while actual movement is prevented by the obstacle.

Programming for the timing of muscle activity in agonist and antagonist can be seen in Fig. 1.3 for the briefest (and also fastest) movement shown (a skilled ballistic movement), as well as for one of moderate speed and duration, termed a continuous movement. The name "continuous" is derived from the bell-shaped velocity profile with only a single peak, indicating that no adjustments were necessary to correct for undershoot or overshoot and bring the limb to the desired final position or posture. Simple continuous movements typically are propelled by a triphasic agonist–antagonist–agonist pattern of EMG activity (which is exaggerated in Fig. 1.3), as opposed to the biphasic agonist–antagonist pattern of the skilled ballistic movement. The initial agonist burst in ballistic and continuous movements is centrally programmed, because it is not altered by

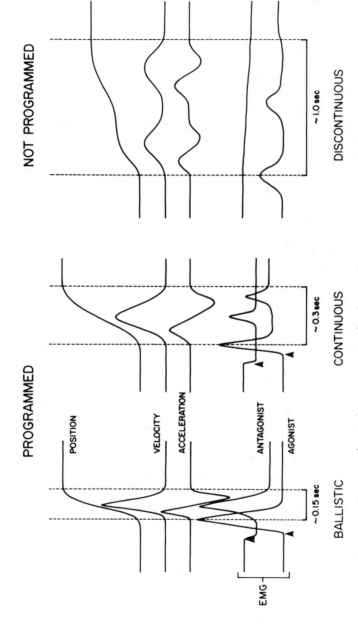

Fig. 1.3. Programs for simple movements often betray their presence by a virtual lack of corrections of movement parameters and by smooth transitions between "hold" and "move" phases. Skilled ballistic (very fast and controlled) movements and continuous movements (of moderate speed) are most programmed, while discontinuous (slow) movements are least programmed. Movement amplitudes are about 30 to 20 deg. *Arrowheads* mark onset of EMG changes. (From Brooks, 1983)

sudden changes of the load against which the muscle is working. Simple continuous movements of moderate speed are common components of natural, programmed movements.

Most movements depend on sensory information that is fed back from peripheral sense organs e.g., muscle spindles, joint receptors and cutaneous receptors) to the spinal cord and brain. (Think of familiar routines such as getting dressed, eating a meal or writing.) If no sensory guidance is used for either agonist or antagonist commands, the mode of control is called "feedforward" or "open loop" (Fig. 1.4). The advantage of open-loop control is speed of adjustments, but its disadvantage is the lack of sensory guidance, present in closed-loop control. In a closed-loop system the feedforward (programmed) commands are remembered or "stored" and compared with the information arriving from sensory organs in the periphery. Thus, the codes for intended movements can be compared to information about the movements as they actually occur. Any mismatch between the intended and the actual events can be corrected for by intended as well as by automatic adjustments, demonstrating the advantage of the closed-loop, feedback mode of control.

Figure 1.3 describes arm movements that "step" from one stationary target to another. Another kind of intended movement (not illustrated here) is made in pursuit of moving targets. "Pursuit" movements are also made by estimating the initial boosting impulse required to catch up with the target, correcting residual errors, and making an estimated final braking impulse to halt the movement. They are thus made as a sequence of small steps, much like discontinuous movements. This is discussed further in Chap. 7.1.

As has been discussed, when making planned, programmed movements, we normally use sensory feedback for adjustment of the speed and path taken to optimize accuracy, but we can execute the task without feedback if it is not available or if

speed is the critical element. This option of ignoring feedback does not apply to movements that have not yet been learned and therefore cannot be planned. These movements are feedback-dependent and not programmed (as labeled in Fig. 1.3) or are at best minimally programmed. These are the movements we use when we are uncertain how to proceed. A novice golfer might move the club in that uncertain way slowly back and forth during his first lesson on how to get a measure of the distance between club and ball before swinging. The beginner at any skilled motor action must start by making the movements in such a way that feedback about the evolving movement can be used to adjust the path of motion to achieve the desired result. In the case of a tennis swing, for example, it is to have the racquet head contact the ball.

Two-way communication between sensory and motor systems is essential for normal behavior and particularly for the learning of new tasks, and vision is one of the most important senses. Only after practicing the swing can the player stop looking at the ball and use the now programmed movement to direct the shot to the desired spot, without that visual aid. Learning to "touch-type" is another familiar example where visual aid is used throughout learning. Even though vision is an important guide, it is not always sufficient in itself. The cerebellar patient in Fig. 1.2B watches helplessly as his unwilling fingers miss the mark despite slowed movements. He suffers from loss of proprioceptive guidance. Proprioception is the most important sense from inside our bodies (as opposed to "exteroceptive" senses, which monitor the environment). It is the sense of what the muscle itself (proprio-) is doing. Sense organs in the tendons signal how hard the muscles are pulling, and sense organs within the muscles signal how much and how fast the muscles are being stretched. Proprioceptive feedback assists the CNS in calculating, for instance, how much the triceps brachii muscle is stretched when the biceps brachii muscle contracts to flex the elbow. In addition, we orient our limbs with the aid of *kinesthetic* input from receptors in the joints and *somatic* input from skin sensors for touch, temperature or pain. In programmed movements, the expectation of what sensory inflow will occur is taken into account to preserve the programmed ("intended") action. Other senses such as hearing and the sense of balance are also important. In a later chapter we will explore the responses to "vestibular" inputs, the reports from the inner ear about head position in relation to gravity and about head movement. The influence that expected sensory signals would have is modified by internal ("corollary") signals according to the expectation, which dampens down possible unwanted reactions of, for instance, the stretch reflex. Internal adjustment of sensory inflow (not shown in Fig. 1.4) is part of movement programming and will be taken up in Chap. 6.

3. Learning and Motor Skill

We earlier discussed the concept of comparing intended with actual or evolving movements. Information about the progress of evolving movements comes directly through sensory peripheral feedback, as has been outlined, and also through internal feedback from neurons in the brain and spinal cord that integrate information from several inputs. (Some spinal interneurons, for example, can signal changes in posture because they receive inputs about several joints.) All the information about the evolving movement is fed back to centers in the brain that compare what is happening with what should have happened and on this basis make compensatory adjustments. The better the movements have been learned, the fewer the corrections that are needed. Such movements acquire the continuous velocity profile illustrated in Fig. 1.3. They are faster and can be strung together into smoother compound movements and postures; in other words, they add skill to natural movements. Motor skill thus is the optimal use of programmed movements.

How does this learning of movements and programming optimize motor skill? Clearly, learning of any kind depends on experience. If a motor task is executed successfully and this success is recognized (i.e., we *make* a good shot in tennis and we *know* it is a good shot), then the neural and muscular activity associated with that movement is committed to "motor memory" as subprograms. Continued use of the same programs for the performance of the

Fig. 1.4. Regulation diminishes disturbances of the regulated output variables. In the (fast) feedforward mode, regulation by the controller is based directly on sensed disturbances. In the (slower) feedback, or "servo" mode, regulation is based on the sensed effects that disturbances have on the regulated variables. (From Houk, 1980)

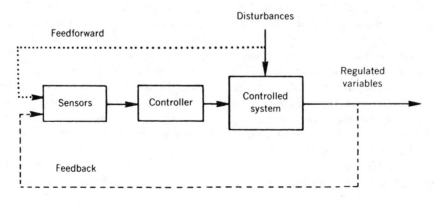

task to be learned increases the accuracy of the memory, and therefore that of movement execution. Thus learning uses both the sensory and the motor systems: we remember both how we made the successful movement and how it should feel if it is proceeding as intended.

We can gain a better understanding of these ideas by considering an actual example of motor learning. Figure 1.5 describes the learning process for the simple task of turning a handle in the horizontal plane and holding it for a few seconds in "target" zones at one end or the other before the return movement (Fig 1.5A). The subjects were monkeys that were given *no* special incentive to make movements of any particular kind or speed; they were merely expected to move the handle to the alternate target within a couple of seconds after the target display switches from one place to the alternate one. Similar results are now also being obtained with human subjects.

Figure 1.5B shows a striking result: as training progresses, the discontinuous movements made by an untrained animal are replaced by continuous ones. This result is representative of the progress of many animals. Learning to make continuous movements means learning to *plan the starts and stops together*—that is, to program accelerations and decelerations together so that postures and movements can follow one another without the need for corrections (Fig. 1.3). The bottom line in Fig. 1.5B shows that, in fact, partially programmed movements remain uncommon; in other words, the animal does not plan accelerations without planning decelerations. This means that the brain learns to estimate the "move" programs together with (i.e., in relation to) the "hold" programs for arm postures before and after arm movements. Getting set for take-off, making a correct flight, and bracing for landing are all learned together. When these subprograms are matched properly, the velocity profile is bell-shaped (continuous), with only minimal discontinuities.

Why do humans and animals adopt this strategy when they are not required to do so? Since the need is not imposed upon the subjects, it must be found within the subjects, in the "wisdom of the body," which, after all, includes the brain. The need seems to be economy of planning the effort, how to optimize various aspects of the movement to suit them best to the prevailing circumstances. Continuous velocity profiles turn out to be versatile from that point of view (Chap. 7.2).

Another important aspect of motor learning is revealed by Fig. 1.5C. Motor skill, that is the use of programmed movements, increases rapidly only after the animals gain *insight* into the behavioral requirements. This is documented by the abrupt rise of the skill learning curve to make accurately programmed movements after the beginning of understanding, when the subjects begin to make behaviorally correct responses by deliberate choice rather than randomly, which gets half of them right and half wrong. The transition to insight is marked by the dotted circle and line as "50% behavioral sureness." The behavioral requirements were to make moves that were related purposefully to the target indicators, that is, to move at the right times and in the right directions. Figures 1.5B and C show that some programmed movements were made right from the beginning of training, but that neither of the two trainees increased their use ("know-*how*") much until they showed signs of understanding *what* it was that they were expected to do. The result means that individuals improve their motor skill through the use of programmed movements only after they have properly understood the behavioral goal for which the movements are to be used.

Movements are learned from past experience if they are recognized as having been successful (Fig. 1.5C). How is such reinforced experience converted into motor memory? This amounts to asking how neurons can be adapted so that they are more likely to respond to previously useful inputs, that is, how neural centers are made to generate subprograms. This process, which will be discussed in Chaps. 11, 13, and 14, rests on the recognition of the usefulness of successful motor behavior, and that this recognition is communicated from higher to lower brain centers. Learning from previous experience thus depends on sensing and moving, not just on sensing. The two processes are facilitated by unceasing communications between the sensory and motor systems. One example where this is of great importance is "active touch," or handling objects. Their shapes and textures are perceived better when the objects are actively explored than when they are passed over the passive hands and fingers. As a consequence, manipulation of such objects becomes more adroit with continued practice. Retention and improvement of skill depends on continued use of appropriately adjusted programs. Maxims such as "try, try, try again" and "practice makes perfect" express the common knowledge that continued practice improves learned movements. Another maxim, "use it or lose it," reminds us that the most skillful use of motor programs tends to fade unless the programs are actively refreshed.

Most of our movements and postures, no matter how casual, contain programmed components. These programs can be learned and applied in a vast variety of situations, because the central nervous system adapts to its environment. We use the well-developed sensory images of our bodies and those of our motor capabilities. Spinal motoneurons, for instance, are adapted to (they "know") the properties of

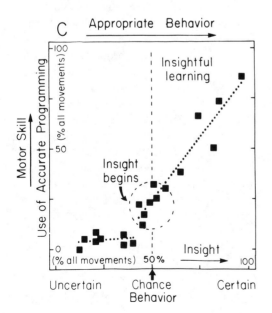

Fig. 1.5. This figure teaches two points about motor learning. First, starts and stops are learned together for programmed movements (A, B). Second, Motor skill, i.e. use of accurately programmed movements, depends on the insight gained about appropriate behavior for the task (C). (A) *left:* monkey performs task of turning a handle into alternate targets by flexing and extending the elbow. *right:* position and velocity traces of non-programmed and programmed movements (see Fig.1.3). (B) During motor learning continuous movements supplant discontinuous ones, but partially programmed movements remain unchanged. (C) Motor skill grows from the beginning of insight about appropriate behavior for the task (*circled area*) in direct proportion to the progress of insight towards certainty. [(B) based on flexions and extensions of a monkey, (C) on extensions only; All data and A, B from Brooks, Kennedy and Ross, 1983; C from Brooks, 1986]

the muscles to which they are connected, and more generally, *the brain knows the body that it resides in,* after all they grew up together. To this we could add that they "grew up together" in the gravitational field of the earth, implying that many of our antigravity efforts are likely to have been learned. There is much evidence that reflexes are adjusted to move and hold limbs according to the gravitational effects as well as to the equal and opposite mechanical effects exerted by limb movements on the body and by the body on the ground. For instance, we have to *learn* to overcome postural illusions when raising or lowering our bodies by muscular effort in abnormally strong or weak gravitational fields. The point here is that, since the central nervous system is adapted to the body as its environment, motor tasks may be learned by concentrating on the overall objective and letting the hierarchy of motor centers coordinate the execution.

Thinking of the brain and body growing up together is not merely a quip; it reflects the clinical finding that slowly growing brain lesions do not necessarily betray their presence by early signs of dysfunction, because the brain learns to *adapt* and to *compensate* for them in movements and postures. It is the suddenly inflicted lesion that can produce immediate, catastrophic consequences.

An urgent problem for therapists is to learn how to help patients replace motor programs that have been lost after brain damage, for example by a stroke. The inactive tissue disconnects remaining cortex and subcortical centers from their programmed inputs; consequently, the capacity to make voluntary movements is impaired. Unwanted, disabling postures are "released" and take over as the remaining inputs become predominantly inappropriate. New, unwanted influences are probably also created by invading, new neural connections. These pathological influences will generate unwanted programs, leading to abnormal postures and limited

movement capability. Just as repetition of good programs leads to good results, repetition of poor programs leads to bad results and the need to "unlearn" them. It may be possible to thwart this sequence by early efforts to help patients acquire more desirable programs through occupational and physical therapy.

4. Summary

Motor control is the study of posture and movements that are controlled by central commands and spinal reflexes, and it is also the name given to the functions of mind and body that govern posture and movement. The two modes interact extensively during the execution of motor plans comprising sets of feedforward commands for complex motor actions learned from successful, previous motor performance. Behavioral plans are made up of programs for various parts of the performance. Subjects develop motor skill (use of accurate programs) only after they have gained insight into the appropriate task-behavior. Programs, in turn, are composed of subprograms that encode even smaller details of the execution of planned motor acts. Postures and movements are guided by a mixture of programs and sensory feedback, because calculations made ahead of time in the central nervous system are always corrected after comparison to central and peripheral reports about reality. The central nervous system succeeds in bringing about planned actions because it adapts its neural commands according to the prevailing circumstances, for example, whether the movement is being resisted or not. The skill of natural (compound) movements, which involve many muscles and joints, depends on how well their component simple movements are fitted together in the planning. This integrative fitting includes the postural tensions before and after movements. For practically all movements, the forces of agonist and antagonist muscles are planned and timed ahead of movement onset. This also applies to skilled ballistic movements, which are characterized by a rapid rise, and calculated fall, of muscle tension.

References

The reference list for this introductory chapter contains general background reading at various levels for this entire book. It is not meant to be a comprehensive list. Specialized monographs are cited at the ends of appropriate chapters.

General Textbooks

Barr, M. L., and Kiernan, J. A. 1983. *The human nervous system.* 4th ed. Philadelphia: Harper & Row. (a text for health science students, 412 pp.)

The Brain. 1979. A *Scientific American* book (September 1979 issue). San Francisco: W. H. Freeman & Co. (general readership)

Brodal, A. 1981. *Neurological anatomy.* 3rd ed. New York: Oxford University Press. (a reference work for graduate students and professionals, 1053 pp.)

Kandel, E. R., and Schwartz, J. H., eds. 1985. *Principles of neural science.* 2nd ed. New York: Elsevier/North-Holland. (a text oriented toward health science students, 731 pp.)

Mountcastle, V. B., ed. 1980. *Medical physiology.* 14th ed. St. Louis: C. V. Mosby Co. (an extensive text for health science and graduate students. Vol. 1, on the nervous system, 947 pp.)

Nieuwenhuys, R., Voogt, J., and van Huizen, Chr. 1981. *The human central nervous system.* 2nd rev. ed. Berlin: Springer Verlag. (a text for graduate students and professionals, 253 pp.)

Schmidt, R. F., ed. 1978. *Fundamentals of neurophysiology.* 2nd ed. New York: Springer Verlag. (an outline for health science students, 339 pp.)

Schmidt, R.F., and Thews, G., eds. 1983. *Human physiology.* Berlin: Springer Verlag. (a text for health science students. Part I, on the nervous system, 328 pp.)

Shepherd, G. M. 1983. *Neurobiology.* New York: Oxford University Press. (a text for undergraduate students, 611 pp.)

Somjen, G. 1983. *Neurophysiology: the essentials.* Baltimore: Williams & Wilkins. (a brief text for health science students, 551 pp.)

Stein, J. F. 1982. *An introduction to Neurophysiology.* Oxford: Blackwell Scientific Publications. (an outline for undergraduate and health science students, 386 pp.)

Some Books about Motor Control

Bernstein, N. 1967. *The coordination and regulation of movements.* Oxford: Pergamon Press. (for graduate students and professionals)

Eccles, J. C. 1973. *The understanding of the brain.* New York: McGraw-Hill Book Co. (general readership and for undergraduate students)

Evarts, E. V., Shinoda, Y., and Wise, S. P. 1984. *Neurophysiological approaches to higher brain functions.* New York: John Wiley & Sons. (for graduate students and professionals)

Granit, R. 1970. *The basis of motor control.* New York: Academic Press. (for graduate students and professionals)

Granit, R. 1977. *The purposive brain.* Cambridge, Mass.: The M.I.T. Press. (for all levels)

Kelso, J. A. S., ed. 1982. *Human motor behavior: an introduction.* Hillsdale, N.J.: Lawrence Erlbaum Associates. (for beginning undergraduates)

Kelso, J. A. S., and Clark, J.C. 1982. *The development of human movement control and coordination.* New York: John Wiley & Sons. (for graduate students and professionals)

Kots, Y. M. 1977. *The organization of voluntary movement.* New York: Plenum Press. (for professionals and graduate students)

Lance, J. W. and McLeod, J. G. 1981. *A physiological approach to clinical neurology.* 3rd ed. London: Butterworths. (for graduate and professional students)

Matthews, P. B. C. 1972. *Mammalian muscle receptors and their central actions.* London: Edward Arnold. (for graduate students and professionals)

Phillips, C. G., and Porter, R. 1977. *Corticospinal neurones: their role in movement.* New York: Academic Press. (for graduate students and professionals)

Schmidt, R. A. 1982. *Motor control and learning: a behavioral emphasis.* Champaign, Ill.: Human Kinetics Publishers. (for undergraduates)

Handbooks and Symposia

Brooks, V. B., ed. 1981 *Handbook of Physiology.* Sect. 1, Vol. 2. *Motor control.* Bethesda,

Md.: American Physiological Society. (33 chaps., 1514 pp.)

Darian-Smith, I., ed. 1984. *Handbook of Physiology*. Sect. 1, vol. 3. *Sensory processes*. Bethesda, Md.: American Physiological Society. (25 chaps., 1217 pp.) The "Handbook" series of the APS presents a critical, comprehensive presentation of physiological knowledge and concepts.

Desmedt, J. E., ed. 1983. *Motor control mechanisms in health and disease*. Vol. 39. *Advances in Neurology*, New York: Raven Press. (more clinically oriented than the "Handbook" volumes above; 67 chaps., 1200 pp.)

Edelman, G. M., Gall, W. E., and Cowan, W. M., eds. 1984. *Dynamic aspects of neocortical function*. New York: John Wiley & Sons. (22 chaps., 718 pp.)

Lynch, G., McGaugh, J. L., and Weinberger, N. M., eds. 1984. *Neurobiology of learning and memory*. New York: Guilford Press. (34 chaps., 528 pp.)

Schmitt, F. O., and Worden, F. G., eds. 1974. *The neurosciences, third study program*. Cambridge, Mass.: M.I.T. Press. (93 chaps., mostly detailed. 1091 pp.)

Stelmach, G. E., ed. 1976. *Motor control: issues and trends*. New York: Academic Press. (9 fairly theoretical chaps., 230 pp.)

Stelmach, G. E., and Requin, J., eds. 1980. *Tutorials in motor behavior*. Vol. 1. *Advances in psychology*. Amsterdam: North-Holland. (41 short essays, some rather detailed, 680 pp.)

Towe, A. L., and Luschei, E. S., eds. 1981. *Handbook of behavioral neurobiology*. Vol. 5. *Motor coordination*. New York: Plenum Press. (general, well-balanced overviews with less detail than the APS volumes; 11 chaps., 640 pp.)

Willis, W. D., Jr., and Rosenberg, R. N., eds. 1982. *The clinical neurosciences*. Vol. 5. *Neurobiology*. New York: Churchill Livingstone. (basic neuroscience for clinically oriented readers, fairly detailed, 626 pp.)

Illustrations in Chapter 1

Brooks, V. B. 1983. Motor control: how posture and movements are governed. *Phys. Ther.* 63:664–673. [Figs. 1.1 and 1.3]

Brooks, V. B., Kennedy, P. R., and Ross, H. G. 1983. Movement programming depends on understanding of behavioral requirements. *Physiol. Behav.* 31:561–563. [Fig. 1.5A, B]

Brooks, V. B. 1985. How are "move" and "hold" programs matched? In *Cerebellar functions*, eds. J. R. Bloedel, J. Dichgans, and W. Precht. Berlin: Springer Verlag, pp. 1–21. [Fig. 1.5A, B]

Brooks, V. B. 1986. How does the limbic system assist motor learning? *Brain. Behav. Evolution*. In press [Fig. 1.5C]

Houk, J. C. 1980. Homeostasis and control principles. In *Medical physiology*, ed. V. B. Mountcastle. 14th ed. St. Louis: Mosby Co. [Fig. 1.4]

2

Implementation by the Central Nervous System

In this chapter we acquaint ourselves with some functions and structures of the brain concerned with motor control. How much of the brain is needed at any one time for motor control? I can think of no better way to answer this question than to quote from Denny-Brown's introduction to *Neurophysiology* in the 1960 edition of the *Handbook of Physiology.*

First, every motor reaction has an adequate stimulus, immediate or remote; and second, all that is known of motor function indicates that the nervous system as a whole contributes to each motor act. It is not possible to indicate separate mechanisms for posture and movement. Postural reactions are fundamental in neural organization, and movement in its most elementary form is seen as modifications of postural responses. There is a similar difficulty in defining "function" which can be used only in a general sense equivalent to activity. The operative physiological term is "performance" which from spinal to cortical levels can be traced in various grades of refinement and in more appropriate relation to the whole organism and finally the whole environment. A segmental reflex may be perfectly performed in terms of the segmental structures it serves, but for its integration into behavior we have to examine higher and higher levels of neural activity.

To gain an overall impression, we will take a quick tour through the brain. We take in the view from a height of land that lets us identify the general features of the landscape without obscuring it with too much detail. All statements and diagrams are purposely oversimplified; we will encounter the finer points in later chapters, particularly in Chap. 5. and 11–14. For general orientation we begin with some major landmarks. Figure 2.1 identifies the main areas of the cerebral mantle, the locations of the cerebellum, the thalamus, basal ganglia, hypothalamus, brain stem (medulla oblongata) and its relation to the spinal cord. We will refer to this overall contour map as we go along.

1. The Sensorimotor and the Limbic Brain

We learned in the preceding chapter that posture and movement are controlled by the mind and the senses, which together are used to make plans and to execute them. In addition, we must consider the influence of the emotions that are brought to bear on the sensorimotor machinery through the cooperation of two brain systems. The locations of their main constituent parts are indicated in Figs. 2.1 and 2.2. The sensorimotor system consists of the sensory, motor, and their associative connections. The limbic system is an old set of structures surrounding the brain-stem, branching out through their more modern cortical connections. Both systems influence the mind in important ways.

The sensorimotor brain deals with (non-limbic) sensations and their perceptions, and with motor functions. The limbic brain deals with species-typical behavior and the resulting emotional needs, based on biological drives like feeding, drinking, reproduction, and other life-, and species-preserving activities such as maternal behavior and socialization, which includes fight-or-flight decisions. Last, but not least, the limbic system is essential for another capability crucial for species survival: that is to learn from experience (see Chap. 13.7, later). The sensorimotor and limbic systems are defined by their *functions* rather than by their anatomical parts, as they are grouped into neural "task systems" according to functional demands of the moment (Chap. 2.2). Each of the systems can adjust its own output by comparing what is needed and what is happening. At least, this is a well-known method of control for many parts of the brain in the nonlimbic system, and seems a reasonable way to think about the limbic part.

Figure 2.2 is a starkly oversimplified "circuit diagram" of the connections of the main parts of the brain. The figure, though just a cartoon, teaches us the anatomical reality of the limbic and sensorimotor systems and some of their connections. The basal ganglia and the cerebellum are both pictured as side-loops to the nonlimbic cerebral cortex. The basal ganglia receive only cortical input, while the cerebellum is also connected with the spinal cord. The thalamus, linked reciprocally with the cortex, is depicted as containing relays for all sensory (afferent) and motor (efferent) paths as well as the two side-loops.

The limbic system is a construct to denote a set of forebrain structures that are interconnected with the hypothalamus and parts of the midbrain. Limbic connec-tions converge on and are distributed from the hypothalamus (Fig. 2.1C). The hypothalamus regulates many vital functions such as body temperature, heart rate, blood pressure, water and food intake, and others. It helps maintain homeostasis by adjusting mechanisms within the body and also through interaction with the external environment. If we are thirsty, for instance, we preserve body water through internal control devices, but we may also institute a search for water through use of the sensorimotor system. The hypothalamus and limbic system are also involved in sexual and emotional behavior. Basic biological needs with regard to the internal state of the body are regulated by the hypothalamus through the autonomic nervous system and the neuroendocrine pituitary system. The autonomic connection is shown schematically in Fig. 2.2 as reaching the brain stem. The same arrow also denotes limbic influence on centers in the brain stem (and midbrain) whose far-flung projections modulate cellular activity throughout most of the brain.

The hypothalamus communicates through the anterior thalamic nuclei with the most "associative" limbic structure—the cingulate gyrus of the cerebral cortex—which forms part of the mesial rim around the corpus callosum (Figs. 2.1C and 2.3A). The cingulate gyrus projects to the hippocampus, an essential structure for the formation of memories, which in turn projects back to the hypothalamus. This circuit, drawn in Fig. 2.3B, was proposed 50 years ago by Papez to account for the ability of emotions to reach consciousness, and for that of conscious, rational thought to influence the emotions. The hypothalamus receives reports from senses basic to these biological drives, and it also receives feedback about their implementation from the limbic system (so named by MacLean; Figs. 2.2 and 2.3A, B). The hypothalamus exerts its controls through loops of various complexities, some short and some long. Limbic short loops are comparable to spinal segmental reflexes, and long loops

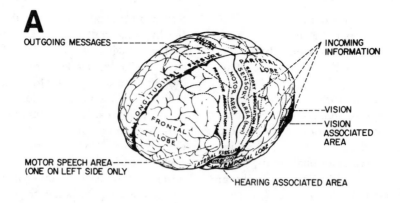

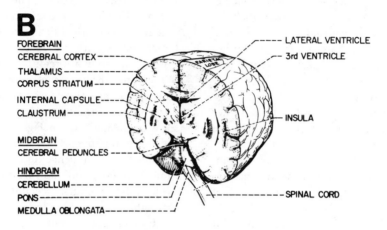

Fig. 2.1. Four views of the human brain. (A) Surface view; (B) coronal section; (C) vertical, sagittal section; (D) horizontal section. (From McNaught and Callander, 1983)

are comparable to their controls through supraspinal systems.

An ancient core pathway, the medial forebrain bundle (Fig. 2.3C), connects many limbic structures with the lateral hypothalamus, from the cerebral cortex down to the midbrain (mesencephalon), including the most ventral part of the basal ganglia. The medial forebrain bundle (MFB) also connects with a very old cortical complex in the medial wall of the base of the temporal lobe, the amygdala. This complex, located close to the hippocampus and connected to the hypothalamus, is involved in the modulation of aggressive behavior, and is in general concerned with the emotional connotations of memory. The structures connected by the medial forebrain bundle (as first shown by

Nauta) are related to the life- and species-preserving functions mentioned above, because they elicit related behavior when stimulated (as first shown by Hess), and they contain neurons that discharge in relation to such behavior (cf. reviews by Mogenson and by Rolls). For instance, recognition of an object of interest is reflected in the discharge of neurons in the medial (inferior) temporal visual association cortex (Fig. 2.1A), but this discharge is concerned with identification rather than with its significance for need-directed behavior. The crucial property of feeling the *need* to act is added by the limbic system, yielding the recognition of significance of a stimulus in terms of that need through neural activity in the amygdala and the lateral hypothalamus, as well as the caudate nucleus

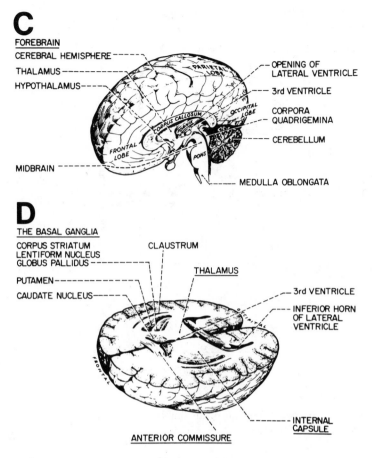

C

FOREBRAIN
CEREBRAL HEMISPHERE
THALAMUS
HYPOTHALAMUS

OPENING OF
LATERAL VENTRICLE

3rd VENTRICLE

CORPORA
QUADRIGEMINA

CEREBELLUM

MIDBRAIN

MEDULLA OBLONGATA

PARIETAL LOBE
OCCIPITAL LOBE
CORPUS CALLOSUM
FRONTAL LOBE
PONS

D

THE BASAL GANGLIA

CORPUS STRIATUM
LENTIFORM NUCLEUS
GLOBUS PALLIDUS

PUTAMEN

CAUDATE NUCLEUS

CLAUSTRUM

THALAMUS

3rd VENTRICLE

INFERIOR HORN
OF LATERAL
VENTRICLE

INTERNAL
CAPSULE

ANTERIOR COMMISSURE

FRONTAL

Fig. 2.1 (*continued*)

of the basal ganglia, to which the inferotemporal cortex projects.

Neurons in these structures and in the limbically innervated, most ventral output component of the basal ganglia, the substantial innominata, respond for food and drink, for instance, *if* the monkey is hungry or thirsty. (Significantly, these are the same sites that upon (self-)stimulation lead to eating or drinking behavior.) These areas are connected with the n. accumbens in the most ventral part of the basal ganglia (Fig. 2.3C), which can lead to limbically motivated locomotion by activating midbrain locomotor centers. Need-sensing limbic projections are integrated in the association cortex, which can instruct the projection system to the spinal cord to initiate appropriate motor activity. In other words, limbically induced, "need"-directed motor activity is transmuted by the high-level association cortex into overall plans for "goal"-directed motor actions. When a previously meaningful stimulus becomes irrelevant, perhaps because it has failed to elicit meaningful action, neurons in the temporal cortex (and its subcortical targets) cease to respond. The subject now no longer pays attention, it has become "habituated," and the gates to motor action are closed. MacLean points out that interactions served by the limbic cortex assist species survival through socialization. Loss of limbic cingulate cortex, for instance, deprives mother animals of maternal behavior needed to rear their young, and of play which is essential in forming viable family relations.

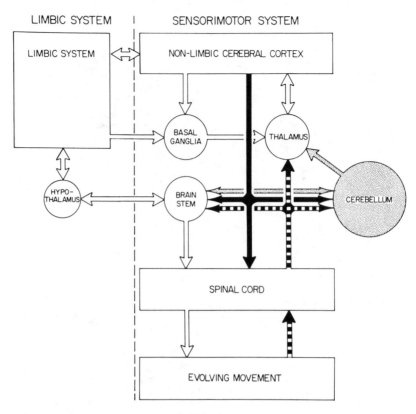

Fig. 2.2. Diagram of major components of the limbic and sensorimotor systems (separated by *broken line*). (From Brooks, 1983)

Discoveries of this sort are important because they reveal successive stages of decision making in the initiation of goal-directed behavior. Limbic drives evolve from general "ideas" into motor goals (general plans) through corticocortical processing in the higher association cortex. Figures 2.3 and 2.4 posit "drive-reduction" as the mainspring for action, but we must realize that in some cortical areas and in some subcortical centers these drives become mixed until one can substitute for another, or that other drives, more related to the social environment of the subject, can substitute for them. Integration by means of branches from afferent systems reaching subcortical centers (e.g. in the midbrain) has long been proposed by Penfield, who called it the "centrecephalic" system. Life- and species-preserving drives are "sublimated" into culturally oriented behavior

through the control exerted by the higher association cortex over the limbic system. Fulfillment of biological (or sublimated) drives is coordinated by means of returning loops between the limbic system, the midbrain and the middle level, and the association cortex. Major components of the brain, as indicated in Figs. 2.2 and 2.3, operate together, making the whole brain one neural task system. For motor performance set in the emotional context, the limbic and nonlimbic parts of the brain are essential and inseparable partners. Details of the interactions are discussed further in Chaps. 11 and 14.

The limbic and nonlimbic systems are linked also with respect to memory and motor learning. Figure 2.2 indicates the connection between high-level association cortex and limbic cortex, and Fig. 2.3 that

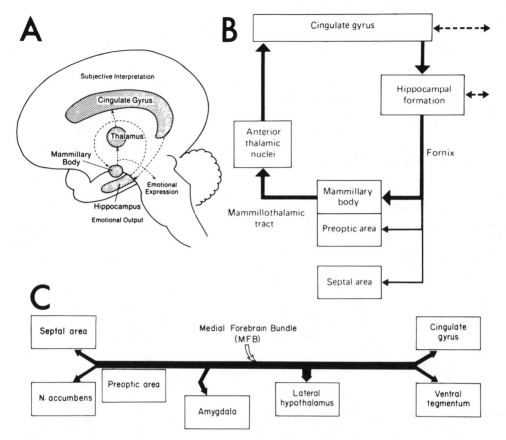

Fig. 2.3. The main components of the limbic system. (A), (B) Modified diagram of neural circuit proposed by Papez *(heavy arrows)*. *Light arrows* indicate known projections of the fornix to the hypothalamic regions (mammillary bodies and preoptic anterior hypothalamic area) and to the septal area (which probably corresponds to a region near the anterior commissure of the human brain). *Dotted lines* indicate some connections to sensorimotor structures of the nonlimbic brain. (C) Nauta's "continuum" of components connected to the medial forebrain bundle. Compare to Fig. 2.2. [(A) From Shepherd, 1983; (B) modified from Kupfermann, 1981; (C) adapted from Mogenson, Jones and Yim, 1980]

between limbic (e.g., cingulate) cortex, the hippocampus and thence the thalamus. The corticolimbothalamic pathway is essential for quick, insightful learning and its preservation in memory. Both the hippocampus and the amygdala are essential as shown by Mishkin. The drive and its reduction are necessary conditions for learning. An example would be the quicker learning after the insight of having made behaviorally correct responses (e.g., starting in the circled area of Fig. 1.5C). In contrast, the previous, slower "rote" learning by mere repetition is less dependent on limbic function and is lower in the hierarchy of learning modes proposed by Thompson. When motives fuel the formation of memories, their storage involves the amygdala–hypothalamic system and its closely associated cortical areas (e.g., orbitofrontal and cingulate cortex). Memory and motor learning are discussed further in Chaps. 11, 13, and 14.

An important component of the limbic system is the hippocampus, which is involved in laying down memories, giving them their emotional connotation through a circuit that leads from the hippocampus through the amygdala to the thalamus. Thus, *all goal-directed motor activities begin with appropriate "enabling" commands for the cortical areas to which they are connected.* (Fig. 2.7). The limbic (e.g., cingulate) cortex is connected with all of the association cortex, which provides the neural substrate for recognizing, selecting, attending to, and acting on relevant sensory information in the awake state. Motor programs are learned through spatial memories that are laid down upon neocortical commands to the hippocampus, which in turn stimulates the thalamus. This circuit is separate from that for the emotional content of memories, which is linked through the amygdala, as mentioned above. The limbic system might thus be involved in the storage and processing of all associative memories.

In wakefulness, one other general brain system must be active, although it is not illustrated in this chapter. To function properly, the brain has to be in a state of arousal which is controlled by projections from the midbrain ascending reticular formation that, among other things, facilitates cortical output neurons. During sleep, particularly the rapid eye movement (REM) phases of deep sleep, cortical inhibitory interneurons are facilitated, causing inhibition of output neurons such as corticospinal, corticothalamic and corticopontine cells.

General motor plans (e.g., for making a golf swing as in Fig. 1.1) are fashioned into specific motor acts (e.g., of the arms, trunk and legs) by the middle level that organizes and supervises the operation of the required, sequential simple motor programs. Examples of handwriting (Fig. 2.6) carried out in three grossly different sizes and therefore with entirely different muscles and joints, demonstrate how an overall plan is preserved even when it is carried out by different programs. Motor plans are scaled as a whole, for amplitude of execution, by a special part of the basal ganglia (the putamen), and the components of the plan are optimized by the cerebellum for execution by the motor cortex and its subcortical targets. We are familiar with having to string successive components together one after another from experiences such as "getting stuck" sometimes when making a previously learned sequence of knots, or playing a piece on the piano, or reciting a memorized poem. The basal ganglia are instrumental in running sequences of motor programs automatically to complete a motor plan (according to a proposal by Marsden.)

Some obvious, common human experiences show the importance of the brain systems discussed above. The activities of limbically innervated "reward" and "satiety" centers in the forebrain and midbrain (along the medial forebrain bundle, Fig. 2.3C) are related to the subject's feeling of need to fulfill the drives or of having done enough to satisfy them (Fig. 2.4). Motivation and the emotional state of mind influence learning and performance of any task. Neither a balky child nor a disinterested adult learns easily or improves motor skill. This may well be caused by inadequate limbic support of sensorimotor processing. Motivating trainees or patients can be of great assistance in establishing motor programs to acquire motor skill.

2. Command Hierarchies

The flow of information through the neural centers shown in Figs. 2.2–2.7 depends on the nature of the task to be carried out, the emotions of the subject, and very importantly on previous experience. For example, detailed instructions for a task become very much more useful, particularly for a novice, if the trainee first forms a general mental scheme of what he or she is supposed to do in a particular situation. What is true for this example of motor behavior applies also to programming in the brain: general plans have to come before specific programs. For instance, the decisions to perform a task in a certain way (through particular behavioral uses of the trunk and limbs as in Fig. 1.1) are choices of strategy based on understanding and associating many factors, including where the ball is located, the lay of the land, the wind, and others.

Figure 2.4 is a cartoon of the essential functions of the limbic and sensorimotor parts of the brain. The arrows indicate information flow, that can also form neural task systems. The demands expressed as "needs" by the limbic system are analyzed and integrated by the association cortex (e.g., prefrontal, parietal, and temporal lobes, Fig. 2.1A), which also selects the best plans of action to take and so informs the "projection" system indicated in Fig. 2.5. The projection system consists of the sensorimotor cortex, cerebellum, part of the basal ganglia, and associated subcortical nuclei. This system guides the spinal cord how and when to give orders for specific motor actions to the skeletomuscular system. Some parts of the projection and spinal systems—that is, the middle and the lower levels of the motor hierarchy—receive only indirect limbic connections (thin arrows in Fig. 2.4). Feedback lines course from some areas of the higher association cortex to the amygdala and from there back to the mainspring of limbic drives, the hypothalamus. These points are illustrated as block diagrams in Fig. 2.8 and are discussed in more detail in Chap. 11.2.

One of the crucial functions of the highest level is to *select what is relevant* within the context of the task before communicating with centers lower down in the motor hierarchy. Relevance with regard to biological needs is first posited by the limbic system, and secondly endorsed as appropriate for motor action. Figure 2.5 shows that association cortex operates at the "highest" level of the motor hierarchy. High, middle and low centers are terms coined by the great neurologist Hughlings Jackson on the basis of his clinical observations. These terms still serve a useful purpose today, although they are used in a less strict sense than they were in the last century. Most arrows of communication in Fig. 2.5 are drawn in only one direction merely as a first introduction. In fact, communication proceeds in both directions, up and down, in the sensorimotor hierarchy. The cerebral association areas not only send instructions outward, but also receive and assess diverse inputs consisting of processed sensory information and of internal feedback sent out from the lower and middle levels of the motor system. Some association areas relate the orders they have issued to the limbic demands and the sensorimotor progress made by the entire system. The latter is fed back to the limbic

Fig. 2.4. Cartoon summary highlighting the motivational function of the limbic system in motor control. Direct and indirect connections indicated as *heavy* and *light arrows*. Feedforward connections (A) and feedback between equivalent systems in (B).

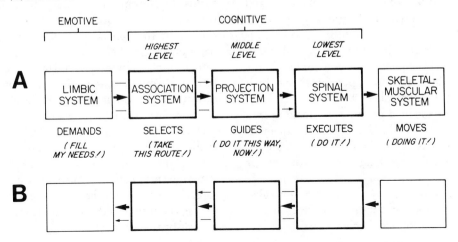

system, which adjusts the nuclei, referred to above, that modulate the subject's feeling whether the "needs" fueled by limbic drives have been adequately satisfied ("rewarded").

Now let us take a look at the sensorimotor system. The association cortex operates at the highest level, forming perceptions and concepts of motor action, that is, "plans" or "strategies" (called "instructions" at the top of Fig. 2.5). These are conveyed to the sensorimotor cortex through corticocortical connections, for instance from the prefrontal and parietal areas to the premotor cortex that is one of the "projection areas" of Fig. 2.5). Conveyance is assisted by two other structures that belong to the middle level: the putamen loop of the basal ganglia and the cerebellum, which are explained below (not shown in Fig. 2.7). Nonlimbic sensory, motor and association cortex are drawn as one combined box in Fig. 2.2. The entire (neo)cerebral cortex projects to the basal ganglia (whose input stage is called the striatum because of its striate appearance when stained to reveal the myelinated fiber bundles that penetrate it). The striatum consists of two nuclei, the caudate and putamen, which are separated by an internal highway of fibers called the "internal capsule" (Fig. 2.1A, D). The basal ganglia deal with a wider range of functions than the cerebellum; they adjust complex, simple, and semiautomatic functions. Examples of simple functions are the direction and force of muscular exertions in postures and movements by stabilizing joint stiffness through spinal and supraspinal mechanisms. Complex functions include the preparation for motor performance, which Denny-Brown called "behavioral set," and plans (explained below) for engaging in a repertoire of simultaneous or sequential motor acts. These could be, for example, doing different things with each arm or making purposeful changes of posture while carrying out some other intended act with the arms. Entire sequences of purposeful motor acts (each consisting of sev-

eral compound movements) are planned together ahead of time as motor plans. This planning involves the high-level association cortex, together with the caudate nucleus to which it projects. It is for this reason that caudate lesions destroy the ability to coordinate simultaneous or sequential motor acts and to make delayed responses to choices (which are also consequences of lesions of the high-level prefrontal association cortex). The putamen is linked to sensorimotor cortex and probably deals with scaling, adjusting, and updating simple programmed actions.

The cerebellum (see Figs. 2.1C, 2.2 and 2.7), motor cortex, brain stem and putamen circuit of the basal ganglia (in contrast with the caudate circuit and the association cortex) operate at the middle level, dealing with tactical planning how to carry out the movements needed for a given strategy. Strategies prescribe the general nature of plans, and tactics give them particular specifications in space and time, enabling their practical execution as part of kinematic tasks, which include the participation of all forces bearing on the active joints. Cerebellar contributions lie in the tactical "packaging" of the movements and postures needed for planned motor acts, that is, by making up appropriate programs for sequencing and composing intended, compound movements and their constituent simple movements. The lateral part of the cerebellum performs this "programming" task by adjusting cortical and subcortical structures that project to the spinal cord. More medial parts of the cerebellum adjust and update, rather than program, movements based on feedback from the spinal cord. An example of lost integration at the middle level was provided in Chapter 1.1: decomposition of learned compound movements during cerebellar dysfunctions into consecutive, dysmetric simple movements. Tactical instructions may call for adjustments (e.g., of force, speed or mechanical stiffness of joints), according to the kinematic circumstances of the moment.

There is little evidence that the central nervous system (CNS) controls any of these particular variables in an always fixed manner. Instead there is much evidence for control of any and all variables flexibly so as to achieve the required adjustments. Higher centers generate less specific commands that lower ones. Descending paths carry tactical instructions to the spinal cord, the lowest level in Figs. 2.2–2.5 and 2.7, where they are coordinated and finally translated into properly timed commands for muscle tensions. Adjustments are made by means of regulating the threshold and gain of spinal reflexes that govern muscle tension. The *threshold* is the level at which reflex corrections, of muscle length for example, are set to begin. An analogy might be the house temperature at which the thermostat turns on the furnace. *Reflex gain* is how much correction is supplied for a particular level of muscle stretch. In the furnace analogy, gain would be the intensity of heating that the furnace puts out, once it has been switched on at threshold. Another important example of a reflex property under de-

scending control is the relative strength of opposing muscles. Strong reciprocal inhibition allows the limb to swing loose, that is, to be compliant. We saw in Fig. 1.3 that joints become more compliant before the onset of planned movements. Weak reciprocal inhibition, in contrast, permits cocontraction of opposing muscles, which stiffens the joint. The golfer in Fig. 1.1 holds his arms fairly stiff during the hold before the swing, makes them compliant during the swing, and then stiffens them once more before impact. The ever-changing interplay between brain and spinal cord in modulating reflexes was the reason for the warning in Chap. 1 against making too rigid a distinction between reflex and voluntary actions.

Therapists can increase or decrease existing reflexes by appropriate touch, pressure, applications of hot or cold packs, or imposed postures. These maneuvers, which are based primarily on manipulations of securely conducted interactions within the spinal cord, or those connected by "long loops" between it and higher centers, can build up helpful responses or decrease unwanted ones. These procedures can improve degraded motor programs, because the brain can use proffered inputs and may even learn new ways to trigger particular subprograms. Repetition, and understanding by the patient of what is wanted, can call forth increasing supraspinal support of the therapeutically evoked responses.

Move programs are triggered by the cerebellum at appropriate times to activate lower levels, guiding movements in a planned manner from one intended, programmed hold situation toward another (e.g., Fig. 1.5). The cerebellum performs its programming functions after the higher level association cortex has created the overall motor plan. In summary, the hierarchical actions of motor performance are based on functions of identified parts of the brain, whose interactions lend it the subtlety of feelings and of acquired skill.

The specifications for detailed, skillful

Fig. 2.5. Diagram of levels in the hierarchy of motor control. Note that information flows both up and down and in loops. See text for explanation. (Modified from Phillips and Porter, 1977; in Shepherd, 1983)

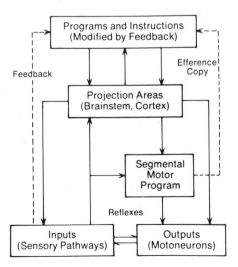

motor execution can be committed to memory through often repeated use. As mentioned above in relation to Fig. 2.3, such rote learning of motor habits does not need the limbic hippocampus and amygdala, but may depend on the cooperation of parts of the middle level that all address the same targets at the lower level—that is, that share a common "topographic" organization. (This is illustrated in Fig. 2.8, to follow). Versatile motor commands can be constructed out of the convergences from many cell assemblies that receive different combinations of inputs. They are usually fashioned at the middle level from several "somatotopic body maps" for various adequate stimuli. This reshuffling of the cards, this integration of many somatotopies into various topographic combinations, is taken up further in Chaps. 11–14.

The three levels of control (higher, middle and lower) do not operate as a rigid hierarchy, with orders going only from the top downward, because most structures are connected through internal feedback loops (i.e., within the CNS), to correlate ascending and descending messages. Such loops are indicated by the arrows in Fig. 2.5 (also in Figs. 2.2 and 2.7). At all levels of the nervous system, correlation is achieved by *comparison* of the intended (i.e., "expected") effects of commands that have been sent to lower levels in the hierarchy with the actual effects that they have produced. This method of accounting requires internal feedback of "reference" copies of outgoing commands from one level to be filed with its superior level. Reference copies are called "efference" copies (because they are copies of efferent messages destined for other places; Fig. 2.5) or "corollary" discharges. For instance, central commands to start or stop movements (destined eventually for spinal motoneurons) distribute corollary start or stop discharges to other central structures. One important function of these corollary copies of efferent commands ("reefference") is to prevent sensory systems from interfering with the intended movement. Thus, preparations are made not to overreact to sensory messages generated by movements during their execution. These peripheral sensory signals and their centrally relayed "feedback" and its integrated representations ("reafference") are used, however, to assess the progress of the movement. Sperry, and later von Holst, proposed that copies of the efferent messages could cancel the sensory consequence (reafference) of expected movements. Alternately, the sensory systems could be adapted (made insensitive) to their occurrence, as proposed by Mackay.

Sensorimotor centers interact at many levels, distributing the power to start, stop or modify programs. For instance, a program that depends on discharge of cortical neurons can be held up by a "not ready" signal from, say, the spinal cord, until the entire system is in an appropriate state of readiness. Figure 2.5 indicates that feedback even from the periphery and the lowest hierarchical level (broken lines) can adjust high-level programs to ensure their success. The sensorimotor centers of the middle level (cf. Figs. 2.2 and 2.5) coordinate the head, trunk and limbs. These centers translate such items as movement direction, force and timing into patterns of muscle action with the aid of the lowest level. We should note that instructions to the spinal cord for most postural muscles are mediated by paths different from those for fine control of finger movements, that is, by the pyramidal tract. The descending tracts are not drawn separately in Fig. 2.2, but Fig. 2.5 denotes projections from the motor cortex to interneurons as well as directly to spinal motoneurons.

Execution of motor tasks is set in train by commands (subprograms) that are parceled out to centers of the middle level and thence to the lowest motor centers, the "spinal output stages" consisting of motoneurons and interneurons, which are the agents that connect output stages with their central as well peripheral inputs. The output stages specify intensities and durations of action for particular muscles, but they never act in isolation. Muscles are coordinated in the spinal cord by connecting systems of spinal interneurons and supraspinally by paths descending from the brain stem after mutual interactions with middle-level centers (trace the arrows in Fig. 2.5).

How are neural centers assembled to function as a system for a particular motor task? Figure 2.2 provides an example for paths descending from the motor (precentral) cortex. They are represented together with other descending paths in the one black arrow that gives off branches to brain stem and cerebellum, and continues down to the spinal cord. In addition, fibers descending in the pyramidal tract from sensory (postcentral) cortex connect with ascending systems, which enables the sensorimotor system to control its own inputs. Of course, there are actually many paths descending from cortex and brain stem. Most of them engage spinal interneurons, which are critical links in the creation of functional, temporary "task systems" by imposing their own special coordinating instructions. The spinal cord acts like a "smart terminal" for descending commands, because it can provide versatile subroutines leading to suitably task-oriented outputs. In fact, this is a general property of neural centers: connections for subroutines are provided by genetic inheritance and are then adjusted for easy access by frequent usage. Each level thus helps the others by taking over the ability to make local decisions through its own neural linkages. Thus, intent is conveyed by repeated translations from the highest brain levels to the spinal cord, and by means of these "long loops," course corrections are finally sent to the muscles. Here we glimpse how a neural task system harnesses the machinery of the muscles to serve the mind. How remarkable that this is possible when the individual parts of the system cannot read the meaning of the mind!

By making general decisions first and leaving details to be fitted later into the circumstances of the moment, the CNS is able to produce the same effects over and over again, though never in exactly the same way. The types of movements illustrated in Figs. 1.1 and 1.2 provide examples. For another, think of how we sign our names and how similar is that signature whether written on paper or on the blackboard. Yet, we use different sets of muscles in the two cases. An example of this sort is reproduced in Fig. 2.6, where the "motor plan" for writing familiar words is clearly preserved, no matter whether the main writing fulcrum is the wrist, elbow or shoulder.

Motor programs are ready-to-use models of motor actions. They are put into effect by activation of their many subprograms, which enables the replay of previously learned acts. A "model" resides in

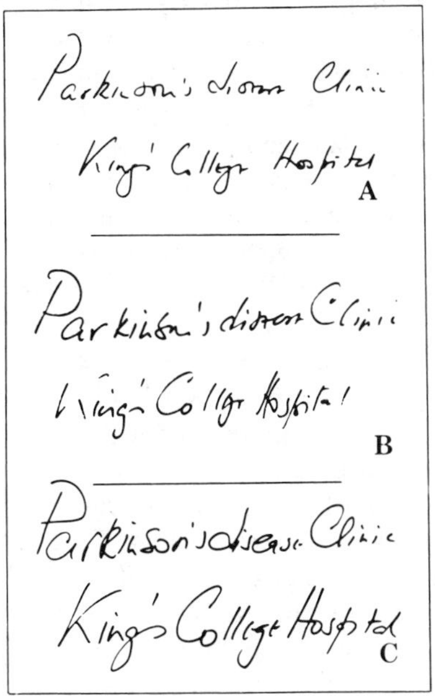

Fig. 2.6. Handwriting retains its character even if undertaken with major use of three different joints. (A) Normal; (B) using the elbow as fulcrum; (C) using the shoulder joint as fulcrum when writing with the outstretched and unsupported arm. Writing reduced photographically to same size after different sizes of felt-tipped pens had been used. (From Marsden, 1982)

distributed fashion in several parts of the brain, which are connected by paths that are activated more easily in a particular context, like the interplay between practiced actors in a long-running play. Any one actor can start the chain of interactions. Easy interaction at cell junctions (synapses) is acquired by frequent use. Programs of the middle level (e.g., sensorimotor cortex, cerebellum, and the putamen circuit of the basal ganglia) function as subprograms of the motor plans of the higher level. Spinal programs can be subprograms of those in the middle level. We already know from Chap. 1.1 that preservation of programs means retention of motor memory. Small subprograms trigger activity that may be confined largely to one brain center, for instance to motor cortex in response to cerebellar prompting (see Figs. 2.2 and 2.7). Repeated motor acts like the coordinated movements of the body and limbs in Fig. 1.1, or the apposition of the index fingers in Fig. 1.2, are re-created through the concerted action of many subprograms, each of which encodes only parts of the whole motor task. The re-creations are never exactly the same, however, because the brain adapts to changes in the environment and also in our feelings. It is not easy, for instance, to appose two fingers gently when we are tense or upset; the limbic system is also involved. So, if we are asked for the locations of plans and programs in the many interactive loops, we must reply that they are distributed throughout the system.

It is important to realize that "knowledge" of overall purposes contained in motor plans is not shared by the parts of the brain that carry them out. What is shared are secure channels of communication. Subprograms can function for a particular purpose because the task system has established especially secure synaptic linkages in preferred paths. They can be triggered by signals with only limited significance for the overall task. The participating neurons are not informed about overall significance. This is therapeutically

relevant because it offers the opportunity to start up unused programs. Therapists can trigger programs with stimuli that are unusual but effective. For instance, nonwalking (akinetic) patients with Parkinson's disease can be made to walk with visual, auditory or vestibular cues, such as bouncing a ball or rocking their shoulders back and forth, or tilting them forward. In some situations, the brain can adapt and learn new cues for existing motor programs. Preferred paths for motor programs are thought to be created by modificatons of some synapses on those paths.

It is believed that most parts of the CNS contain modifiable synapses whose efficiency can be altered by inputs of special significance, for instance feedforward information about sensory events or feedback from higher centers about success. According to Kandel's studies of transmission in invertebrate *Aplysia,* frequent message traffic through synapses increases the amount of transmitter released from their presynaptic endings, giving their transmission greater "synaptic security." Secure synapses are the essence of how neurons are assembled into functional groups. Unused synapses wither away and are replaced by active ones. A current theory (by Edelman) proposes that all active neural lines compete for available synaptic spots on neurons. The most active ones are envisaged to win out and thus lay down ready lines of communication for further messages of the same sort. According to this theory, the fittest cell assemblies (or groups) survive in a dynamic, rather than a permanent, static equilibrium that is maintained by the volume of their message traffic. The rule "use it or lose it" applies here, much as for a trader in the stock market whose importance depends on his volume of trading, but who can maintain his post only as long as he can pay for his transactions. One might therefore guess that the products of modifiable synapses, namely very small subprograms, are distributed throughout the CNS. Programs do not reside clustered in particular nuclei but instead are formed by subprograms that are distributed in the CNS. The size of the distributed system is determined by the number of CNS centers that participate in a particular programmed task. The (self-) selection, or self-organization, of neuronal groups would thus follow the rule that "the squeaky wheel gets the oil," or put more politely, that preferred lines of communication are maintained in the nervous system as use-dependent refinements of the genetically inherited connections.

3. Task-related Systems

The term "task system" is meant to describe those anatomical centers that are most actively involved in a task at any given time. Task systems can include practically the entire CNS for various phases of complex motor acts, or they can be restricted to high activity in fewer centers for specific episodes of postures and movements. The systems function with a mixture of feedforward commands and feedback adjustments (see Figs. 1.4 and 2.5).

Compound arm movements, as in Figs. 1.1 and 1.2, provide good examples of the operation of middle-level centers as a task system. Movement direction is thought to be programmed by motor cortex, with special monitoring of relevant events by association cortex. The motor cortex also specifies the mechanical joint stiffness as well as the velocity and end points of movements. The spinal cord implements these by setting the angles and mechanical stiffness of joints. Joint stiffness, which is determined by the degree of contraction of opposing muscles (co-contraction), governs the force needed to move a joint through a given angle. Appropriate muscular actions for this task are specified for the spinal cord by the cerebellum, cerebrum, and putamen loop of the basal ganglia. The connections of these structures are drawn with different emphases in Figs. 2.2 and 2.7. In Fig. 2.7, the limbic origin of the motor drive is indicated as preceding the generation of an "idea" for the behav-

ioral motor act. That loosely defined term, idea, is meant to denote the unready quality of the emerging behavioral motor plan. The dotted lines in Fig. 2.7 denote indirect limbic connections to the association cortex, the basal ganglia, and the lateral cerebellum, as well as the relatively direct return path from the higher association areas to the amygdala and thence to the hypothalamus. The grossly oversimplified scheme of Fig. 2.7 will be made more real by Figs. 2.8–2.10 and with detail to be supplied in Chaps. 11–14.

Let us take a look at a more limited motor task: the spinal reflexes that operate on the golfer's arm during a swing (Fig. 1.1). Even this involves more than a purely spinal task system because of unceasing supraspinal involvement, varying only in degree and timing. For the whole swing of the arm we must include all centers. However, even for the more limited task of "inflight" management of arm muscles, spinal reflexes alone cannot compensate adequately for unexpected perturbations.

It has only recently been recognized that the two input structures of the dorsal basal ganglia, the caudate and the putamen (Fig. 2.1B,D), lead into two separate circuits. As mentioned in Chap. 2.2, the caudate loop of the basal ganglia is involved in setting up behavioral acts and coordinating overall motor plans by virtue of its connections with the higher association cortex, while the putamen loop probably updates programs for postures and movements to carry out the task appropriately by virtue of its connections with the sensorimotor cortex. We also remember that the cerebellum acts as a composer for intended motor acts, fashioning them out of compound and simple movements as well as their supporting postures. Furthermore, the cerebellum coordinates their starts, their progress and their stops. Here we are concerned with how the basal ganglia and the cerebellum interact with the cerebral cortex. Somatosensory inputs activated by the movement are shown in Fig. 2.7 as lines deriving from "move," feeding back to the spinal cord, which is labeled "motor servo," a term that denotes spinal ("servo") control by negative feedback (see Fig. 5.1 later).

The cerebellum operates in a manner that might also apply to the basal ganglia, and in fact, to many brain systems. Figure 2.7 indicates that the cerebellum is connected as a side-loop, which provides it with copies of, for example, commands for the cerebral cortex. The cerebellum also receives copies of the cortical output, which permits it to compare the original orders with their execution. (This is discussed further in Chap. 13.) It is conceivable that the basal ganglia loops might, like the lateral cerebellum for instance, also appraise the success of corticocortical processing, which they then might modify through use of their particular subcortical inputs, including their limbic inputs. The caudate loop, for example, might compare hypothalamic commands (which it receives through the amygdala), with their processed output from limbic cortex to association cortex. (The caudate loop also receives copies of these signals.) The putamen loop of the basal ganglia might act in a related manner on the "supplementary"

motor cortex. The putamen loop is thought to adjust the execution of patterns of intended motor acts, appropriate to the overall goal, while preserving the relations between the parts of the patterns (Chaps. 11 and 14). The proposed actions of these loops may have great practical significance for motor training and learning, because comparison is always made of *ongoing activity*. The proffered view of motor control implies that only active trials can improve performance, lead to adaptation, and result in motor learning. In contrast, passive postures and movements imposed on the subject, or even worse, just mere mental consideration of exercises without active follow-up, are of no practical value. This line of reasoning fits that enunciated by Pribram, who summarized learning as a sequence of tests and evaluations of their consequences, or, as he put it: "test, operate, test, and exit." Our view offers a neural basis for this insight and for the recognition that motor learning must include the "knowledge of results," mentioned in Chap. 1.

The caudate circuit of the basal ganglia is an important member of the task system for enabling behavioral motor acts, for

Fig. 2.7. A simplified view of information flow for voluntary movements. The components are explained in the text and in previous figures. Thalamic and other nuclei are omitted, and only some limbic connections are shown *(broken lines)*. The hypothalamus (H) is not part of the "highest level" of the motor hierarchy. Reflections of somatosensory input from the evolving movement are indicated by *interrupted arrows*. Compare to Figs. 2.3–2.5 CX, Cortex; BG, basal ganglia; Cb, cerebellum. (Derived from Allen and Tsukahara, 1974; Paillard, 1983; Delong, Georgopoulos and Crutcher, 1983)

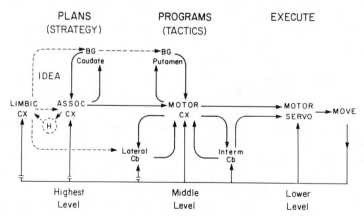

"packaging" them for automatic runs of previously learned behavioral performance routines. A well-known example is that of greeting a person by the successive acts of standing up and proffering a hand. Doing several things at once, or in routine sequence, depends on normal caudate function. The strategy of integrated use of programs was referred to in Chap. 1.1 as a motor plan or complex program, which is formed on the basis of previously successful experience. Although the use of the memories for these plans requires the activity of the nonlimbic sensorimotor system, unconscious, motivational limbic influences are needed to enact motor plans and to assemble their programs and subprograms. To let the limbic system influence the sensorimotor system in complex, integrated functions, "gates" have to be opened from the limbic system to various structures, including the basal ganglia and the cerebellum. The immobile patient with Parkinson's disease may be an extreme example of deficient "gating," since the basal ganglia cannot function because of missing support by their substantia nigra (something like a power supply failure). This can lead to decomposition of behavioral sequences, such as that of greeting a friend, into successive motor acts. The putamen circuit of the basal ganglia is thought to scale the intensity of motor patterns such that their appropriate identities are preserved. The samples of handwriting in Fig. 2.6 are a good example. Parkinsonian patients retain the ability to execute motor patterns, but they make the constituent movements too small. Hence their writing is small and their speech is slurred and rapid, just as their stride is a shuffling sequence of short steps.

When any part of the brain fails in its function, the intent cannot be carried out except in a degraded manner. We saw an example of degraded arm movements in Fig. 1.2. No part of the brain ever works in isolation, yet local lesions can degrade performance by influencing particular functions. For instance, stroke victims and patients with Parkinson's disease or with cerebellar damage correctly appreciate their environment and plan their movements correctly, but can govern neither the correct execution of intended movements nor their adaptation to changing conditions. In contrast, patients with lesions in any part of the loop linking association cortex with the caudate nucleus cannot coordinate sequential or simultaneous motor acts, although they can correctly execute individual movements.

We conclude the description of task-related systems with reference to motor learning by expanding the diagram of Fig. 2.7. Fig. 2.8A is a block-diagram of information flow through some cortical areas, in conjunction with their respective thalamic nuclei, that participate in repetitive, rote learning of motor responses to sensory inputs. Various inputs are integrated in the higher association cortex. Outputs from prefrontal and parietal cortex return to premotor cortex (labeled in Fig. 1A) and thence to the motor cortex which issues commands for motor responses to the lower level. The connected cerebellar and striatal circuits indicated in Fig. 2.7 have been omitted as a simplification although their participation is essential for normal motor function. They are considered in Chaps. 11–14.

Limbic influences are brought to bear on special parts of the cerebral cortex (Fig. 2.8B) as well as on the cerebellum and the basal ganglia (not shown). (Limbic connections are indicated by broken lines as in Fig. 2.7). Limbic drives ascend from the amygdala to limbic cortex which projects to the association cortex (Fig. 2.8B), whose output circles back to the amygdala directly, as well as indirectly through the entorhinal cortex to the memory-encoding hippocampus. These connections are essential for insightful learning. (The entorhinal cortex, hippocampus, and subiculum form part of the inside wall of the temporal lobe that is labeled in the side view of the brain in Fig. 2.1A. The inwardly curving inside wall borders on the lateral ventricle and is visible, but not labeled, in the horizontally sectioned brain in Fig. 2.1D).

The circuit of Fig. 2.8A (plus the non-illustrated connections of the cerebellum and basal ganglia) might suffice for repetitive, slow learning as in the left half of Fig. 1.5C. While this goes on, however, the subjects orient themselves, probably by creating preferred paths through the limbic and non-limbic circuits shown in Figs.

2.8A and B, as well as through connections to area 24 (not illustrated). When they are sufficient, the subjects experience insight into the task-requirements, which enables them to improve their motor skill through rapidly increasing use of "continuous" movements that are programmed predictively by the middle level, as indicated in the right half of Fig. 1.5C. Exactly how the limbic system engages the cerebellum and the basal ganglia is still uncertain. Some

Fig. 2.8. (A) Simplified diagram of information flow from sensorimotor areas of the cerebral cortex to higher association areas for elaboration of motor outputs in response to sensory inputs. Cortical areas are shown as interacting units with their respective thalamic nuclei. (B) Similar scheme as in (A) for elaboration of motor outputs (not labeled) in response to limbic drives. The limbic circuit from the amygdala to the limbic cortex (area 23) and back is indicated by broken lines, as in Fig. 2.7 (connections with area 24 not shown). Normally, motor responses are elicited by combinations of sensory and limbic inputs.

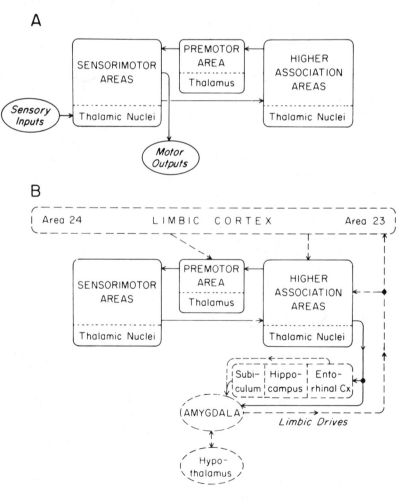

possibilities are mentioned in Chaps. 11–14.

4. Summary

Each side of the brain contains two interwoven and interactive parts, consisting of limbic and nonlimbic structures. The limbic system governs basic biological drives and emotional behavior by controlling the neuroendocrine and autonomic systems through the hypothalamus. This part of the brain also generates emotional motivation, the "need" for action, and it influences (and is influenced by) the sensorimotor, nonlimbic part of the brain. The latter deals with (nonlimbic) sensations, their perceptions and sensorimotor functions. It consists of the sensory, motor and their associative systems. The sensorimotor and limbic systems are defined by their functions rather than by their anatomical parts, as they are grouped into neural "task systems" according to functional demands.

Control of postures and movements is exerted through a command hierarchy that can be thought of as having highest, middle, and lowest levels. The highest level operates in the association cortex, which elaborates perceptions and overall motor plans (strategies). This planning function is achieved by selection and use of information that is relevant in the task context. The limbic system denotes what is relevant to the perceived needs of the body, and enables the nonlimbic brain to convert needs into goals. Life-preserving limbic drives can be sublimated in the higher association cortex. The basal ganglia help enable and coordinate goal-directed behavior. The caudate loop of the basal ganglia controls the efficiency of processing in the higher association cortex.

Strategy is converted into motor programs (tactics) at the middle level, which consists of the sensorimotor cortex, the cerebellum, the putamen loop of the basal ganglia, and the brain stem. At the middle level, programs are made to determine and correlate body equilibrium, movement directions, force, and speed, as well as mechanical stiffness of the joints, that is, move programs and hold programs. The putamen circuit of the basal ganglia enables intended simple movements probably by updating their programs to keep them appropriate for the task purpose. Since the basal ganglia, like the cerebellum, are located on side-loops to chains of corticocortical links, it is conceivable that the basal ganglia, like the cerebellum, exert their control functions as comparators of the input–output relations of corticocortical processing. This view fits the experience that only active participation produces motor improvement or learning, while passive imposition of postures and movements can have no practical value. Locomotion can be enabled by the most ventral component of the basal ganglia, through the nucleus accumbens, by pallidal projection to the midbrain locomotor centers, capable of bypassing the calculations of the cerebral cortex. All need-directed motor activity is channeled by the limbic system to the appropriate level of the nonlimbic system.

Natural movements, which always involve several joints, are composed of simple movements that affect only one joint. The lowest level, the spinal cord, translates its commands into muscular activity, which it (servo-)regulates through stretch reflexes. Motor execution is guided by task-related parts of the hierarchy. Some may be more important than others at different stages of a motor task, but none ever works in isolation. The cerebellum is a very important coordinator of goal-directed action, which it initiates and guides as complex and simple, intended motor acts. The cerebellum helps to establish, and triggers the timing of, move and hold programs. It also guides and improves their use by updating them with information about how well they are being carried out. The hierarchy correlates and adjusts its actions by means of two kinds of feedback. The actual states of limb force, speed, position, and joint stiffness, as signaled from the periphery, are monitored by various levels of the CNS. In addition, there is internal feedback: reference (reefference, or corollary) copies of commands for lower levels are used to modify the sensory feedback (reafference) created by the movement, and are also fed back up to higher centers for comparison of their intended (expected) effects with the actual motor performance. The higher association areas of the cerebral cortex project back to the mainspring of limbic drives, the hypothalamus, suggesting that the limbic system also monitors and adjusts its action through its own comparator loops.

Motor learning occurs at two levels, through the acquisition of motor habits and of associative knowledge. Habits of detailed motor execution probably depend on the middle level of the motor hierarchy. Associative, insightful, knowledge depends on higher association cortex, and for its motivational and spatial aspects depends on the hippocampus and the amygdala, as part of the limbic system.

References

Allen, G. I., and Tsukahara, N. 1974. Cerebrocerebellar communications systems. *Physiol. Rev.* 54:957–1006. [Fig. 2.7]

Brooks, V. B. 1983. Motor control: how posture and movements are governed. *Phys. Ther.* 63:664–673. [Fig. 2.2]

Delong, M. R., Georgopoulos, A. P., and Crutcher, M. D. 1983. Cortico-basal ganglia relations and coding of motor performance. In *Neural coding of motor performance*, eds. J. Massion, J. Paillard, W. Schultz, and M. Wiesendanger. *Exp. Brain Res.* Suppl. 7, pp. 30–40. Berlin: Springer Verlag. [Fig. 2.7]

Denny-Brown, D. 1960. Motor mechanisms—introduction: the general principles of motor integration. In *Neurophysiology.* Sect. 1, Vol. 2. *Handbook of physiology,* ed. H. W. Magoun, pp. 781–796. Washington, D.C.: American Physiological Society.

Eccles, J. C. 1977. Cerebellar function in the control of movement (with special reference to the pioneer work of Sir Gordon Holmes). In *Physiological aspects of clinical neurology,* ed. F. C. Rose, pp. 157–178. Oxford: Blackwell Scientific Publications.

Edelman, G. M., and Finkel, L. H. 1984. Neuronal group selection in the cerebral cortex. In *Dynamic aspects of neocortical function,* eds. G. M. Edelman, W. E. Gall, and W. M. Cowan, pp. 653–695. New York: John Wiley & Sons.

Evarts, E. V. 1975. Changing concepts of central control of movement (The Stevenson Lecture). *Can. J. Physiol. Pharmacol.* 53:191–201.

Gentile, A. M. 1972. A working model of skill acquisition with application to teaching. *Quest* 17:3-23.

Hess, W. R. 1954. *Diencephalon, autonomic and extrapyramidal functions.* New York: Grune and Statton.

Kandel, E. R. 1979. Cellular insights into behavior and learning. *Harvey Lect.* 73:19-92.

Kupfermann, I. 1981. Hypothalamus and Limbic System I: peptidergic neurons, homeostasis, and emotional behavior. In *Principles of neural science,* ed. E. R. Kandel and J. H. Schwartz. pp. 433–449. New York. Elsevier/North-Holland. [Fig. 2.3B]

MacKay, D. M. 1973. Visual stability and voluntary eye movements. In *Handbook of sensory physiology.* Vol. 7, part 3. *Central visual information,* ed. R. Jung, pp. 307–331. Berlin: Springer Verlag.

MacLean, P. D. 1970. The triune brain, emotion and scientific bias. In *The neurosciences. Second study program.* ed. F. O. Schmitt, pp. 336–349. New York: Rockefeller University Press.

Marsden, C. D. 1982. The mysterious motor function of the basal ganglia: The Robert Wartenberg Lecture. *Neurology (NY)* 32:514–539. [Fig. 2.6]

McNaught, A. B., and Callander, R. 1983. *Illustrated physiology.* 4th ed. Edinburgh: Churchill Livingstone. [Fig. 2.1]

Mishkin, M., Malamut, B., and Bachevalier, J. 1984. Memories and habits: two neural systems. In *The neurobiology of learning and memory,* eds. J. L. McGaugh, G. Lynch, and N. M. Weinberger, pp. 65–77. New York: Guilford Press.

Mogenson, G. J., Jones, D. L., and Yim, C. Y. 1980. From motivation to action. Functional interface between the limbic system and the motor system. *Progr. Neurobiol.* 14:69–97.

Mountcastle, V. B. 1979. An organizing principle for cerebral function: The unit module and the distributed system. In *The neurosciences. Fourth study program.* Cambridge: The MIT Press, pp. 21–42.

Murphy, M. R., MacLean, P. D., and Hamilton, S. C. 1981. Species-typical behavior of hamsters deprived from birth of the neocortex. *Science,* 213:459–461.

Nashner, L. M. and Grimm, R. J. 1978. Analysis of multiloop dyscontrols in standing cerebellar patients. In *Cerebral motor control in man: long loop mechanisms,* ed. J. E. Desmedt. *Progr. Clin. Neurophysiol.,* Vol 4, pp. 300–319.

Nauta, W. J. H. 1971. The problem of the frontal lobe: a reinterpretation. *J. Psychiat. Res.* 8:167–181.

Paillard, J. 1983. The functional labelling of neural codes. In *Neural coding of motor performance,* eds. J. Massion, J. Paillard, W. Schultz, and M. Wiesendanger. *Exp. Brain Res.* (Suppl. 7) pp. 1–19. Berlin: Springer Verlag. [Fig. 2.7]

Papez, J. W. 1937. A proposed mechanism of emotion. *Arch. Neurol. Psychiat.* 38:725–743.

Penfield, W. 1975. The Mystery of the mind. Princeton, N.J.: Princeton University Press.

Phillips, C. G., and Porter, R. 1977. *Corticospinal neurons. Their role in movement.* New York: Academic Press. [Fig. 2.5]

Pribram, K. 1972. *Language of the brain.* Englewood Cliffs, N.J.: Prentice-Hall.

Rolls, E. T. 1981. Processing beyond the inferior temporal visual cortex related to feeding, memory, and striatal function. In *Brain mechanisms of sensation,* eds. Y. Katsuki, R. Norgren, and M. Sato, pp. 241–269. New York: John Wiley & Sons.

Shepherd, G. M. 1983. *Neurobiology.* Sect. V. *Central systems.* New York: Oxford University Press. [Figs. 2.3A and 2.5]

Sperry, R. W. 1950. Neural basis of the spontaneous optokinetic response produced by visual neural innervation. *J. Comp. Physiol.* 43:482–489.

Thompson, R. F., Clark, G. A., Donegan, N. H., Lavond, D. G., Lincoln, J. S., Madden, J., Mamounas, L. A., Mauk, M. D., McCormick, D. A., and Thompson, J. K. 1984. Neuronal substrates of learning and memory: a "multiple-trace" view. In *Neurobiology of learning and memory,* eds. G. Lynch, J. L. McGaugh, and N. M. Weinberger, pp. 137–164. New York: Guilford Press.

3

Information Processing

The business of the brain is to process information, and our task here is to learn how it does so. It is important first to understand what the brain is trying to achieve, what information it has to work with, and what the end products of its calculations are. This chapter deals with two aspects of motor control: how we begin and how we conclude skeletomuscular adjustments. First, we see how we act because of what situations we perceive ourselves to be in, that is, how motor adjustments are spawned from sensorimotor perceptions. Second, we see how the calculations for motor adjustments are based on the properties of what they adjust: the lengths and tensions of muscles.

The brain processes information about the world around us, about the state of our bodies, and about the brain itself. Since all information for long-distance transmission is coded as all-or-none neural discharges, the various possible origins of the many messages that each central neuron receives cannot be discriminated. The identity of origins may be preserved to some degree by the identities of the paths through which the messages arrive, if these paths are well "labeled" as major trunk lines by secure synaptic connections. Messages from multiply connected networks probably are "anonymous calls," except that neural systems seem to orga-

nize the information content of their many inputs through comparisons of reference messages of the sort discussed in Chap. 2. Deciphering the information content of neural message traffic therefore seems to depend on experienced use of inherited, prewired connections and of learned new connections.

The codes of receptors and of muscles can be unraveled because their discharge frequencies reflect the intensities of their actions. This also applies to neurons with direct connections to them, but as we have seen above, too many messages converge on central neurons to let their discharge rates reveal their origins. Central sensorimotor codes will be more fully understood when we have a better grasp of the operating principles of the CNS, which are emerging from three sources of knowledge: (1) the correlations being made between cell discharges observed in various parts of the brains of behaviorally active animals; (2) the analysis of the disabilities of patients with lesions of known parts of the CNS and of their experimental replications in animals; and (3) the continued study of neural connections, which relates to the first two sources. At this time, neuroscientists still labor to unravel the mysteries of the CNS "computer" that was delivered without explanations about its construction or operation!

1. Sensorimotor Models and Reality

Sensorimotor integration is the key to motor control, and yet we know that personal sensory perceptions do not always reflect the quality or the intensity of the sensory inputs. Instead, perceptions are based on "edited" versions of those inputs. For example, as city dwellers we cease to be aware of constant noise if it holds no meaning for us. Such "habituation" is brought about by blocking of transmission between cells at various levels of the CNS, perhaps with guidance by a limbic structure, the hippocampus. Another example is failure to recognize people when we meet them out of context. Conversely, patients who know they have lost a limb still refer pain from the severed nerve endings to the phantom limb. These examples impress on us that sensory perceptions are context-oriented, and that they function as models against which our brains match sensory signals about reality.

Understanding subconscious sensory editing is important for the study of motor control, because motor behavior and the details of its execution usually depend on perceptions that reflect the sensorimotor context of *greatest relevance*. An oft-quoted example is the vigor with which we pick up a heavy-looking suitcase. If it turns out to be empty, the excessive force that we have applied (because of the wrong perception) will topple us over backwards. But suppose the suitcase really is very heavy. Concentrating on the task of lifting and carrying it will reduce the discomfort felt from tired muscles and squeezed hands, so that we ignore it. Pain is depressed partly by descending sensorimotor paths that modulate the brainward ascent of proprioceptive and painful ("nociceptive") sensory inputs. In some situations, sensations from the trunk and limbs are accentuated rather than depressed, in the context of planned or ongoing movements. An example would be the heightened skin sensitivity of the fingers during gentle exploration of the surface of an object (active touch). The contribution of skin receptors to kinesthesia of the hand depends on the position of the fingers and their direction of movement. These thoughts highlight the possibilities of improving motor performance through carefully selected biofeedback.

The perception of the positions of our limbs is based largely on messages to the CNS from the "spindle" muscle sense organs. This has been established in human subjects whose tendons could be pulled on during surgery while patients were protected from pain by local anesthesia. All patients reported the sensation of rotation of the joints to which those muscles attach. In an extraordinary procedure, McCloskey confirmed these reports by having himself made an experimental subject by transection of the tendon of the big toe extensor. The sensation of joint rotation was always in the direction that would normally stretch the test muscle. Stretches were detected with acuity comparable to that demonstrable for the detection of movements imposed on the intact toe. Vibration of the tendon evoked an illusion of plantar flexion at the terminal joint of the toe, that is, as if stretch had been applied to the extensor hallucis longus muscle (see also Fig. 3.1). Voluntary isometric contraction of the muscle produced no sensation of movement (Fig. 3.2).

Spindles signal muscle length and, therefore, muscle stretch (or lengthening) when they are stretched along with the muscle in which they are embedded. This occurs because they are anchored on the same tendons: they lie "in parallel" with the fibers of the muscle (see Fig. 4.8 later). These sense organs tend to keep muscle length constant by activating alpha MNs to cause contraction of stretched muscles (This action is indicated by a + symbol in the diagram of the stretch reflex arc in Fig. 3.3.) The stretch reflex thus shortens the stretched muscles and their spindles, which is an example of *negative feedback*. The discharge of alpha MNs (the "efferent" signal or reflex "output") cancels the input, which was the original muscle stretch (cf. Fig. 1.4). Muscle spindles measure muscle length and its rate of change. The messages from opposing muscles, when combined, add up to information about joint position and speed of movement (cf. Figs. 3.3 and 3.4). Control systems that operate on the principle of negative feedback are called *servo mechanisms.*

Perceptions based on the stretch reflex can be distorted if there is interference with the feedback. Illusions result, for example, if spindles are stimulated artificially, as by vibration of the muscle (to which their primary endings happen to be very sensitive). Vibration makes spindle discharge levels rise and reflexly excite alpha MNs of the vibrated muscle. The resulting involuntary contraction is called the "tonic vibration reflex." The brain does not understand that this is an artificially caused occurrence, and consequently the meaning of messages on the previously well-labeled afferent line can no longer be identified properly by the brain. Since spindle discharge ordinarily means muscle stretch, the subject now experiences an *illusion* of limb movement in the direction that would normally stretch the muscle that is being vibrated.

For instance, as shown in Fig. 3.1, vibrating biceps (or its tendon) creates the illusion of elbow extension and a corresponding error of position sense of the forearm in the extension direction. Such errors can be as large as 30 deg! The brain cannot distinguish between these false position data and real ones, and therefore adds them in position estimates. Most subjects experience "hyper"-extension if their forearm is slowly moved toward extension by the experimenter during vibration, because the arm already feels displaced toward extension. If it is moved beyond the *illusory* point of full extension, subjects report sensations ranging from their arm being bent backwards to being broken. Although no pain is felt, the brain reacts to the illusion by causing overt signs of pain, such as writhing, sweating and gasping. In some subjects the brain may fail to intengrate the false and the real position data, in which case subjects give bizarre reports about their arm being in two positions, either at once or alternately. Some even report their arm in positions that they know are anatomically impossible!

The tonic vibration reflex (TVR) has diagnostic and therapeutic applications. It can be used to assess the functionsl state of stretch reflex paths and to uncover latent

Fig. 3.1. Posed photograph to illustrate the perception of the extended position of the arm of a blindfolded subject (lower position) while the biceps brachii is being vibrated (upper position). Each mark on the scale is 10 deg. (From Goodwin, McCloskey and Matthews, 1972)

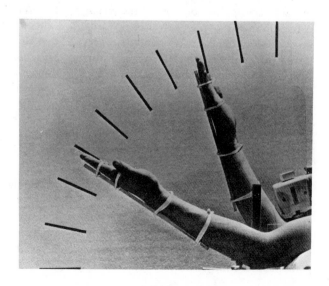

dysfunctions of the basal ganglia and the cerebellum. For the former, writing becomes smaller during vibration of wrist muscles (because fewer joints need then be controlled?); for the latter, it can reveal the inability to make rapid alternating movements. Therapeutically, the TVR can be used to assist rehabilitation of hemiplegic patients, because its application helps them regain control over flaccid limbs by facilitating onset and strength of voluntary contractions. Vibration can also be used to inhibit spastic motor patterns of antagonistic muscles. Finally, the TVR can be used for biofeedback to assist patients with reduced skin sensations to reacquire an internal "contact" with the affected part, as a precondition for regaining motor control over that part.

The best-known example of task-oriented editing of sensory information is the control exerted by gamma MNs over the sensitivity of muscle spindles (Figs. 3.3 and 4.8B). Gamma MNs control the length of the small (intrafusal) muscles that can pull on the sensory endings of the proprioceptive afferent fibers that are anchored on them, in parallel with the extrafusal fibers of the main muscle (Fig. 4.8A). Thus, gamma (fusimotor) MNs keep spindles sufficiently stretched to maintain their sensitivity, which would be lost during shortening of the muscle in which the spindles are embedded. In this way, gamma MNs assist the servo function of the stretch reflex. This assistance of spindle sensitivity operates during all but the quickest contractions in isolated experimental tissue preparations, but it strengthens the stretch reflex only moderately in intact animals. This puzzle is put into perspective below and in the following chapters.

A theory proposed by Matthews in 1964 holds that for intended movements, the brain sends programmed command signals to gamma MNs to modulate the "fusimotor system," which "biases" spindle sensitivity according to the needs of the *expected* movement. This is an example of how internal (corollary) use is made by gamma motoneurons of efferent motor commands destined for external, muscular adjustments through the action of alpha motoneurons (Chap. 2.2). In this way, a model of the expected movement would be lodged in the programmed spindles. The functioning combination of gamma MNs and spindles would enable spindles to detect any mismatch between movement programs and actual, ongoing movements. Control through gamma MNs is a subprogram, which in Matthews' theory, impresses models of the intended movement onto the spindles. This makes spindles act as "error detectors," that is, of errors of departure from the model.

Spinal alpha MNs can respond to error messages by adjusting the length of the main muscles through the stretch reflex, but it is effective only for small adjustments of postures and slow movements. This is in accord with Sherrington's original definition of his term "proprioception," that the deep receptors measure the actions of the organism itself, not those imposed by the outside world. The reflex "gain" (the output that results from a given input) appears to be insufficient to cope with large changes of muscle length. As already discussed in Chap. 2.2, afferent messages from the spindles, presumably dealing with muscular adjustments, are relayed to the cerebrum and cerebellum: the middle level of the motor hierarchy (Fig. 2.1). This cerebrocerebellar circuit adjusts motor output as required by changes in external circumstances. One way it does so is by controlling the degree to which alpha and gamma MNs are activated together, or "coactivated." Expected levels of alpha-gamma coactivation are established during motor learning, which begins with adaptation of the activation levels of either alpha or gamma MNs, or both (Chap. 4.2).

According to the *servo-assistance theory* outlined above, programmed movements are monitored by muscle spindles that signal departures from the movement program (model), which is impressed on them by centrally modulated gamma bias.

These spindle signals are supposed to evoke motor adjustments through stretch reflex responses of alpha MNs. The theory, which is currently being placed in perspective by experimental verification, proposes that the CNS "knows" whether the planned movement is proceeding according to plan or not. Stretch reflexes can be increased by fusimotor action but, as we will see in the following chapter, this only works for slow and small alignments when tested in human subjects or in behaviorally active animals. The proprioceptive system seems to be designed to cope with small, slow changes produced by muscles one on another, but not with large changes imposed by perturbations. For our orientation we note here that gamma MNs do not turn on spindles sufficiently to change the gain of the stretch reflex and to recruit significant numbers of alpha MNs by this means. Instead, the large-scale recruiting of alpha MNs is managed by supraspinal commands. (These points are explored further in Chap. 4.2.)

How does the CNS know what the muscles are actually doing? This information is decoded from the combination of four input sources: (1) the peripheral sensing of the joint angles and skin deformation, (2) the peripheral sensing of muscle forces generated by the tendon organs, (3) the peripheral sensing of muscle lengths and their changes by muscle spindles, and (4) the reference (corollary) copies of the instructions sent by the CNS middle level to spinal alpha and gamma MNs. It is important to stress that corollary discharges by themselves, however, cannot generate central perception of voluntary movements, although they are important in letting us sense our efforts. Figure 3.2 illustrates this point. The index finger of the left hand (marked with a circle) had been ring-blocked by injection of lignocaine at its base. The blindfolded subject was asked to extend all digits of the left hand, starting from a flexed position. Immediately afterwards the subject was asked to indicate his perception of the positions of the fingers of the left hand by positioning those of the right hand. The assumed positions of the right hand fingers in Fig. 3.2 show that the subject perceived his insentient left index finger *not* to have extended at all joints, when in fact it had actually done so. ("Sense of effort" is considered further in Chap. 7.3.)

With regard to gamma bias, we remember that it changes the sensitivity of muscle spindles. Here is an analogy for the need to decode the bias: imagine that you are pulling a load up by a rope slung over a pulley, and that you are asked to determine the weight of the load by the effort you are making, that is, the force with which you are pulling on the rope. Unless you know what kind of pulley is used, how many times the rope goes around to divide the weight, the load cannot be determined. But once the mechanical efficiency of the pulley is known, the force applied by you

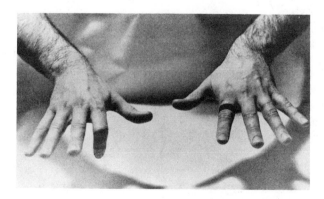

Fig. 3.2. Photograph to illustrate, by the positioning of the fingers of the right hand, the perception of a blindfolded subject of the nonextended position of the left index finger *(circled)*, which had been ring-blocked by injection of lignocaine at the base. (From Goodwin, McCloskey and Matthews, 1972; in McCloskey, 1981)

can be interpreted and the weight of the load becomes known.

The brain can decode the difference between the effects on muscle spindles produced by stretch of extrafusal muscle fibers and by contraction of intrafusal muscles. The instructions to gamma MNs are taken into account in the decoding of the ongoing movement. The brain can also tell the difference between alpha–gamma coactivation and separate activation of alpha MNs, without gammas. In other words, the brain can decode to what extent stretch effects on muscle spindles are produced by extrafusal muscle stretch or by gamma bias on intrafusal muscle fibers (fusimotor bias). *For movements that have been experienced previously, the brain seems to expect levels of alpha–gamma coactivation that were appropriate in previous, successful trials.* When this expectation is not fulfilled, decoding becomes faulty and illusory movements are perceived.

An example is provided by the common motor act of pressing our fingers against an unyielding surface. It is known that we perform this, like most motor acts, with the use of alpha–gamma coactivation. Here is how we know that the brain distinguishes the level of incoming spindle activity caused by stretch of the muscles in which they are embedded, as distinct from that caused by contraction of their intrafusal muscles. Although coactivation raises spindle sensitivity in our finger muscles, we do not experience hyperextension of the fingers, as was the case for the subjects with artificial, vibratory input to spindles that the brain could not include in its calculations. Hence we do not experience an illusory backward bending of the fingers, or a backward movement of the surface against which we press. Therefore, the brain presumably extracts the true peripheral message about muscle stretch by subtracting the effects of its own, central fusimotor bias on the spindles.

How the CNS receives peripheral sensory information about muscle tension (i.e., force) is shown in Fig. 3.3. This information comes from tendon organs of the main muscle. They signal how much force is being actively exerted by the muscles, which they can sense because they are inserted at the ends of the muscle fibers ("in series": see Fig. 4.8 later). Although inputs about force and joint angles are not edited by the gamma system, they are subject to other descending influences and to censor-

Fig. 3.3. Block diagram of a muscle control system. Muscle and the weight it pulls *(load)* are regulated by "feedback" from tendon organs and from spindles that project to spinal neurons as shown, as well as farther centrally into the brain (not shown). Descending "feedforward" central controls reach all spinal interneurons, not only those indicated in the diagram. Excitation and inhibition are denoted by + or −. (Modified from Houk, 1974)

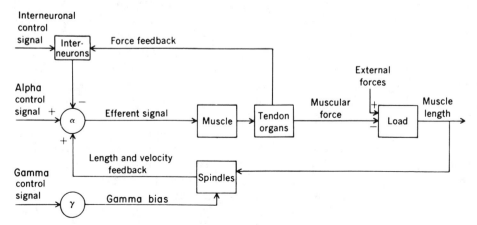

ship by "presynaptic inhibition" from other incoming fibers. (This is explained in Chap. 4.1, Figs. 4.9 and 4.10.) So far we have ignored what role the joint receptors might play, that are active over the whole range of joint movement. They provide the CNS with information about limb postures, information that is independent of muscle receptors and thus serves to back up the information base for the creation and correction of movement programs. The examples considered in this chapter make it clear that for motor control the brain does not use sensory or motor models separately, but instead combines them in the sensorimotor context of the task to be carried out.

2. From Neurons to Muscles

The preceding section described the conditions in which movement programs can be implemented by one or the other of two ways. When large force changes are called for, discharges of spinal alpha MNs can be programmed directly by supraspinal systems. Smaller changes can be obtained by alterations of the activation of gamma MNs (the fusimotor system). In what "language" does the brain address spinal neurons? The brain does not reckon motor actions in terms of particular muscles, let alone their properties. Such calculations are the task of the spinal cord, whose output stages specify the tensions of particular muscles. *What* to do is translated into *how* to do it by the middle level of the motor hierarchy that specifies the desired postures and movements, that is, movement end points and the path, as well as the speed with which to move from one such point to another (the "trajectory"). This we know from the performance of human subjects and of behaviorally active animals ("move" and "hold" programs; Fig. 1.5). The middle level of the motor hierarchy breaks down general motor plans created by the association cortex (complex programs) into end point and path programs. They, in turn, are translated into subpro-

grams that deal with the actions of joints; that is, *the external world is translated into coordinates of the internal world, the body.* Successive specifications go down to the level of lower motor centers that control single joints through the "final common path" (Sherrington's famous term) from spinal motor nuclei to individual muscles. In sum, the intent of a subject is translated into motor action by the middle level and the spinal cord. The middle level programs for intended direction, trajectory, and the stiffness with which a limb is maintained at the specified movement end point. The spinal cord, in contrast, speaks the languages of joint stiffness and muscle tension.

This realization opens the way for us to decode the languages of the brain because we can measure the properties of muscles and how they are governed by the spinal cord. This unit, and the following chapter, spell out the essentials of these properties. Subsequent chapters delve into how far the properties of other parts of the brain relate to the external or internal descriptions of posture and movement. If speed of an intended movement is unimportant, limb postures (i.e., joint angles) can be changed by simple adjustments of steady muscle tensions. Steady tension is maintained by *nonsynchronous* firing of motoneurons at low rates, causing nonsynchronous contractions and relaxation sof the muscle fibers that they innervate, the "motor units," resulting in "tonic" levels of tension and EMG. Changes of tonic EMG can be seen in Fig. 1.3, leading to changes of tonic muscle tension, since that is proportional to the integrated EMG activity. Most smooth movements are generated by combined control of tonic tension levels with that of "phasic" changes that rise and fall in a short time as in Fig. 1.3, because of *synchronous* activation of motor units. Phasic muscle bursts of activity affect the trajectory, that is the speed in relation to the traversed path, but not the end point of the movement. The forces that produce the movements are scaled to allow for contraction and relaxation times of the muscles and for mechanical properites of the limb and its joints, such as mass, inertia, momentum, viscosity and friction. Smooth force scaling is based on the discharge patterns of spinal motoneurons. These patterns are well adapted to the mechanical properties of the muscles they innervate. (After all, they grew up together!) (See Chap. 1.3.)

We are now ready to study how information passes from neurons to muscles, beginning with a look at some important properties of muscle as a tissue. Muscle tissue is elastic; it springs back when stretched. The restorative spring force, consisting of passive tissue elasticity and active contractile force, depends on the length to which the muscle has been stretched (Hooke's law). These relations can be visualized conveniently as muscle length–tension curves, illustrated in Fig. 3.4. When muscle lengths are regulated by weak tonic stretch reflexes, motor units are activated nonsynchronously at low rates. This allows muscle fibers to relax before reactivation. Length–tension relations for those rates have the same general shape as those of non-innervated, inactive muscle tissue, except that they are at a higher level than those of neurally inactive ("passive") muscles. Stretch reflexes are generally weak; they do not recruit many spinal motoneurons in response to muscle stretch (i.e., they have low "gain"). Their normal range of action is confined to small, slow length changes, and thus to small, slow movements. Note that the number of active motoneurons, and therefore muscle motor units, is essentially constant for any one length–tension curve. It is the spring-like properties of muscle that let the fibers generate greater force when stretched to greater lengths. Weak, low-level tonic stretch reflexes produce low muscle "tone." (The definition of tone is based on the readiness to resist imposed stretch by means of "passive" muscle properties and "active" tonic stretch reflexes: see Chap. 8.1.)

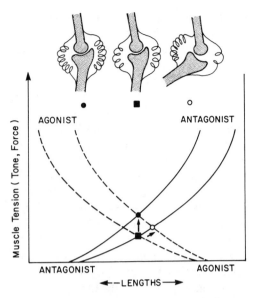

Fig. 3.4. Comparison of three limb postures that differ in joint angle and/or joint stiffness. Two sets of length–tension curves are shown for muscles that act in opposition to each other (antagonists), as sketched in the diagrams above, where springs represent muscles. Curves for agonists and antagonists, and directions of their length changes, are shown as broken and solid lines. Agonist *(broken line)* is at greatest length on the left when the antagonist *(solid line)* is shortest, and vice versa. *Upward arrow* (from *filled square* to *filled circle*) indicates increased co-contraction of antagonists, which increases joint stiffness without change of muscle lengths; *sloping arrow* (to *open circle*) indicates increase of agonist tone, creating a postural equilibrium at a new position, that is, at new muscle lengths. Equilibrium at the filled circle can support most weight, at the open circle less, and at the filled square least. (Modified from Brooks, 1983)

Figure 3.4 presents length–tension curves for opposing muscles at two levels of tone. (The curves for non-innervated muscle tissue would be even lower: they have not been drawn in the figure.) The muscles are not moving: the curves are at a particular moment in time (i.e., time is not an axis for the graph). The abscissa is labeled as lengths of muscles and the ordinate is labeled in terms of their force, which is the tension that the muscle can maintain at a particular length, given a particular level of neural activation. In other words, when a particular number of motoneurons drive the muscles to a particular tension, that tension will vary along the length–tension curve according to the mechanical stretch imposed on that muscle.

At equal levels of tension, the curves of opposing muscles cross, marking where agonist and antagonist muscles balance to maintain a steady joint angle. The *ratio* of the tensions generated by the agonist and antagonist determine the equilibrium point of the limb (see the diagrams of the muscles acting on the joint in the upper row of Fig. 3.4).

How much opposing muscles co-contract at their point of equilibrium is also defined as a property of the limb posture at equilibrium. Much co-contraction steadies the joint to resist imposed loads. As stated earlier, high resistance makes the joint mechanically stiff, and low resistance makes it compliant. The mechanical joint stiffness is the result of the sum of the tensions of the opposing muscles at their particular lengths: that is, ("positional") stiffness is the *sum* for the opposing muscles of their ratios of tension/length. The limb postures marked in Fig. 3.4 by the filled square and filled circle have different joint stiffnesses at the same joint angle, because the steady tensions of both muscles have increased equally. The muscle contractions have been *isometric,* that is without external change of length, and the joint has not been moved. When the passive (viscoelastic) muscle properties or the active tone of the opposing pair are unequal, one muscle shortens and the other is stretched, rotating the joint to a new angle where their tensions are once more equal. This has occurred in the posture defined by the open circle, when only agonist tone increased. This kind of length-changing contraction is called *isotonic.* Observations of human and animal performance suggest that the CNS programs limb postures in terms of length–tension relations of muscles acting on the joints of the limb. These relations are specified by spinal output stages that

regulate (maintain) the thresholds and gains of tonic stretch reflexes under the control (for new values) of supraspinal commands. These concepts were mentioned in Chap. 2.3 and also Chap. 3.1 with reference to Fig. 3.3 The behavior of muscle suggested in Fig. 3.4 is referred to as the "mass-spring" model. The viscoelastic properties of opposing muscles are equal at the "neutral" joint position (for the elbow it is near 85 deg, that is, 5 deg toward flexion from the 90-deg position shown in Fig. 7.4A). Other angles are maintained by tonic muscle discharge of one or the other of the pair to make up the difference between their passive properties at the particular length. The springlike property of muscle tissue amounts to about 15% of maximal voluntary tension against stretch. (This is discussed further in Chaps. 4.1 and 8.1; see Fig. 8.1.)

During maintenance of high muscle tone, tonic stretch reflexes reactivate muscle fibers before they have had time to relax fully, which fuses the nonsynchronous, individual contractions (twitches) into sustained (tetanic) contractions. Each incomplete relaxation leaves a residue of unresolved tension that appears as an unevenness on the length–tension curve of that muscle at a particular moment in time. Muscle tissue is slow to contract and to relax: that is the rate-limiting factor here. How this develops at different rates of activity can be studied by controlled, nonsynchronous stimulation of several branches of the motor nerve of a muscle. Length–tension relations can be measured when the joint is held at various angles, that is when the muscles develop force without changing their length ("isometric" contractions, as marked on the abscissa). These length–tension curves mimic those produced by muscles at various levels of tonic stretch reflex activity. Figure 3.5A illustrates the transition from a smooth, concave curve (at 3 stimuli/second) to the appearance of unevenness at 5 stimuli/second to a force "hump" at 10 stimuli/second. These representative curves were obtained in trials with the soleus muscle of the anesthetized cat. At high levels of tone, nonsynchronous contractions follow one another quickly and their unresolved tension leftovers sum into a force "hump." The higher the tone, the faster the nonsynchronous contractions follow one another, until they contract nearly synchronously, making their force humps resemble those produced by "phasic" contractions. These artificial trials approximate physiologically normal conditions in which muscles usually contract in unfused tetani (of which examples are illustrated in Fig. 4.3). The largest tension in the experiment of Fig. 3.5A is produced at the peak of the hump, which occurs at the angle at which the joint is usually held in nature (about 60 deg for the cat's ankle). Muscle length at this angle is called the "resting" length, at which muscle cells also work optimally because the active sites of the thick and thin filaments overlap most for greatest contractile efficiency. Figure 3.5A *thus demonstrates how muscles exert their greatest tension at those joint angles which have to be manipulated most often.* (compare these experimental graphs later to the graph obtained for the flexors of the human elbow; Figs. 4.10 and 8.1.)

Figure 3.5B draws our attention to another asymmetrical muscle property, namely that the contractile muscle machinery is activated more effectively at long rather than short lengths. After contracting isometrically (Fig. 3.5A), the muscles were lengthened or shortened at constant velocities (Fig. 3.5B). The graphs on the left demonstrate that contractile tension is well maintained during muscle lengthening, which occurs physiologically, for instance, during stretch of antagonists. However, during shortening (shown on the right) contractile tension falls off sharply below the isometric values marked on the central ordinate scale. Both lengthening and shortening effects are greatest at high tensions (e.g., the uppermost curve), because energy is stored in the elastic muscle elements in line (in "series")

with the actively shortening contractile parts of the muscle. Figure 3.5B demonstrates that forces developed during muscular contractions, and thus during joint movements, depend on the direction of movement. This means that *in order to generate a particular force about a joint, the CNS must specify both the speed and direction, that is the velocity, of all muscles acting on that joint.* The directional ("vector") properties of muscles thus shape the central commands needed to drive them functionally. We will meet applications of this principle throughout this book: the properties of each hierarchical level determine how it is controlled by the CNS.

Let us visualize how the properties illustrated in Fig. 3.5 work together. An example of a length–tension curve with a typical phasic force hump is illustrated in Fig. 3.6A, superimposed upon the "tonic" curve beneath it. The upper curve, with the force hump, represents a contraction during a particular moment, and the lower curve the momentary tone from which the muscle started. Both curves plot one important property of a contraction against muscle length: the *tension* (or force) generated. An equally important property for the control of movement is the *velocity*.

In Fig. 3.6B, tension as well as velocity are plotted against length, in a three-dimensional description of properties of a muscle at a particular moment. At a single velocity this relation is a length–tension curve as in Figs. 3.5A and 3.6A, and at a single length it is a force–velocity curve as in Fig. 3.5B. What force the muscle can actually generate depends on both length and velocity, and is therefore defined for a given moment by the intersection of two such curves. In Fig. 3.6B this intersection is drawn at the normal, resting length of the muscle, which it maintains at the most common angle of the joint that it acts on. We can see that at this length the force hump is at its peak. We see again that the muscle generates maximal, or near-maximal, tension at its resting length, which

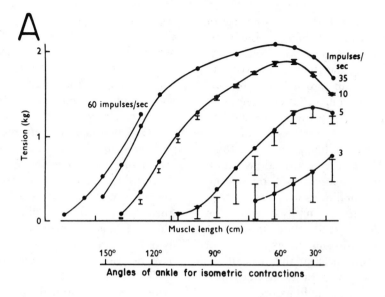

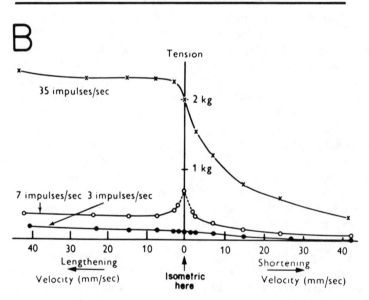

Fig. 3.5. Contractile muscle force depends on limb position, its rate of change, and direction. (A) Length–tension curves of isometric (soleus) muscle at different rates of nonsynchronous supramaximal stimulation of five branches of the motor nerve of an anesthetized cat. Force "humps" develop at nerve frequencies that nearly fuse tetanic contractions at joint angles indicated in lower abscissa. *Bars* indicate range of mean values. (B) Muscle force is maintained during lengthening but falls during shortening below isometric values [at *vertical arrow,* measured at ankle position of 70 deg as in (A)]. [(A) From Rack and Westbury, 1969; (B) from Joyce, Rack and Westbury, 1969; both in Lewis, 1981 and in Rymer, 1983]

provides the most powerful control at the most usual joint angle, that is the most usual limb "posture."

Excitation of the motor nerve from the spinal cord determines how frequently the muscle is excited, but how it actually contracts and relaxes is determined by the properties of the muscle tissue. One of those properties is that muscles can generate more contractile force while being stretched (lengthening) than while they are shortening. These conditions are labeled in Fig. 3.6B on the velocity abscissa, which increases in either direction from the middle (where the length–tension curve, transferred from Fig. 3.6A, is drawn at zero velocity). Let us examine the interactions of the three variables in Fig. 3.6B. We must remember that the two graphs are drawn just for resting length and zero velocity, at one particular level of neural excitation from the spinal cord. The force–velocity graph (going to the left) shows that maximal force can be generated over a wide range of velocities during "lengthening contractions." An example of a lengthening contraction would be that of the elbow extensor, triceps brachii, during a "stiff" elbow flexion when it co-contracts with the antagonist, biceps brachii. In contrast, the force that can be produced (at resting length) falls off rapidly when the muscle shortens unopposed (as shown in the velocity graph going to the right). This would be the case for the elbow flexor, biceps brachii, during a "loose" elbow flexion. The faster the shortening, the less force is generated.

We can gain a better impression of the relations of length, tension and velocity by drawing not just two intersecting curves as

in Fig. 3.6B, but a family of each, and again as in Fig. 3.6B, at one particular level of activation by the spinal cord. Figure 3.6C combines these conditions to describe the state of the muscle for one particular moment. The force hump is now a hill rising above the sloped length–tension sheet of the tonic state. The illustration gives just one example of phasic and tonic ten-

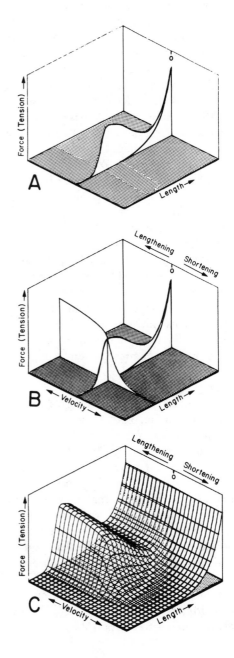

Fig. 3.6. Muscle length, tension and velocity are interdependent properties of muscle tissue. (A) Upper and lower length–tension curves describe tension levels for different muscle lengths at a particular moment during phasic and tonic contractions, respectively. Compare to Fig. 3.5. (B) Length–tension curve as in (A), and force–velocity curve define possible momentary force by their intersection (at resting length and at zero velocity). (C) A family of curves as in (B) generates two surfaces that describe the muscle at equivalent times in two different states of activation. The upper one, with the force hill, defines a particular intensity of phasic activation of the muscle by the spinal cord. The lower surface describes a level of muscle tone. (From Brooks, 1983, modified from Partridge and Benton, 1981)

sions; either could be lower or higher than those shown, depending on the intensities of neural activity emanating from the spinal cord. Different intensities produce different EMG tonic levels and bursts, and consequently different movements. (That was illustrated in Fig. 1.3.)

There is only one point where the length–tension curve of Fig. 3.6A intersects the velocity–tension curve of Fig. 3.6B to produce a particular velocity at a given combination of muscle length and tension, at one moment in time. When we consider the family of curves to which Fig. 3.6A and B belong, we obtain the "surface" drawn in Fig. 3.6C. There is only one particular surface that combines a set of lengths, tensions and velocities obtained at a particular level of neural activation, at a given moment in time. The brain can control length or tension or velocity, but it cannot control all three at once independently. If lengths and tensions are controlled, velocity is not an independent variable. Conversely, if the brain calls for a particular velocity, then either the length or the tension can be specified; the third variable is determined by the properties of the muscle. The adjustments of length and tension can be made by the spinal cord, if needed. This integrative ability frees supraspinal levels from having to consider the properties of muscles, and simplifies the control of one level of the CNS by another.

Muscles can only maneuver on the force hill shown in Fig. 3.6C in those ways that combine *compatible muscle lengths, tensions and velocities.* Because of these constraints, plans for movements must include properties of the particular muscles to be used and of the loads that they will encounter. If unexpected conditions arise, they have to be dealt with in the evolving movement on the basis of feedback information (see Fig. 2.1). The spinal cord and some supraspinal centers handle the information relevant for muscles, and are the final arbiters to determine exactly how muscle force is to be applied by cooperat-

ing agonists (synergists) and by their antagonists. The time factors in movements call for more complicated computations than are required for static postures. The CNS must now manipulate length, force and speed for all muscles acting on a joint. (We will examine the force hills of opposing muscles juxtaposed as a hill and valley in Fig. 4.6C in Chap. 4.1.) To these factors we must add another, timing, which was left out of Figs. 3.4–3.6 but was stressed in Fig. 1.3. Movements, like skiers, choose their paths on the slopes according to what speed they can manage with what force at their particular stage of exhaustion or control. There is an important consequence to the relations graphed in Fig. 3.6B and C, namely that lengthening muscles generate more tension than shortening ones. It means that lengthening muscles store up more viscous and elastic force, which is available for release as contractile force; in other words, lengthening muscles contract more *efficiently* than shortening muscles. We will find that this is important for locomotion and for learning of all motor skills (Chaps. 10.4 and 11–14). Muscle properties thus provide the variables for the most elementary output "language" of the spinal cord in the computation of posture and movement.

3. Summary

The CNS generates motor actions on the basis of correlations of peripheral sensorimotor information with central models based on past experience. Limb positions and movements are encoded as afferent messages by receptors in muscles, skin and/or joints. Muscle sense is very important. For instance, the tonic vibration reflex leads to illusory limb positions (as if the vibrated muscle had been stretched), because it is elicited by direct, vibratory stimulation of primary spindle endings, which the brain does not include in its reckoning. In contrast, spindle discharges evoked by intrafusal muscle contraction are interpreted correctly, presumably because the brain has corollary information about the degree of fusimotor bias. The brain decodes where the limbs are in space by combining external afferent sensory input and internal corollary discharges. Sense of position and effort cannot be established by corollary discharge alone.

Motor commands from the highest level of the hierarchy encode postures as positions in external, extrapersonal space. The middle level translates the commands from coordinates relating to the external world to those relating to the internal world of the body. It specifies how stiffly positions are to be maintained (hold program), and encodes movements in terms of their paths and the speeds at which they are to be traversed (trajectory, move program). The spinal cord encodes the commands into activity of alpha and gamma motoneurons. The final joint angle depends on the ratio of the tensions generated by the opposing muscles. The mechanical stiffness with which the joint is held at that angle is determined by the sum of the tensions of the opposing muscles. The tonic stretch reflex operates as a servo mechanism, that is in the negative-feedback mode, to cancel the reports about muscle stretch by muscle spindles through stretch-evoked activity of alpha MNs. The gain of the stretch reflex is low, appropriate for coping with the relatively small tension changes generated between the muscles acting on the same joint. The reflex gain does not suffice to make alpha MNs respond to large, imposed changes of length or load.

Matthews proposed that gamma motoneurons (MNs) assist spinal servo action not only by increasing spindle sensitivity during muscular contractions, but also by modulating spindles according to the programs of expected movements ("servo-assistance"). The programs are thought to be supplied by the cerebrum and cerebellum, which also adjust the degree of alpha-gamma coactivation. This mode of operation would make spindles act as detectors of errors with reference to programs (or models) for intended postures and movements. We note for our orientation, however, that the gain of this gamma route would only be sufficient to cope with slow, small load changes. Large tension changes are brought about by supraspinal adjustment of the number of active alpha motoneurons. (This is discussed further in Chap. 4.2.)

Length-tension curves of inactive (passive) muscle tissue and active ones with low levels of tonic stretch reflex activity have smoothly upward-rising shapes. Muscle fibers exert greater tension when stretched than when they are relaxed because of the spring-like properties of muscle tissue. The tension exerted by a muscle at a particular level of neural activation is greater at greater lengths, i.e. without change of the number of active spinal motoneurons. When muscles are activated at faster rates, the fibers cannot relax quickly enough and leave unresolved force humps on the previously smooth curves. Length-tension curves of opposing muscles define, at their intersection, the angle of the joint on which the muscles act. The joint can be made loose or stiff at the equilibrium position by using only a little or much antagonist co-contraction. Muscles generate maximal tension at their resting lengths, which provides the limb with the best control at the most commonly assumed postures (hold program). The movement trajectory is encoded separately from position, and has to take account of the fact that muscles generate more force while being stretched than during unopposed contraction. Move programs can therefore take advantage of the greater elastic energy of lengthening muscles. Stretch reflexes are adjusted according to peripheral feedback about muscle length from spindles, about muscle force from tendon organs, and about joint angles from spindles and joint receptors. The output of the spinal "final common path" is encoded as muscle force. How it is patterned for each muscle depends on the properties of that muscle tissue. Muscle lengths and tensions are interdependent, as defined by length–tension curves. At any moment in time, the combinations of lengths and tensions are interdependent with the velocity of muscle shortening or lengthening. Thus, the brain can control any two of these variables for a given level of neural activation, but the third must assume suitable values to permit the muscle to function. These determinations can be made at the spinal level because discharge patterns of spinal MNs become adapted to the properties of the muscles that they innervate. This segmental capability simplifies the operation of the CNS because it reduces the calculations necessary for supraspinal control.

References

Bizzi, E., Accornero, N., Chapple, W., and Hogan, N. 1981. Processes underlying arm trajectory formation. In *Brain mechanisms of perceptual awareness and purposeful behavior,* eds. O. Pompeiano and C. Ajmone-Marsan, pp. 311–318. *Int. Brain Res. Org. Monogr. Ser.* vol. 8. New York: Raven Press.

Brooks, V. B. 1983. Motor control: how posture and movements are governed *Phys. Ther.* 63:664–673. [Figs. 3.4 and 3.6]

Burke, R. E., and Edgerton, V. R. 1975. Motor unit properties and selective involvement in movement. *Exercise Sports Sci. Rev.* 3:31–81.

Cooke, J. D. 1980. The organization of simple, skilled movements. In *Tutorials in motor behavior,* eds. G. E. Stelmach and J. Requin. *Advances in psychology,* vol. 1, pp. 199–212. Amsterdam: North-Holland.

Craske B. 1977. Perception of impossible limb positions induced by tendon vibration. *Science* 196:71–73.

De Domenico, G. 1979. Tonic vibratory reflex. What is it? Can we use it? *Physiotherapy* 65:44–48.

Goodwin, G. M., McCloskey, D. I., and Matthews, P. B. C. 1972. The contribution of muscle afferents to kinesthesia shown by vibration-induced illusions of movement and by the effects of paralysing joint afferents. *Brain* 95:705–748. [Figs. 3.1 and 3.2]

Hayes, K. C., and Marteniuk, R. G. 1976. Dimensions of motor task complexity. In *Motor control: issues and trends,* ed. G. E. Stelmach, pp. 201–228. New York: Academic Press.

Houk, J. C. 1974. Feedback control of muscle: a synthesis of the peripheral mechanisms. In *Medical physiology,* ed. V. B. Mountcastle. 13th ed. St. Louis: C. V. Mosby Co. [Fig. 3.3]

Joyce, G. C., Rack, P. M. H., and Westbury, D. R. 1969. The mechanical properties of cat soleus muscle during controlled lengthening and shortening movements, *J. Physiol* (Lond.) 204:461–474. [Fig. 3.5B]

Keele, S. W. 1981. Behavioral analysis of movement. In *Motor control.* Sect. 1, vol. 2. *Handbook of physiology,* ed. V. B. Brooks, pp. 1391–1414. Bethesda, Md.: American Physiological Society.

Lewis, D. M. 1981. The physiology of motor units in mammalian skeletal muscle. In *Motor coordination.* Vol. 5. *Handbook of behavioral neurobiology,* eds. A. L. Towe and E. S. Luschei, pp. 1–67. New York: Plenum Press. [Fig. 3.5]

MacKay, D. M. 1966. Cerebral organization and the conscious control of action. In *Brain and conscious experience,* ed. J. C. Eccles. New York: Springer Verlag.

Matthews, P. B. C. 1981. Evolving views on the internal operation and the functional role of the muscle spindle. *J. Physiol. (Lond.)* 320: 1–30.

McCloskey, D. I. 1981. Corollary discharges: motor commands and perception. In *Motor control.* Sect. 1, vol. 2. *Handbook of physiology,* ed. V. B. Brooks, pp. 1415–1447. Bethesda, Md.: American Physiological Society. [Fig. 3.2]

McCloskey, D. I., Cross, M. J., Honner R., and Potter, E. K. 1983. Sensory effects of pulling of vibrating exposed tendons in man. *Brain* 106:21–37.

McMahon, T. A. 1984. *Muscles, reflexes, and locomotion.* Princeton, N. J.: Princeton University Press.

Miles, F. A., and Evarts, E. V. 1979. Concepts of motor organization. *Ann. Rev. Psychol.* 30:327–362.

Moberg, E. 1983. The role of cutaneous afferents in position sense, kinesthesia, and motor function of the hand. *Brain* 106:1–19.

Partridge, L. D., and Benton, L. A. 1981. Muscle, the motor. In *Motor control,* Sect. 1, Vol. 2. *Handbook of Physiology,* ed. V. B.

Brooks, pp. 43–106. Bethesda, Md.: American Physiological Society. [Fig. 3.6]

Rack, P. M. H., and Westbury, D. R. 1969. The effects of length and stimulus rate on tension in the isometric cat soleus muscle. *J. Physiol. (Lond.)* 204:443–460. [Fig. 3.5A]

Rymer, w. Z. 1983. Muscle afferent contribution to the regulation of muscle length and tension. In *Neurobiology*. Vol. 5. *The clinical neurosciences,* ed. W. D. Willis, pp. 435–469. New York: Churchill Livingstone. [Fig. 3.5]

Sanes, J. N., and Evarts, E. V. 1984. Motor psychophysics. *Hum. Neurobiol.* 2:217–225.

II

The Lower Level of the Motor Hierarchy

This part deals with the mechanisms of some spinal functions, how commands from the middle level engage reflex mechanisms and how neural signals are translated into coordinated muscle tensions. We consider the various means of managing the output of spinal motoneurons, which Sherrington called the "final common path" for commands to muscles. Towards this end we review the properties of motor units and of spinal fusimotor control, of interneurons and their descending controls, and of supraspinal mechanisms that prepare the spinal cord for voluntary movements. These matters are taken up in some detail because they are of great importance in understanding sensorimotor integration and because they afford a glimpse of hierarchical motor control at work. Here we can learn how neural assemblies, though "uninformed" about the wider meaning of higher instructions, can nevertheless harness the muscles to those instructions (see Chap. 2.2).

Understanding this subject opens the doors to numerous practical applications in training workers, athletes, and dancers, as well as patients with motor disabilities. Facilitation and inhibition of "automatic" mechanisms have long been used as therapeutic procedures to assist spastic patients with postural adjustments, weight bearing and independent limb movements. As another example, walking can be triggered off by postural reactions. This trick was used by James Parkinson, who employed small boys to assist patients suffering from the "shaking palsy" in getting around by tipping them forward to trigger walking as a consequence of postural reactions. The juvenile assistants then had to run ahead to stop the walking patients, because they could not do that by themselves either. Another useful approach has been to awaken the patients' "sense of effort" through various sensory stimulations, which seem to function as biofeedback. In this way, we can learn to "concentrate" on performing movements for which we have had no "feel," and motor learning can be aided.

This part completes the transition from the Introductory Overview, which ended with Chap. 3.1, to a more down-to-earth examination of our subject. Students who feel the need for review of the physiology and anatomy of the nervous system should consult suitable texts, of which some are listed at the end of Chap. 1.

4

Spinal Segmental Control

This chapter examines how the spinal cord engages the various kinds of muscles, what their properties are and how they act on the joints they innervate, and how muscular changes are sensed by muscle receptors. The guiding theme is: what are the mechanisms for holding and moving joints?

1. Motoneurons and Motor Units

Motoneurons that innervate a particular muscle (e.g., soleus) form a motoneuron "pool" or "nucleus." Alpha and gamma MNs are mixed together in this assembly, which is located in the ventral horn of one or several segments of the spinal cord. The ability of the cord to carry out its "lower level" functions in motor control is based on a firm rule by which MNs are brought into activity or removed from it. As so often occurs in biology, the rule follows from structural detail, in this case how the MN pool is innervated. All MNs, large and small, in a nucleus receive afferent fibers from all the spindles in the innervated muscle. The easiest way to think of this is to remember that any one Ia fiber gives off a branch to every MN in a pool. When a spindle discharges, its afferent fiber branches have different effects on large and small MNs, because the afferent endings are spaced closer together on the surface of small MNs. This causes more in-

tense current flow across the membranes of small MNs than large ones. Since, in addition, small MNs have higher membrane resistances than large ones, the voltage drops—that is the excitatory postsynaptic potentials (EPSPs) are bigger in small MNs—according to Ohm's law. The basic factor for reflex recruitment is EPSP amplitude: larger EPSPs reach the thresholds of MNs more easily. It follows that small MNs are "recruited" into the active MN pool before large ones, which have higher recruitment reflex thresholds.*

Recruitments of motoneurons progresses from small to large MNs in a stereotyped manner with but little variation of threshold for any particular MN. This size principle (of Henneman) holds for tonic and for phasic stretch reflex responses as well as for other reflex actions and even for intended, voluntary movements. The succession of recruited MNs

*Readers should not confuse this with thresholds to direct *electrical stimulation,* which vary in opposite manner: they are lowest for large cells and fibers. The reason is that synaptic transmitters drive cell membranes to biochemically determined equilibrium potentials, that is, they achieve a certain voltage across the membrane by stimulating with constant current, whereas electrical stimulators usually are a source of constant voltage. Therefore, the effective stimulator current varies inversely to the membrane resistance and thus generates more current for low-resistance, large fibers than for small ones.

provides smooth increases of tension, because large MNs have large axons with many branches, forming large "motor units" of innervated muscle fibers. Despite the differences in motor unit sizes, the tension contributed by any one motor unit is roughly the same *fraction* of the total, because large units add more, but do so at a high background level. Since spindle endings discharge tonically, small MNs (including gamma MNs) are *tonically* active. Large MNs are not tonically active because they are recruited only when tension has risen in the later phases of reflex contractions. Large MNs are therefore *phasically* active. Reflex inhibition also accommodates the size principle and follows the rule: last recruited, first decruited. Phasically active MNs are removed from the recruitment pool ("decruited") first and tonically active MNs last. Henneman's size principle is the expression of a genetically inherited system of connections between cells with appropriate properties. They automatically smooth changes of muscle force by grading them finely against low levels of background force and by making them large when high force levels prevail. In other words, this arrangement that keeps transient changes in proportion to their background levels, defines the working range of spinal adjustments without having to burden higher CNS levels with those details (cf. Chap. 2.2). An arrangement equivalent to this motor output scheme exists on the sensory intake side: we sense transient changes of touch, light, sound, and so forth, in relation to the prevailing steady background of the sensory modality in question. (This is known as the Weber–Fechner rule.) Thus, sensory as well as motor parts at different levels of the nervous system set their own working ranges, which buffers them against abrupt, large changes. The ranges can be changed (i.e., scaled) by interaction with other parts of the brain. The operations of different task systems are scaled to appropriate levels to facilitate predictive programming and ongoing control. Other chapters will

show that this principle applies to the organization of most aspects of the central nervous system.

The physiological properties of the muscle fibers in small and large motor units are adapted to their tonic and phasic functions. The main histological and metabolic properties of muscle fibers in motor units of different sizes are listed in Fig. 4.1. The histogram spans the range from the plentiful slow, small red fibers (Henneman's type C, on the left side of the histogram) through intermediate fibers (type B), to the smaller number of fast, large pale fibers (type A), on the right side of the histogram. All muscle fibers of a motor unit have the same properties. Since the branches of a motor unit are widely distributed in a muscle, their admixture places muscle fibers of types A, B and C next to each other. This is illustrated in Fig. 4.2, where different densities of mitochondrial stain reflect concentrations of enzymes (ATPase) for aerobic metabolism. When tonic motor units are active at low rates, they do not produce and accumulate large, unresolved tension humps, as we saw in Chap. 3.2 with regard to Fig. 3.6A. Even when they are active at higher rates, their tetanic tensions are smaller than those of large phasic fibers, which contract more quickly. The table beneath Henneman's histogram (Fig. 4.1) lists some of the metabolic adaptations. Tonically active, small fibers can maintain high levels of aerobic (red) myoglobin metabolism, based on a rich capillary supply line for oxygen. This makes them fatigue resistant. The phasic activity of large, pale fibers is based on anaerobic breakdown of stored glycogen, which upon its exhaustion leads to quick fatigue.

Slow muscles, driven by small alpha MNs, receive more input from spindle afferent fibers of Ia diameter than fast muscles driven by large MNs. (The names of afferent and efferent fibers are reviewed in Fig. 4.8.) This makes stretch reflexes of Ia origin especially important for postural adjustments (Fig. 4.3) through the modulation of viscoelastic (stiffness) properties

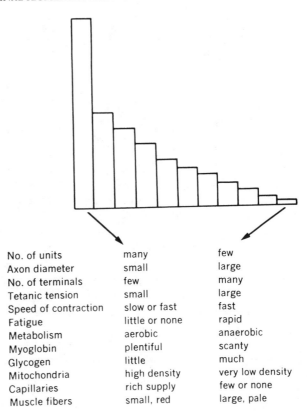

No. of units	many	few
Axon diameter	small	large
No. of terminals	few	many
Tetanic tension	small	large
Speed of contraction	slow or fast	fast
Fatigue	little or none	rapid
Metabolism	aerobic	anaerobic
Myoglobin	plentiful	scanty
Glycogen	little	much
Mitochondria	high density	very low density
Capillaries	rich supply	few or none
Muscle fibers	small, red	large, pale

Fig. 4.1. Distribution of motor unit properties according to their sizes are plotted in histogram. Below is a list of characteristics of motor units and their muscle fibers for the two ends of the histogram. An approximately continuous gradation between these limits is assumed. (From Henneman, 1980)

of tonically active antigravity muscles. There have been many attempts to find exceptions to the recruitment order according to neuron size in stretch reflexes (i.e., Henneman's principle), but no convincing ones have been found as long as muscle functions are considered within their main task contexts. Some exceptions for multi-task muscles are described further below. The recruitment order includes the amplitudes of monosynaptic input to MNs (from Ia EPSPs) and the equivalent scaling

Fig. 4.2. Muscle fibers of different motor units are mixed together. Appearance of large, pale type A fibers, small, dark type C fibers, and intermediate type B fibers in a cross section of medial gastrocnemius muscle of the cat. (From Henneman, 1980)

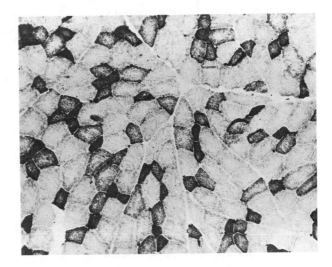

of polysynaptic input for excitation of flexors and inhibition of extensors (from the flexor reflex afferents, or FRA, Chap. 5.1).

A similar classification of motor units to that of Henneman was reached by R. E. Burke on the basis of fatigue resistance and twitch tensions as the main indicators. Figure 4.3 summarizes the main results for the much-studied cat's medial gastrocnemius (MG) muscle. Henneman's type A is equivalent to Burke's fast-contracting, fast-fatiguing type (FF, low fatigue index) that can generate high tetanic tensions. Type B probably corresponds to the fast-contracting, fatigue-resistant (FR) type, and type C to the slow-contracting S type that generates only low tetanic tensions and is extremely fatigue resistant (high fatigue index). Type FF is shown in the top line of Fig. 4.3A as being suitable only for phasic activity because it fatigues in 1 to 2 minutes. The properties of this group are plotted in the left corner of the three-dimensional display in Fig. 4.3B. The fatigue index classifies motor unit responses to intracellular stimulation of their MNs (every second at 40 stimuli/second for 0.3 second). The index is the ratio of tension produced during 2 minutes of this stimulation compared to that during the initial stimulation. Records giving these values are reproduced for three motor units in the left-hand (a) column of Fig. 4.3A. The right-hand (b) column presents the unfused appearance of the ("tetanic") contraction responses of all three units. Note that the tetanic tension "sags" after about 0.4 second for groups FF and FR, but not for S. FF and FR are plotted in Fig. 4.3B with open circles and S with filled circles. These three types of motor units have also been demonstrated as distinct groups in the posturally active human medial gastrocnemius by intramuscular microstimulation of single motor axon branches (not illustrated).

In more phasic muscles, such as those in the human hand, motor units are separated less clearly into three type groups. Figure 4.4A illustrates the distribution for the first dorsal interosseus muscle, plotted in the same manner as in Fig. 4.3. The method of sampling the force developed by single motor units by "spike-triggered averaging" is shown in Fig. 4.4B. The EMG is recorded (extracellularly) with needle electrodes during voluntary isometric contractions made by this abductor of the index finger against a strain gauge. Action potentials of a single muscle fiber trigger an averager of the tension developed by the motor unit to which that fiber belongs. Several hundred repetitions reveal the average tension record of the motor unit, because these time-locked signals stand out from the random background noise. Figure 4.4C illustrates operation of the size principle in this muscle by relating the recruitment of individual motor units to their particular threshold tensions.

Tests of the size principle have revealed that the innervation of motor units by Ia fibers is arranged according to the main physiological functions of each muscle. For example, the illustration for the first dorsal interosseus shows no exceptions to the principle when tested during its prime function, abduction of the index finger (Fig. 4.4A,B). About 10% of the motor units do not conform to the same rule, however, when the same units are tested during their participation in a secondary function where that muscle is only a synergist: flexion of the index finger. This demonstration (by Denny-Brown, and later by Desmedt, not illustrated here) that the Ia innervation of spinal motor nuclei is organized according to the primary functions of muscles is important, because postural adjustments are grasped best at present by considering the action of muscles with double functions, across two joints (Fig. 9.9). It seems likely that more "exceptions" to the size principle will be found. Their very presence will alert us to new aspects of functional organization for special uses in postures and movements.

The main, currently known, apparent

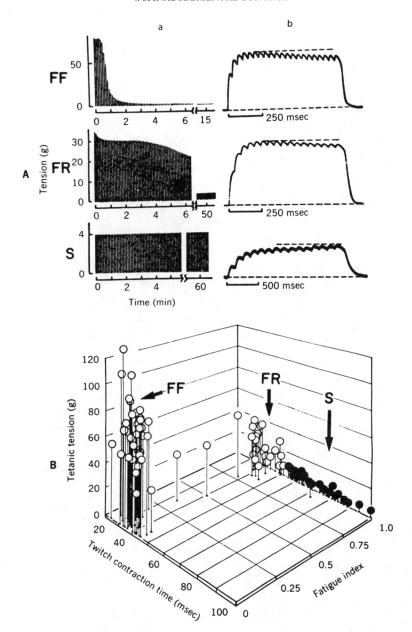

Fig. 4.3. Classification of motor units by muscle contractile properties, into types FF (fast-fatiguing), FR (fatigue-resistant) and S (slow) in medial gastrocnemius of the cat. (A) Tension records show onset of fatigue in column a, and in column b "sag" of tetanic tension below maximum marked by dashed line. (B) Three-dimensional plot relates tetanic tension (ordinate) to twitch contraction time and to fatigue index on left and right abscissae, respectively. (From Burke et al, 1973; in Henneman, 1980; and Burke, 1981b)

exception from Henneman's size principle is a reversal of the usual recruitment order of MNs in human voluntary movements, which is set in train by some non-noxious skin inputs. This has been demonstrated for abduction of the index finger by the first dorsal interosseus muscle (as in Fig. 4.4) and also for extension of the knee. In

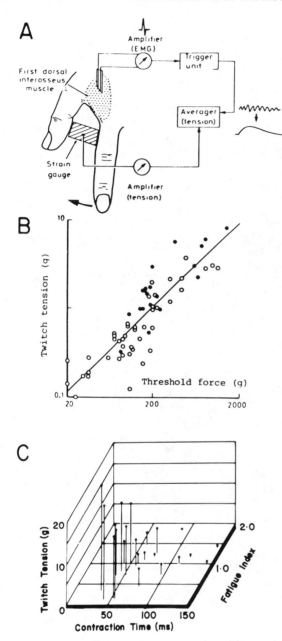

Fig. 4.4. Properties of human motor units during voluntary contractions of the first dorsal interosseus muscle, an abductor of the index finger, determined by "spike-triggered averaging." (A) Diagram of a method to obtain tension developed during finger abduction (see *arrow*) by a single motor unit using the action potential of one of its muscle fibers as a time-locking trigger to average many trials (see text). (B) Demonstration of Henneman's size principle for twitch tensions (ordinate) produced by single motor units at their particular threshold force levels (abscissa). All data from one subject, obtained as in (A), at different times (*open* and *filled circles*). (C) Relations for single motor units between twitch tension [ordinate, as in (B)], contraction time and fatigue index, plotted as in Fig. 4.3. [(A) From McComas, 1977; (B) from Milner-Brown, Stein and Yemm, 1973; (C) from Stephens and Usherwood, 1977; (B,C) in Burke, 1981a,b; (A,C) in Stuart and Enoka, 1983]

both cases, high thresholds of motor units fall while low ones rise, leading to preferential recruitment of large, phasic units. Since this change occurs in relation to voluntary movements, it is likely that the non-noxious skin stimulation alters the effectiveness of descending commands to the MNs. A centrally controlled mechanism that does just that is described in the next chapter (flexor reflex afferents, or FRA; Fig. 5.6). Findings such as these will probably turn out to be examples of central guidance of peripheral sensitivity, all organized in the context of the movement intent (Chap. 3.1). Departures from the size principle, which is based on the cellular properties of MNs, should alert us to possible new interpretations of the functional context in which the muscles are functioning.

Such opportunities are arising from related animal experiments. FF- and FR-type MNs in the MG pool of the cat (see Figs. 4.3 and 4.5A) can be excited *before* S-type units by polysynaptic skin input from the foot and ankle. Again we may be seeing the action of the FRA on a muscle with double function (ankle flexion, knee extension). This may be a fragment of some adjustment of a "long-loop" action (a form of intent-related supraspinal employment of MNs; see Chaps. 2.2 and 6.2), because the same MNs are preferentially excited by stimulation of certain descending paths (from the red nucleus, discussed later in relation to Fig. 13.12). Skin input has also been found to facilitate "long-loop" responses to stretch of thumb muscles, which will be discussed in Chap. 6.2. It seems likely that the reversals of the usual order are brought about by spinal interneurons. Interaction of peripheral, afferent inputs and of descending, supraspinal commands are the topic of Chap. 5.1.

Small and large motor units work together in the maintenance of posture and execution of movements. Those initially active in posture and in slow contractions usually also participate in stronger, faster actions when large MNs have been recruited. This has been shown for hindlimb muscles of the cat and for isometric voluntary contractions of human finger muscles. Figure 4.5A shows that in an animal that is standing still or walking or running at ordinary speeds, most of the force is generated by the red, slow soleus, but during extra efforts such as galloping or vertical jumping it comes mostly from the pale, fast medial gastrocnemius. During these extra efforts the soleus continues to contribute as much as before. The first-recruited half of the cat's MG population (Fig. 4.5A) consists almost entirely of fatigue-resistant units (S, FR and fast, intermediate). Note on the left ordinate that they are used for standing, walking and running, although they together produce

only about one-quarter of the maximum force available from the MG unit population (as marked on right ordinate). We should note how little energy is used in ordinary locomotion, because it takes advantage of recovering kinetic energy by stretching active muscles (see once more the uneven length–tension–velocity relations in Figs. 3.5 and 3.6).

The "recruitment model" of Fig. 4.5A aligns units on the right abscissa as percentages of the total pool recruitment according to their size, as judged by their Ia EPSP amplitudes. (This display is a rearrangement of data as in Fig. 4.3.) These data are related on the left abscissa to the maximal tension output of each unit during fused isometric tetani. The plot of motor unit discharge rates of human m. extensor indicis proprius (Fig. 4.5B) shows that most low-threshold units (starting on the left half of the abscissa) are still firing when high-threshold units have joined in for their steeper, more limited ranges of active tension (right half of the abscissa). The rate (but not the size sequence) with which MNs are recruited one after another is determined by the basal ganglia. Their dysfunction slows recruitment, and hence the summation of tension, which depresses acceleration and prolongs the duration of movements.

In conclusion, we should note that changes of MN frequencies can provide fine gradations of tetanic contractions, as in Fig. 4.3A. The effective range of this control over muscular force is about 10-fold. Recruitment, as in Fig. 4.5A, provides coarser gradations, but over a 5–10 times greater range. Therefore, muscles with small motoneuron pools, such as those moving the fingers or the eyes, take greater advantage of frequency control than muscles with large motor nuclei.

We saw in Chap. 3.2, with reference to Fig. 3.6, that the properties of muscles and the mechanical consequences for trunk and limbs are the final conditions that have to be met by appropriate spinal output. Muscle properties constrain the calcula-

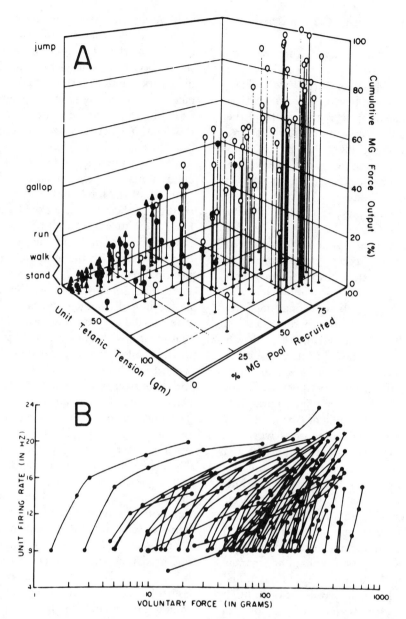

Fig. 4.5. Small motoneurons assist large ones. (A) "Recruitment model" for cat medial gastrocnemius (MG) motor pool, shown as a different plot of same unit distribution as in Fig. 4.3. *Filled ovals* and *triangles,* fatigue-resistant (FR), fast (intermediate) and slow (S); *open ovals,* fast-fatiguing (FF) types. (B) Steady firing frequencies of individual motor units in human extensor digitorum communis muscle. All units discharge in the same frequency range (ordinate), but for different ranges of voluntary force (abscissa). [(A) From Burke, 1979; (B) from Monster and Chan, 1977; both in Burke, 1981b; and Stuart and Enoka, 1983]

tions of the CNS, from the most sophisticated strategic plans to the simplest reflexes, because in the end the spinal cord has to encode actions according to muscle

properties. We stressed that the final outcome of CNS motor commands is the generation and management through the final common path of suitable length–tension relations. Therefore, we consider them once more.

Tensions of opposing muscles can be plotted in the same direction on the ordinate (as in Fig. 3.4), yielding the familiar display of intersecting length–tension curves that define angular forces exerted on a lever ("movements of force" or "torque") acting at particular joint angles. This convention serves well to display the ratios of tensions at the postural (hold) equilibrium points. Another convention is to plot opposing muscle tensions in opposite directions. If we "fold down" the curves for either the agonist or antagonist in Fig. 3.4, we obtain Fel'dman's display of length–tension curves of muscle, a display mode that graphically relates the sums of the tensions of opposing muscles at the equilibrium position of the joint. Fel'dman was the first to recognize that the muscle-joint system resembles a mass-spring system with adjustable equilibrium points.

The tension generated by a muscle in response to a given amount of stretch is called muscle "stiffness" and, for the stretch reflex, represents the gain expressed as force change versus length change. When you add the stiffness of opposing muscles as in Fig. 4.6, the result is the mechanical stiffness of the joint, that is the resistance that it offers to a perturbing force. This was related to antagonist co-contraction in Chap. 3.2. Note that when the tensions of opposing muscles are added together at their equilibrium lengths (and are so expressed), then we are in fact adding their stiffnesses. Figure 4.6A presents such curves for elbow flexors and extensors of human subjects who moved a handle rhythmically back and forth in the horizontal plane against various spring loads. If the subject refrained from conscious correction against load changes, as instructed, the arm moved to a new equilibrium point. In Fig. 4.6A and B the subjects held the handle against initial (extending) forces at angles corresponding to the tops of curves 2, 3 and 4, marked by filled circles in Fig. 4.6A. When the loads were re-

duced progressively, the arm flexed to new, stable positions (open circles in Fig. 4.6), which lie on the three torque–angle curves. Without conscious attempts to resist the imposed loads, there were neither changes from one curve to another, nor changes of slope (i.e., there were no changes of gain; no "adaptive" changes as discussed in relation to Fig. 4.14). Changes along torque–angle curves are the net result of changed length–tension curves of the muscles acting on the joint. We know from Chap. 3.2 that these changes reflect the elastic properties of the muscle fibers and do not involve changes of the number of active spinal motoneurons. When changes from one torque–angle curve to another occur, they are made as gradual transitions rather than in abrupt steps, which we will examine further in relation to voluntary movements in Chap. 7.2 (Fig. 7.7) and Chap. 9.6.

Change to another torque–angle curve requires change of the number of active motor units, and thus a new threshold for the tonic stretch reflex. Reflex threshold is defined by where the curve crosses the abscissa (as we have already seen in Fig. 3.4). Steeper length–tension curves of muscles mean greater muscle stiffness. Figure 4.6B depicts three degrees of co-contraction. The upgoing flexor curves (numbers 4, 3, 2) have reflex thresholds at 54, 77, and 91 deg elbow angle, and the downgoing extensor curve (number 1) at 159 deg. The three curves reflect the three levels of motor set assumed by the subject when starting to maintain the arm against three different initial loads. The three broken lines connecting flexor and extensor curves represent the joint stiffness for different combinations of active length–tension curves. Note that each broken line is linear over most of its range, i.e. that joint stiffness is so well regulated during the action of two opposing muscles that it is maintained at a constant ("invariant characteristic") value. Joint stiffness is controlled by the CNS to suit the needs of a motor task, however, by altering the combination of active muscles. Steeper curves for summed muscle stiffness mean increased joint stiffness. The "passive" curves (like the dashed lines in Fig. 4.6A for neurally nonactivated muscle tissue) have been subtracted to yield "active" curves in Fig. 4.6B. The broken lines denoting joint stiffness in Fig. 4.6B plot the equilibrium positions of the joint where they cross the abscissa. The same points can be obtained, of course, by the intersection of agonist and antagonist length–tension curves when plotted as in Fig. 3.4. The balanced equilibrium lengths of suitable opposing muscles constitute the muscular expression of "hold" programs.

Fig. 4.6. (A) Length–tension curves of flexor and extensor muscles of the human forearm, plotted with flexor *upward* and extensor *downward*. *Dashed lines* indicate passive curves. Compare this display to Fig. 3.4. Ordinates, muscle torque (= force × radius, in Newton-meters, Nm); abscissae, elbow *angle* (180 deg = full extension). Flexor lengthening and extensor shortening (i.e., joint extension) is drawn to the right (B), three active flexor curves and a single extensor curve. Their algebraic summation *(broken lines)* represents three levels of co-contraction and hence three levels of joint stiffness. (C) Active response surfaces for opposing muscles that move a hinge joint in opposite directions. Angular velocities increase from zero (at the center) to either side, according to the oppositely directed agonist and antagonist muscles, indicated at the top of the diagram. Compare to Fig. 3.6C and note that for the antagonist pair all coordinate directions are opposite. [(A,B) From Fel'dman, 1980; (C) from Partridge and Benton, 1981]

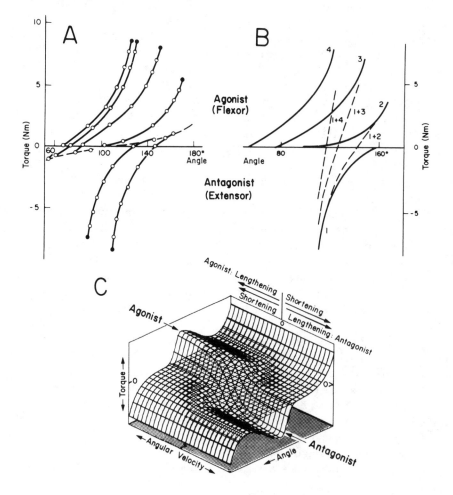

A more lively appreciation of muscle dynamics is obtained by going from the two-dimensional Figs. 3.4 or 3.6A to the three-dimensional display of length, tension and velocity in Fig. 3.6C. The same can be done for two opposing muscles, by going from Fig. 4.6A,B to Fig. 4.6C. Again, the torques of the agonist and antagonist are plotted upwards and downwards; and, as before, angular velocity is plotted to the left for lengthening contractions and to the right for shortening. The force "hills" of the opposing muscles face in opposite directions and are upside-down from each other, because the surfaces for the two muscles represent oppositely directed actions on a hinge joint like the elbow. As one muscle shortens, the other is stretched (lengthened: examine the separate labels for the agonist and antagonist). The joint angle (of the supposed elbow) is shown as becoming more acute during flexor (agonist) contraction and more obtuse during extensor (antagonist) contraction.

Co-contraction is advantageous in several situations. For instance, it can convert a limb into a pillar for weight bearing, or for another, it makes it easier to hold a vibrating object steady, that is to oppose a repetitively alternating torque. When muscles co-contract, their length–tension curves shift toward each other and overlap at the zero–angle joint position (see how the interrupted "stiffness" lines in Fig. 4.6B move toward the middle as you add curve 1 successively with curves 2, 3 and 4). This reduces the extent of joint movement when holding a vibrating object; we manage to hold it in place more firmly. While co-contracting, joint stiffness (indicated in Fig. 4.6B as interrupted lines indicating the sums of the stiffnesses of the participating muscles) can be varied over a bigger range despite more limited variations of the individual muscle stiffnesses.

The display in Fig. 4.6C captures a number of possible combinations at a particular moment in time. This figure makes us appreciate why each level of the motor hierarchy (in this case the spinal cord) must

be able to execute motor commands by drawing on subroutines that coordinate output variables according to established, built-in rules. As pointed out in relation to Fig. 3.6, this occurs because structural constraints, such as properties of muscles and joints, limit the number of possibilities. The angular velocity of the joint, for instance, is constrained by the relative speeds at which opposing muscles contract and relax. This alters the amount of elastic energy that one or the other, or both, can store in their force hills and then release to perform most efficiently and skillfully. The "degrees of freedom" are minimized to ease the burden of calculating motor commands.

This was one of Bernstein's fundamental insights, which led him to postulate that each hierarchical level is capable of fulfilling its limited mission in motor control. Again using the analogy of guided rocket flight (Chap. 1.1), we could describe the coordinations within any one level of the hierarchy as being run by special-purpose computers, at each level. Consider the reentry of the craft from orbital flight. Landing at a given place requires that departure from orbit occur at a certain angle, speed and time. These constraints, which determine re-entry rocket firing, resemble those in Fig. 4.6 shown for muscle action, frozen at a moment in time. Now suppose that the pilot of a returning space shuttle later needs to correct craft attitude during landing. He might transmit the coded command for the intended aim into the computer through some form of "smart" power-steering. The computer can respond quickly because it already "knows" the structural and functional properties of the craft. For example, weight, air speed, action of ailerons and other factors are no longer independent variables. Use of "hierarchical capabilities" for easy management of diverse activities has become commonplace since the advent of cheap microchips for computation. Their use has paved the way for the introduction of "smart" consumer devices, from components in cars to telephones to household appliances, and—most importantly in our context—prosthetic devices.

Adventurous readers can inspect how the agonist force hill in Fig. 4.6C (equivalent to the upgoing flexor curve in Fig. 4.6B) relates to the oppositely oriented antagonist force valley (equivalent to the downgoing extensor curve in Fig. 4.6B). Tunneling from one surface to the other (equivalent to the broken connecting lines in the two-dimensional Fig. 4.6B) would define the joint stiffness at that particular moment in time. The fourth dimension, progress of time, is introduced when we imagine the hills and valleys rising and falling as the muscles go through their contraction cycles. (Chapter 6.2 will afford an opportunity to examine the accompanying time changes of joint stiffness.) Now it remains to consider the natural use of the final common path with regard to participation of the proprioceptors, in terms of the functions of the muscle spindles.

2. Muscle Spindles and Their Fusimotor Control

Muscle spindles are proprioceptive sense organs of the greatest importance; they are as essential for our awareness of the position of our limbs as they are for the fine control of our movements. We retain position awareness after losing the afferent nerves from a joint, but we lose manipulatory control if the stretch reflex is blocked. The finer the muscular control over a joint, the richer is the spindle content of the controlling muscles. The stretch reflex occurs in response to signals from muscle spindles. They contain primary and secondary afferent endings whose messages are conducted to the CNS in nerve fibers of group Ia and II diameter, respectively. Their connections are drawn diagrammatically in Fig. 4.8A. We first consider how muscle spindles function as sense organs, then turn to the properties that they lend to the stretch reflex, and conclude by examining their control by fu-

simotor (gamma) motoneurons in the context of motor control. In this chapter we mostly follow the reviews by Matthews, Burke, Houk, and Loeb (see reference list). Figure 4.7 illustrates the "dynamic" response of a primary ending as well as the "static" one of a secondary ending. Primary fibers discharge more vigorously than secondary ones to (dynamic) length changes and less virogously to (static) maintained length. The lower half of Fig. 4.7 shows the passive, less modulated discharge of both fibers after removal of all fusimotor influence by cutting the ventral root. The dynamic primary (Ia) response was thought to represent velocity pure and simple, but as Matthews' summary in Fig. 4.8 points out, it is now realized that the signal also reflects length, though to an unknown degree.

Primary spindle afferent endings are about 100 times more sensitive to small than to large stretches, which makes their input–output relations very nonlinear. Although their sensitivity falls after a big stretch, it returns within 1 or 2 seconds, ensuring that the spindle can once more respond to small stretches at the new length. (This would occur well beyond the half-second time span of Fig. 4.7.) Secondary spindle afferent fibers (group II) respond more linearly, albeit more modestly, over a wider range of muscle lengths. The differences between the afferent properties are due to different internal structures of the spindle fibers that carry the sense organs, as explained below.

Details of Spindle Structure and Function

Spindles contain "nuclear bag" fibers with a central enlargement enclosing nuclei that are drawn as dots in Fig. 4.8A, and "chain" fibers without such central bags. There are two types of bag fibers, which are distinguished by how nonlinear their responses are to stretch. The less linear responses of bag type 1 fibers derive from their structure. The spirally wound pri-

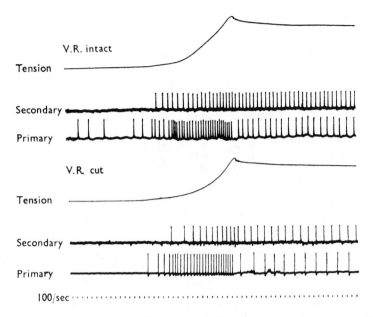

Fig. 4.7. Fusimotor bias sensitizes spindles and makes their discharge less regular. Responses of primary and secondary spindles of cat soleus to 14-mm stretch at about 70 mm/second. *Top,* normal responses, with the ventral root (V.R.) intact. *Bottom,* responses after V.R. was cut to interrupt fusimotor outflow. (From Jansen and Matthews, 1962; in Matthews, 1972, 1981a)

mary endings are in the central regions of all types. Bag type 1 fibers are more elastic (and more viscous) at the sites of their central primary endings than at the more distant site of their secondary endings (see Fig. 4.8A). This uneven consistency gives bag 1 ("dynamic" bag) fibers the odd mechanical property of "creeping" back after a stretch toward their former lengths. Creep reduces the adequate physiological stimulus—deformation of the stretch-sensitive primary endings—and thus blunts their sensitivity from the usual, initial high level. The mechanical properties of their intrafusal muscle fibers helps first to depress, and then to restore spindle sensitivity. During the stretch, the bonds break between the actin and myosin components of the contractile protein actomyosin, which slackens the intrafusal fibers. This "yield" contributes to the sudden drop of sensitivity. (Compare in Fig. 4.7 the lower level and more stereotyped appearance of primary spindle discharges without fusimotor drive with its normal discharge before the

ventral root was cut.) The high sensitivity of bag type 1 fibers is restored in 1 to 2 seconds after intrafusal yield, that is, during and after the creep, when the bonds reform and fusimotor drive resumes.

The physiological range of useful spindle signals is improved by combined "dynamic" and "static" *fusimotor bias.* These actions maintain spindle firing with acceptable variability (signal/noise ratio) in the frequency range of about 50 to 200 impulses per second. Figure 4.8A shows that bag 1 fibers are innervated by *dynamic* gamma MNs, which increase spindle (dynamic) sensitivity and its variability to transient length changes. This exaggerates, rather than improves, their nonlinear properties described above. (Compare once more the upper and lower records in Fig. 4.7.) Dynamic bias therefore creates ambiguous information about muscle length changes, which primary spindles cannot signal accurately anyway because they contract too slowly. Thus, dynamic bias by itself would probably be most suited for

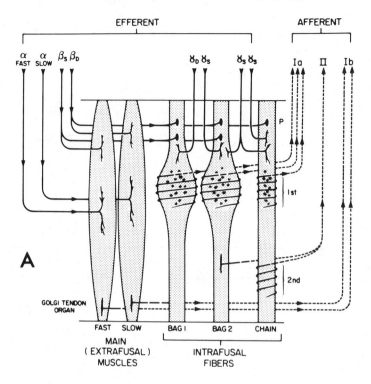

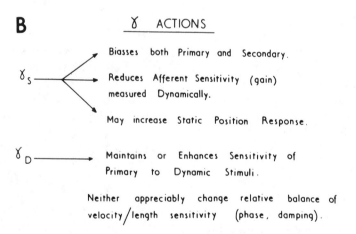

Fig. 4.8. Muscle sense organs. (A) Diagram of sensory and motor connections of mammalian extrafusal (α) muscles and intrafusal (γ) fibers, as well as skeletofusimotor (β) fibers that innervate extrafusal and intrafusal muscle fibers. Static and dynamic β and γ fibers have subscripts S and D, respectively. Plate endings, P; 1st, primary; 2nd, secondary. (B) Summary of static and dynamic fusimotor actions that may be currently deemed to be of functional importance. [(A) From Brooks, 1984; (B) from Matthews, 1981b]

maintaining spindle sensitivity during small postural adjustments (below 1% of muscle length), when its enhancement of primary gain is unopposed by gamma static bias (see Matthews' summary in Fig. 4.8B).

Bag 2 fibers are innervated by *static* gamma MNs (some of which in addition also synapse on chain fibers as shown in Fig. 4.8A). Static gamma MNs increase static position responses, but they decrease dynamic sensitivity. Thus, gamma static bias by itself can raise overall responsiveness of primary *and* secondary spindles so that they can shorten in parallel with the main, extrafusal muscle. This support keeps shortened spindles active during small length changes and yet prevents their saturation during large changes, which helps maintain their calibration. Static support can maintain spindle activity even during rapid shortening of the main muscle, because it keeps bag 2 and chain fibers taut.

Gamma static activation tends to reduce the velocity dependence of gamma dynamic activity, particularly for small movements. The combined actions of primary and secondary endings and of their fusimotor controls thus yield the most accurate reports over the widest range of length changes. The summary in Fig. 4.8B indicates that static and dynamic gamma MNs control different aspects of spindle responsiveness but that neither controls their responses to one distinct physical variable. They alter the emphasis of reports to the CNS about maintained versus changing lengths and about small versus large changes. The cooperative blend of static and dynamic fusimotor actions is under the control of descending paths that affect them differentially. For instance, dynamic gamma MNs are facilitated by the dorsolateral reticulospinal tract and static gamma MNs by the lateral vestibulospinal tract (Chaps. 5.2 and 13.1).

Figure 4.8A also indicates the connections of *beta* (skeletofusimotor) MNs that innervate both extrafusal and intrafusal muscle fibers. The widespread existence in mammalian CNS of these small alpha MNs, called "beta" because of the relatively small diameter of their axons, has been recognized only recently. Beta MNs differ from the even smaller gamma MNs in that they participate in the stretch reflex. This is an important difference, be-

cause beta stretch-reflex activity supports the actions of muscle spindles by guaranteeing a fixed, unvarying measure of coactivation of extrafusal and intrafusal fibers, which is less flexible than the controllable mammalian alpha–gamma coactivation. (Have another look at Fig. 4.8A: beta fibers innervate fibers of the main muscle as well as interfusal fibers. Beta fibers are a retention of the inflexible alpha–gamma linkage in reptiles and amphibians.) The diagram indicates that "dynamic" beta fibers supply slowly contracting extrafusal muscles, while "static" beta fibers supply fast muscles. This helps to preserve spindle sensitivities at low tensions for postural purposes, before recruitment of static beta MNs during movements when they can assist in keeping up spindle discharges, particularly during muscle shortening.

At this point it is useful to relate *spindle function* and *reflex timing*. Reflex responses of active muscles are reasonably symmetrical to application and to release of stretch. This can be seen by following the outside lines (labeled "reflex") of the upper part of Fig. 4.9A. This functional symmetry is achieved by reflex action (so labeled), because the passive, nonreflex, "mechanical" response of the muscle is quite asymmetrical. The shaded area represents the reflex contribution (of a soleus muscle of a decerebrate cat, stretched at 12.5 mm/second). The response is greater to stretch (upwards) than to release (downwards), although they proceeded at the same rates, as shown in the lower part of Fig. 4.9A. The asymmetry of the reflex appears to result largely from asymmetrical dynamic responses of primary spindle endings, of which an example (obtained under similar conditions) is shown in Fig. 4.9B. Primary spindle endings respond far more vigorously to application of stretch than to its release.

Fig. 4.9B is interpreted most easily by comparison to the records in Fig. 4.7, which were obtained under similar conditions. The asymmetrical properties of the spindle help offset the opposite mechanical asymmetry of muscle tissue, which responds more to release from stretch than to its application. The reason is that muscle fibers "yield" (i.e., become less stiff) when stretched more than about 4% of fiber length. The process has an even lower threshold (1.5%) in the common physiological situation where we tense muscles before moving, that is when muscle fibers go from isometric to isotonic contraction. We referred above to muscle yield, also called "short-range elasticity," and we saw that it is related to breaking of the actomyosin bonds. Muscle yield is offset by stretch-reflex action occurring just at that time. Altogether, the stretch reflex thus makes the reactions of innervated muscles more symmetrical to application and release of stretch.

Comparison of the increment of force with and without the reflex during stretch (Fig. 4.8A) indicates that the force per unit length (i.e., the muscle stiffness) is raised by stretch much more quickly with reflex action than without it. This is made plain by comparing the force graphs, above, with the length graphs below, and noticing how the "mechanical" action of muscle tissue parallels the length changes, whereas the "reflex" line rises more quickly than that indicating muscle length. This caused Houk to propose that the reflex stabilizes muscle stiffness (cf. discussion of Fig. 4.6A).

Figure 4.9 compares the efficacies of the stretch reflex during shortening and during lengthening, and shows that the spindles send information to the CNS more readily during stretch than during shortening. Thus, the CNS receives more information about joint movements from lengthening antagonists than from shortening agonist muscles. A glance back at Fig. 4.6C indicates (in the labels for angular velocity) how these roles could go back and forth between opposing muscles when the direction of joint movement reverses. Efficient stretch-reflex action is important for damping oscillations at the end of movements. Early responses of primary spindle afferents (Fig. 4.9C) provide phase-advance, which is enhanced by dynamic gamma bias. Phase advance readies the system for impending change, which helps to prevent tremor.

The message of this chapter so far has been that the spinal cord regulates muscle lengths and tensions in response to proprioceptive information. Sherrington defined proprioceptors as receptors that provide the organism with information arising from the actions of the organism itself (*proprio,* itself). How is proprioception scaled, considering the differing resting lengths of various muscles and the deformations they undergo under physiological conditions? Figure 4.10 shows that the common denominator for muscles inserted on the fingers or on the elbow is the percentage change of the length of muscle fascicles, that is the physiological unit measured by the muscle spindles. This was established by scaling the detection responses of 10 subjects to imposed joint movements with measurements of the length changes (of the fascicles) of each muscle that was stretched during joint displacement.* Assessed in these terms, proprioceptive performance was found to be similar at the elbow and the finger joint, particularly over the range of optimal performance.

Integrative Action of Gamma Motoneurons

How does the fusimotor system fit into the control of intended movements? Gamma MNs have been regarded as tools for central instructions since their discovery, because they respond well to supraspinal stimulation but poorly to most peripheral inputs. The question is: what are the in-

---

*These measurements could not be made on the test subjects and were therefore added from measurements made on the muscles of a fresh cadaver, expressed as alterations in muscle fascicle lengths per degree of angular rotation of the joints when positioned as they were for live testing.

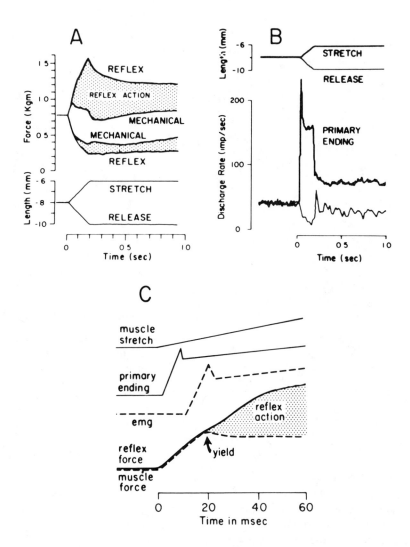

Fig. 4.9. The stretch reflex acts in time to equalize muscle responses to stretch and release: a predictive mechanism of the spinal motor servo. (A) Mechanical response of muscle tissue to stretch (upwards) is smaller than that to release (downwards). This is balanced by inversely sized reflex actions *(dotted areas)*. (B) Asymmetrical reflex actions derive from greater changes of firing rate (dynamic responses) of primary spindle afferent endings to stretch (up) than to release (down). (A) and (B) show the same imposed length changes with the same time course. Compare the plot of discharge rates of the primary ending to the records in Fig. 4.7. (C) The dynamic response of the primary ending (B) is drawn diagrammatically in the second trace on an expanded time scale (speeded up 25 times). It develops in advance of "yielding" of muscle force—that is, of the failure of muscle stiffness *(interrupted line, bottom trace)* to withstand muscle stretch *(top trace)*. This yield is compensated for by the preceding, spindle-evoked, EMG *(middle-level broken line)* generating force by reflex action *(dotted area)*. [(A–C) From Houk, Crago and Rymer, 1981; (A,B) in Houk and Rymer, 1981; and Rymer, 1983]

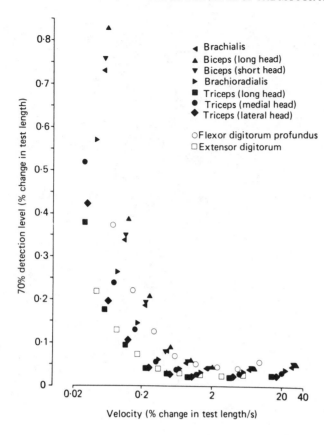

Fig. 4.10. Proprioceptive performance is similar for muscles of various lengths, for example at the elbow and the fingers (particularly in the range of optimal performance) when detection of imposed joint movements is expressed as percentage change of muscle fascicle lengths. (From Hall and McCloskey, 1983)

structions and who is giving them? This is equivalent to asking about the terms of motor programs and about their maintenance during ongoing movements. We do not have answers to these fundamental questions, but new formulations are continually coming forward. The central fact to remember is that fusimotor control maintains the sensitivity of muscle spindles in their optimal range.

Three main schemes have been proposed over the years for the servo-regulation of muscles through fusimotor control of spindles. Each scheme has some advantages and disadvantages, and it is highly probable that they all play some role in particular conditions that can occur in motor control. In addition, there may be other means of control that are not well defined yet. The schemes are summarized in Fig. 4.11, taken from the review by Loeb. Figure 4.11A represents Merton's original length follow-up servo in which the central commands are directed entirely to gamma MNs. This arrangement, which keeps muscle lengths constant against varying loads, predicts discharge of gamma before alpha MNs. Figure 4.11B represents Granit's proposal for alpha–gamma coactivation caused by central commands to both types of MNs, which allows the operation of servo-assistance as proposed by Stein and Matthews. This arrangement, which corrects the intended movement, makes the influence of spindle feedback proportional to the error of the actual movement from the intended movement. It works well for single muscles shortening against a load but not so well for the common situation in which extrafusal muscles act as a stiff spring against a lengthening load (e.g., the triceps brachii acting as antagonist in a stiff, co-contracting elbow flexion; cf. Fig. 3.5B), when alpha and gamma MNs may be driven at different rates. Furthermore, this method of control would be inefficient, because in practice the feedback gain in the reflex loop is very small, as established in deafferented animals (this is discussed in relation to Figs. 7.6 and 9.5). Figure 4.11C represents Houk's proposal that spindles and Gogli tendon organs together stabilize muscle stiffness. Motor commands here provide the basic bias on the membrane potentials of alpha MNs, with a superimposed net excitatory proprioceptive signal to cause recruitment. This arrangement (drawn in Fig. 5.1, together with the muscle, as the "motor servo") serves well when muscles have to maintain a given position against varying loads (i.e., with a variable degree of compliance). It serves less well to explain the recruitment patterns in rapid contractions.

How are we to assess the schemes described above? Fusimotor activity cannot be recorded directly in intact animals or humans, and is therefore usually inferred from changes of spindle discharge that cannot be accounted for by changes of extrafusal muscle length. Records from single Ia fibers have been made in animal preparations during breathing, chewing and induced walking, during walking of freely moving cats, and during slow, small, voluntary ankle or finger movements of human subjects by Hagbarth and Vallbo's "microneurography" (e.g., Fig. 4.13). Such data obtained from human subjects show consistent patterns of spindle function that differ from those gathered from the faster, larger movements studied in behaviorally active animals. In humans, muscles at rest have no fusimotor activity. During muscle function the fusimotor level cannot be changed voluntarily and independently of alpha MN activity. Extrafusal activation of human muscles is always accompanied, but not preceded by, modest intrafusal activation. There is no indication from single-fiber studies that gamma bias changes the gain of stretch reflexes of individual muscles significantly if at all, or that gamma bias changes spindle firing before or during intended slow finger or ankle movements (studied independently by Vallbo and by D. Burke). Most postures and slow movements are made with alpha–gamma coactivation. When does gamma static bias assist dynamic gamma MNs to help implement programs? We

Fig. 4.11. Three servo control systems, using monosynaptic feedback of spindle afferents onto alpha (α) MNs, may be distinguished by the major termination of their input signals: onto gamma (γ) MNs (A), coactivating both alpha and gamma MNs (B), and onto alpha MNs (C). Ia, afferent primary spindle fibers. GTO, Golgi tendon organs. See Fig. 4.8. (From Loeb, 1984)

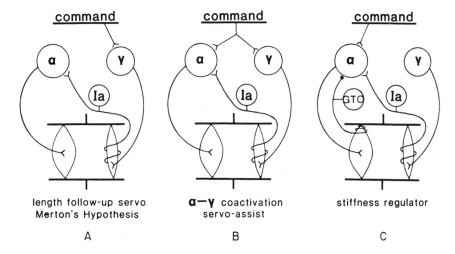

should note that human ankle muscles often act as passive detectors of small perturbations caused by sway during stance (to be discussed in relation to Fig. 9.9). Absent or low fusimotor drive in a quiet muscle leaves spindles highly sensitive to small stretches, which would be useful for alerting the CNS about peripheral occurrences. During muscular corrections of sway, spindle sensitivity would be reset by fusimotor action. (A similarly high spindle sensitivity to small changes appears in Fig. 4.13, which depicts events during slow finger movements by a human subject.)

Records from single spindle primary afferents in behaviorally active animals indicate that central fusimotor drive does not always accompany alpha activity. Gamma drive does not alter spindle firing significantly. In most situations, static bias functions only when the spindle is not dominated by the effects of large stretches (in excess of about 0.01 muscle lengths) and high speeds (in excess of 0.2 muscle lengths per second). If these values apply to the human situation in Fig. 4.10, fusimotor neurons would hardly affect the motor servo at all, because they barely straddle spindle thresholds. Static bias might therefore function in humans during steady postures and in very small, very slow length changes, but servo-assistance could not provide "models" for large, fast movements.

Loeb and his associates have made the closest study of the action of identified spindles in freely moving animals by recording the positions, tensions and EMG of the relevant muscles. Cats were chronically implanted with electrodes in the dorsal roots and muscles, and strain gauges were threaded through the tendons. Data from these devices were correlated to TV images of the animals as they moved about or walked on a treadmill. This permits evaluation of the kinds of action engaged in by the muscle to which the spindle is related (e.g., lengthening contraction, passive extension). They concluded that the mode of spindle firing only changes when a new behavioral state gets under way, for instance when an animal gets up in order to walk. In contrast, perturbations of ongoing, intended movements are not accompanied by changes of spindle firing, as when the cat's leg overcomes an unexpected obstacle during walking.

Loeb postulates that gamma MNs may influence spindles by all three modes shown in Fig. 4.11 as well as by another as yet undefined method of control for fine movements. His concept of a "task group" to accommodate various forms of muscle action is illustrated in Fig. 4.12. The task group consists of alpha, gamma and beta MNs together with spindles and other proprioceptive afferents, which share responsibility for the performance of a kinematically homogeneous task. It is the task-oriented "motor servo" of Fig. 5.1 (minus the muscle itself). Figure 4.12A shows how muscle activity may be divided into independent axes of motion (vertical) and recruitment (horizontal). Figure 4.12B summarizes the three modes of gamma control described in Fig. 4.11. Actively shortening muscle (lower right quadrant in Fig. 4.12A) is best controlled by alpha and gamma coactivation that preserves spindle firing during muscle shortening ($\alpha = \gamma$ in Fig. 4.12B). Passive lengthening (upper left quadrant) requires no coactivation, because passive spindles are best suited to detect the imposed lengthening. Muscles that act like springs by actively lengthening (upper right quadrant) require selective recruitment of alpha MNs and need to avoid simultaneous recruitment of gamma MNs, which would saturate spindle output during muscle stretch ($\alpha > \gamma$). Passively shortening muscles (presumably following movements caused by inertia or external forces) need selective recruitment of gamma MNs to maintain the spindle active ($\gamma > \alpha$). The muscle changes described for the four conditions in Fig. 4.12A are best appreciated by referring once more to Figs. 3.5, 3.6 and 4.6.

Task group action would be of particular interest for bifunctional muscles whose

Fig. 4.12. Concept of "task groups" to control alpha and gamma MNs according to the needs of the task effort. (A) Muscle activity is divided according to motion (along vertical axis) and recruitment (horizontal axis). Symbols, explained in the text, define how central commands access alpha and/or gamma MNs. (B) Patterns of alpha and gamma control described in (A). (From Loeb, 1984)

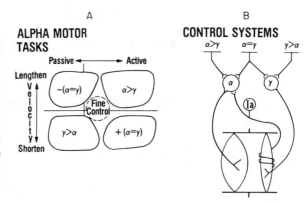

MNs participate in quite different working conditions that require separate alpha and gamma control (e.g., Figs. 4.4 and 9.9). Loeb stresses that *a task group is a functional entity that can only be identified during a behavioral task* by physiological observation. Task groups may be parts of one or of several motor nuclei. The sensory and motor neurons making up the group may participate in other task groups that perform different actions, for instance to stress speed for ballistic movements or to stabilize joints. The participation in movements of components of task groups is orderly and reproducible whenever the task is executed (cf. Chap. 4.1 with regard to Henneman's principle). The task group thus represents the identification by the nervous system of a functional state for which it can usefully optimize sensory information and motor feedback. This state is presumably associated with learning new tasks through plasticity of neural connections and also with maintaining optimization during the continuing development of skeletomuscular structures. Thus, task groups are assumed to be programmed to operate optimally for only restricted ranges of active length and velocity, enabling fast, simple and accurate execution, and ready application of proprioceptive signals to motor control.

Finally, we note that D. Burke and W. T. Thach have both suggested that the most likely use of servo-assistance might be in some form of motor learning. Some indications have been found recently (by Thach) that gamma MNs may deliver commands to set spindle sensitivity in Ia fibers of wrist extensors of monkeys going through very slow alternatively active and passive periods of lengthening and shortening, that is, when the muscle is asked to perform different tasks. Vallbo has shown that fusimotor servo-assistance might function when subjects are uncertain about the load they will have to handle. A suggestion for this idea can be seen in slow, precise movements (that are difficult to make), in which fusimotor activity is disproportionately high. In such an instance, shown in Fig. 4.13, muscle spindle discharge reflects even very small variations in movement speed, which could indeed be useful for signaling mismatches between motor programs and motor execution. The question is considered in relation to cerebellar function in Chap. 13.

The association of task group activity with plasticity of neural connections reflects previous thoughts by others about adaptation of motor programs. The plasticity function of spindles under gamma static bias could be used to *adapt* the feedback control, and thus to modify the reference "model" as well as the movement system. The idea is expressed in Fig. 4.14 with a diagram of a simple "model reference" control system taken from Nashner. The adapted model would give a better and earlier error correction than would be possible by calculation from movement-

ISOTONIC CONTRACTION

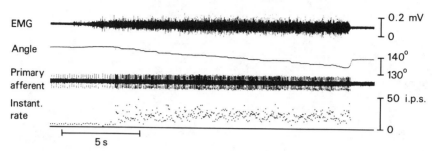

Fig. 4.13. Variations in speed of slow movements are reflected particularly clearly by the discharge rate of primary muscle spindle afferents. Record from single fiber of nerve of flexor digitorum muscle of a normal subject during a slow voluntary flexion of the metacarpophalangeal joint of the ring finger. (Previously unpublished record kindly supplied by Prof. A. Vallbo, 1982.)

generated feedback. (We introduced the concept of adaptive control in Chap. 2.2 and also in Chap. 4.2.) In theory, the system can be tuned so well that it can regulate actual events entirely from the predicted feedback! In practice, it may apply only to a narrow range of movements as judged by the following experiment. It is hard to achieve co-contractions by gain-change of the spinal stretch reflex while consciously trying *not* to resist an imposed load on a joint. The repeatable performances graphed in Fig. 4.6A imply that an individual obeying the "do not resist" (i.e.,

the "yield") command does not adapt the gain of the spinal servo loop. Some individuals do succeed, however, in a similar situation (illustrated in Fig. 6.3), with loads below 10% of the maximal force of the muscles. Thus, adaptive gain changes of the stretch reflex might be implemented by servo-assistance for unloaded, or only slightly tensed, limbs.

3. Summary

Large motoneurons (MNs) have many branches and hence have large motor

Fig. 4.14. Schematic arrangement of a control system that uses *feedback* (i.e., a servo) with two special properties. A comparison is made between the *actual* output of the *system,* and the *estimate* made by the *model.* The resulting *error* information enables the *adaptive control* to adjust the feedback control as well as the model. (From Nashner, 1981; also in Brooks, 1984)

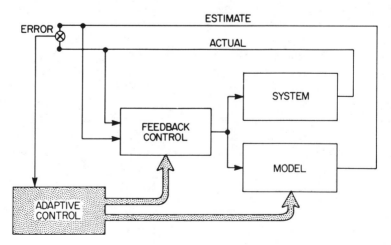

units, while small MNs have fewer branches and smaller motor units. Muscle spindle discharge activates small MNs more efficiently than large ones, and thus recruits them more easily into stretch-reflex activity. The "size principle" of Henneman orders MNs for successive recruitment in stretch reflexes (and decruitment, in reverse order). It applies in voluntary movements as long as the muscle is used in the same function and task context. There is limited, fragmentary evidence suggesting that some descending tracts can modify the recruitment order for fast voluntary movements under certain conditions. Small MNs are tonically active because they receive constant stretch input. Their activity suffices for postures, walking and running. Large MNs participate only phasically, as in galloping or jumping. Discharge rates of MNs are appropriate for the contractile properties of their muscles, and provide gradation of the force of tetanic contractions. Recruitment provides coarser control than discharge rate, but over 5 to 10 times greater range. For muscles with more than one action, size-dependent recruitment applies to the primary function of the muscle. The properties of motor units and the size principle define the working range of the spinal cord, subject to scaling by other parts of the CNS.

The spinal cord coordinates the actions of opposing muscles with due regard to their length–tension relations. Muscles operate much like weights hanging on coiled springs. Control of the tension ratios of opposing muscles, one in relation to the other, determines joint angles and hence static postures, since muscle lengths and tensions depend on each other according to the muscle length–tension curves. The mechanical stiffness at which joint angles are maintained against external perturbations is the sum of the tensions of opposing muscles at their respective equilibrium lengths, that is the sum of the muscle stiffnesses. This can be controlled by the CNS through variation of the active

muscles. Static joint angles and the stiffness at which they are maintained can constitute "hold" programs. Additional commands are needed to set particular trajectories for "move" programs, that is, intended paths and their rates of change, or velocities appropriate for postural changes.

Properties of spindles deduced from experiments with isolated preparations indicate that bias from static, but not dynamic, gamma MNs raises overall position sensitivity of spindles. Only static gamma bias can increase firing of primary and secondary spindles during large muscular contractions. Records from spindles obtained from freely moving animals indicate that the CNS reprograms the fusimotor system in response to stimuli that lead to new behavioral states, thus always assuring a steady flow of sensory information. Dynamic gamma drive may adjust spindle responsiveness during small postural irregularities or small movements. During large length changes, continuous gain control of spindles is provided by simultaneous actions of dynamic and static gamma MNs.

Alpha and gamma MNs are coactivated to maintain the sensitivity of spindle input to the spinal cord. (Some alpha–gamma coactivation is guaranteed at all times by the action of small alpha MNs, called beta, which innervate extrafusal as well as intrafusal muscle fibers.) In very slow movements gamma MNs may be activated independently of alpha MNs. Spinal responses to increases and decreases of muscle length are made more symmetrical by the summed actions of muscle spindles and extrafusal muscles. The CNS relates messages from spindle endings in relation to each other and to the fusimotor drives impressed upon them. The CNS interprets spindle signals in terms of proportional deformation of muscle fascicles, which equalizes messages from short and long muscles. Detection threshold to imposed joint displacement is close to the sensitivity threshold of the spindle receptors.

Servo-assistance by static gamma MNs

might function during isometric (postural) actions and during slow, small movements but not in large, fast length changes. For large movements or corrections, supraspinal descending commands exert their predominant effects on alpha MNs, with subsidiary adjustments of gamma MNs. For small movements or corrections, predominant effects might be exerted on gamma MNs leading to subsequent adjustments of alpha MNs, but there is little evidence that this really occurs in previously learned movements. Servo-assistance could conceivably be more important for learning motor acts than in executing them. Since central commands can access alpha as well as gamma MNs either separately or together, motor programs might assemble appropriate task groups of spinal sensory and motor elements according to the functions to be carried out in the task context.

References

Brooks, V. B. 1984. Cerebellar functions in motor control. *Hum. Neurobiol.* 2:251–260. [Figs. 4.8A and 4.14]

Buchthal, F., and Schmalbruch, H. 1980. Motor unit of mammalian muscle. *Physiol. Rev.* 60:91–142.

Burke, D. 1980. The activity of human muscle spindle endings in normal motor behavior. In *Neurophysiology IV*, ed. R. Porter. *Int. Rev. Physiol.* 25:91-126.

Burke, R. E. 1981a. Motor unit recruitment: what are the critical factors? In *Motor unit types: recruitment and plasticity in health and disease*, ed. J. E. Desmedt. *Prog. Clin. Neurophysiol.* 9:61–84. [Fig. 4.4]

Burke, R. E. 1986. Motor units: anatomy, physiology, and functional organization. In *Motor control.* Sect. 1, vol. 2. *Handbook of Physiology*, ed. V. B. Brooks, pp. 345–422. Bethesda, Md.: American Physiological Society. [Figs. 4.1, 4.3B, 4.4, 4.5, and 4.6]

Burke, R. E. 1979. The role of synaptic organization in the control of motor unit activity during movement. In *Reflex Control of Posture and Movement*, eds. R. Granit and O. Pompeiano. *Prog. Brain Res.* 50:61–67. [Fig. 4.5A]

Burke, R. E., Levine, D. N., Tsairis, P., and Zajac, F. E. 1973. Physiological types and histochemical profiles in motor units of the cat gastrocnemius. *J. Physiol. (Lond.)* 234:723–748. [Fig. 4.3]

Clamann, H. P. 1981. Motor units and their activity during movements. In *Motor coordination. Handbook of behavioral neurobiology*, eds. A. L. Towe and E. S. Luschei, pp. 69–92. New York: Plenum Press.

Desmedt, J. E., and Godaux, E. 1981. Spinal motoneuron recruitment in man: rank deordering with direction but not with speed of voluntary movement. *Science* 214:933–936.

Fel'dman, A. G. 1980. Superposition of motor programs. I. Rhythmic forearm movements in man. *Neuroscience* 5:81–90. [Fig. 4.6A,B]

Freund, H.-J. 1983. Motor unit and muscle activity in voluntary motor control. *Physiol. Rev.* 63:387–436.

Hall, L. A., and McCloskey, D. I. 1983. Detections of movements imposed on finger, elbow and shoulder joints. *J. Physiol. (Lond)* 335:519–533. [Fig. 4.10]

Henneman, E. 1981. Recruitment of motoneurons: the size principle. In *Motor unit types: recruitment and plasticity in health and disease*, ed. J. E. Desmedt. *Prog. Clin. Neurophysiol.* 9:26–60.

Henneman, E. 1980. Skeletal muscle: the servant of the nervous system. In *Medical physiology*, ed. V. B. Mountcastle. 14th ed. St. Louis: C. V. Mosby Co. [Figs. 4.1 and 4.2]

Henneman, E., and Mendell, L. M. 1981. Functional organization of motoneuron pool and its inputs. In *Motor control* Sect. 1, vol. 2. *Handbook of Physiology*, ed. V. B. Brooks, pp. 423–507. Bethesda, Md.: American Physiological Society. [Figs. 4.1 and 4.2]

Houk, J. C., and Rymer, W. Z. 1981. Neural control of muscle length and tension. In *Motor control.* Sect. 1, vol. 2. *Handbook of physiology*, ed. V. B. Brooks, pp. 257–323. Bethesda, Md.: American Physiological Society. [Fig. 4.9A,B]

Houk, J. C., Crago, P. E., and Rymer, W. Z. 1981. Function of the spindle dynamic response in stiffness regulation: a predictive mechanism provided by non-linear feedback. In *Muscle receptors and movement*, eds. A. Taylor and A. Prochazka, pp. 299–309. London: MacMillan. [Fig. 4.9C]

Jansen, J. K. S., and Matthews, P. B. C. 1962. The effects of fusimotor activity on the static responsiveness of primary and secondary endings of muscle spindles in the decerebrate cat. *Acta Physiol. Scand.* 44:376–386. [Fig. 4.7]

Loeb, G. E. 1984. The control and responses of mammalian muscle spindles during normally executed motor tasks. *Exercise Sports Sci. Rev.* 12:157–204. [Figs. 4.11 and 4.12]

Loeb, G. E., Hoffer, J. A., and Marks, W. B. 1985. The activity of spindle afferents from cat anterior thigh muscles. III. Effects of external stimuli. *J. Neurophysiol.* 54: 578–591.

Matthews, P. B. C. 1972. *Mammalian muscle receptors and their central actions.* London: Edward Arnold. [Fig. 4.7]

Matthews, P. B. C. 1981. Muscle spindles: their messages and their fusimotor supply. In *Motor control.* Sect. 1, vol. 2. *Handbook of physiology,* ed. V. B. Brooks, pp. 189–228. Bethesda, Md.: American Physiological Society. [Figs. 4.7 and 4.8B]

Matthews, P. B. C. 1981. Proprioceptors and the regulation of movement. In *Motor coordination.* Vol. 5. *Handbook of behavioral neurobiology,* eds. A. L. Towe and E. S. Luschei, pp 93–137. New York: Plenum Press. [Fig. 4.8B]

McComas, A. J. 1977. *Neuromuscular functions and disorders.* Boston: Butterworths. [Fig. 4.4A]

Milner-Brown, H. S., Stein, R. B., and Yemm, R. 1973. The orderly recruitment of human motor units during voulntary isometric contractions. *J. Physiol. (Lond.)* 230:359–370. [Fig. 4.4B]

Monster, A. W., and Chan, H. 1977. Isometric force production by motor units of extensor digitorum communis muscle in man. *J. Physiol. (Lond.)* 40:1432–1443. [Fig. 4.5B]

Moore, J. C. 1984. The Golgi tendon organ: a review and update *Am. J. Occup. Ther.* 38:227–236.

Nashner, L. M. 1981. Analysis of stance and posture in humans. In *Motor coordination.* Vol. 5. *Handbook of behavioral neurobiology,* eds. A. L. Towe and E. S. Luschei, pp. 527–566. New York: Plenum Press. [Fig. 4.14]

Partridge. L. D., and Benton, L. A. 1981. Muscle, the motor. In *Motor control.* Sect. 1, vol. 2. *Handbook of physiology,* ed. V. B. Brooks, pp. 43–106. Bethesda, Md: American Physiological Society. [Fig. 4.6C]

Proske, U. 1981. The Golgi tendon organ: properties of the receptor and reflex actions of impulses arising from tendon organs. In *Neurophysiology IV.* Vol. 25. *Int. Rev. Physiol.,* ed. R. Porter, pp 127–171. Baltimore: University Park Press.

Rack, P. M. H. 1981. Limitations of somatosensory feedback in control of posture and movement. In *Motor control.* Sect. 1, vol. 2. *Handbook of physiology,* ed. V. B. Brooks, pp. 229–256. Bethesda, Md.: American Physiological Society.

Rymer, W. Z. 1983. Muscle afferent contributions to the regulation of muscle length and tension. In *Neurobiology.* Vol. 5. *The clinical neurosciences,* ed. W. D. Willis, pp. 435–469. New York: Churchill Livingstone. [Fig. 4.9A,B]

Stephens, J. A., and Usherwood, T. P. 1977. The mechanical properties of human motor units with special reference to their fatiguability and recruitment threshold. *Brain Res.* 125:91–97. [Fig. 4.4C]

Stuart, D. G., and Enoka, R. M. 1983. Motor neurons, motor units and the size principle. In *Neurobiology.* Vol. 5. *The clinical neurosciences,* ed. W. D. Willis, pp. 471–517. New York: Churchill Livingstone. [Figs. 4.4A,C and 4.5]

Thach, W. T., Schieber, M. H., and Elbe, R. H. 1985. Motor programs: trajectory versus stability. In: *Cerebellar Functions,* eds. J. R. Bloedel, J. Dichgans, and W. Precht. pp 36–51. Berlin: Springer Verlag.

Vallbo, A. B., Hagbarth, K. E., Torebjork, H. E., and Wallin, B. G. 1979. Somatosensory, proprioceptive, and sympathetic activity in human peripheral nerves. *Physiol. Rev.* 59:919–957.

5

Supraspinal Control

This chapter examines how the central nervous system uses the spinal cord as an interface between the brain and the muscles. First, we learn how spinal interneurons (INs) are controlled and what integrative capabilities they confer upon the use of muscles. Second, we discuss the modes of control exerted by the various paths descending from the cerebral cortex and the brain stem. Continuing from the previous chapter which consolidated our knowledge about motor units, muscle spindles and fusimotor control, we now discover how spinal "microcircuits" assist supraspinal controls by dispatching their commands to coordinated muscles. The spinal cord completes the translation from the language of movements to that of muscles.

1. Control of Spinal Interneurons

So far our attention has been focused on the best-known input and output devices of the final common path: muscle spindles, alpha MNs and gamma MNs. Alpha and gamma MNs are the "final common path" from the spinal cord to the muscles. The MNs adjust the lengths and tensions of muscles with the aid of proprioceptive as well as other sensors that are all coordinated by INs and descending controls. We stress how patterns of IN connections

can create subroutines for motor adjustments.

The balance between the influences of stretch-sensitive muscle spindles and contraction-sensitive Golgi tendon organs is of great importance, because both influence the stretch reflex. Figure 4.8 reminds us how well tendon organs are situated to measure tension changes, because they lie in the tendon "in series" with the ends of muscle fibers. Tendon organs are essentially insensitive to stretch in the physiological range, because stretch is absorbed by the mechanically less stiff muscles before it affects tendons. Tendon organs respond to the active tension of any one of about 10 single muscle fibers inserted near them. These fibers are likely to belong to different motor units, because their fibers are mixed together (see Chap. 4.1). MNs and INs are grouped together as a *spinal-output stage*, which together with the controlled muscle and its sense organs, is called the *motor servo* (delineated by the broken-line boundary in Fig. 5.1). The name, coined by Houk, indicates the self-adjusting nature of the neural circuit (drawn in different ways previously in Figs. 1.4 and 3.3), unless it is directed otherwise by supraspinal control paths whose actions are indicated by arrows in Fig. 5.1. This exemplifies the flexibility of hierar-

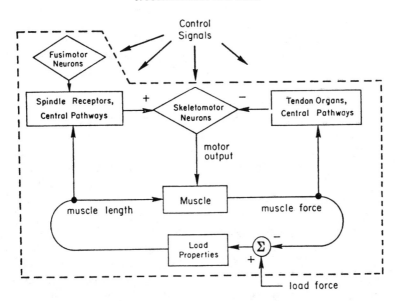

Fig. 5.1. Basic organization of spinal-output stage, enclosed by *broken lines,* called the "motor servo." *Arrows* indicate central control signals (see Fig. 2.6) to fusimotor (gamma) and skeletomotor (alpha) MNs, as well as to interneurons (not shown). Same conventions as in Fig. 3.3. (From Houk, 1974)

chies in motor control, discussed in Chap. 2.2. We note here that supraspinal controls reach alpha as well as gamma MNs. Both are routes for the implementation of motor programs: alpha for fast movements and for adjustments to imposed perturbations, and gamma for postural control and for slow, self-initiated changes (Fig. 4.12).

Supraspinal descending controls engage the motor servo mostly by synapsing on interneurons, although there also are "private" monosynaptic connections with MNs. The following paragraphs and illustrations are largely based on the monumental work of the research group led by Eccles in Canberra, and that in Gothenburg, Sweden, led by Lundberg and Jankowska, and including Grillner, Hultborn, and many others. Since most of their results have been obtained with acute cat preparations, detailed differences between that species and primates have yet to be explored, as well as the full use that the intact body makes of these mechanisms. The description in this chapter follows the reviews by Schwindt and by Baldissera, Hultborn and Illert. Descending control

paths will be taken up in more detail in Chap. 5.2. Hierarchical motor organization, described in Chap. 2, implies that each hierarchical level contains neural circuits that can calculate and carry out their own integrative functions. This was recongnized by Sherrington on the basis of experiments with acute cat preparations and by Bernstein on theoretical grounds.

The neural machinery for spinal function comprises an amazing variety of possible interactions. It is essential to understand their principles, because the contributions made by particular control paths and the spinal interneurons on which they impinge will assume practical importance in the near future. The art of assessing them in the human is advancing rapidly with the use of H-reflex testing. These reflexes, named after their discoverer Paul Hoffmann, mimic the phasic (tendon jerk) stretch reflex to the extent that they are monosynaptic, although the natural stretch stimulus is replaced with electrical stimulation (through the skin) of Ia afferent fibers in motor nerves. Thus a patterned burst of discharges of predominantly group Ia and II fibers is replaced with a single, synchronous volley of Ia, Ib, and group II fibers. Not surprisingly, different patterns of muscles are activated by the two methods. Nevertheless, knowledge of neural interactions obtained with this reflex "model" is beginning to show how we humans use the intergrative capabilities of the final common path. (This is discussed further in Chap. 10 on locomotion.) Remember that the laboratory charts of today become the clinical tools of tomorrow!

The balance between antagonist muscles depends on reciprocal inhibitions, whose actions are strongly influenced by descending supraspinal facilitation (Fig. 5.2). When descending controls are reduced by lesions in the internal capsule, spastic hemiplegia results with marked spasticity in the physiological extensors of the lower limb. Testing with H-reflexes reveals that the hyperactive extensors (deprived of moderating supraspinal controls) tonically inhibit the physiological flexors, which consequently are less spastic and more paralyzed. Normal subjects co-contract opposing muscles to steady, for example, their arm when performing an arm or hand movement that they have not previously practiced. We notice this in everyday experience when making a very slow movement, or a very small movement that must reach a target very accurately. These are feedback-dependent, nonprogrammed movements. Co-contraction is common not only for nonprogrammed movements (cf. Fig. 1.5), but even to some degree for programmed movements whose execution is still being improved. This acquisition of further skill is called movement "tuning" and involves progressively greater relaxation of the antagonist before movement onset ("Hufschmidt" inhibition) while intensified agonist action drives the limb to the well-learned target. A likely route for the inhibition is through the Ia interneuron.

An important segmental capability, which is guided by descending controls, is the coordination of alpha–gamma coactivation of muscles whose actions oppose one another. This could provide a mechanism for implementing motor programs by means of servo-assistance (Chaps. 3.2 and 4.2). Instructions are required for both agonist and antagonist MNs and for their reciprocal linkages through Ia interneurons. Coordinated control is made possible because *alpha and gamma MNs, as well as the interneuron in the reciprocal Ia inhibitory pathway (Ia IN), are reached by the same descending paths* (Fig. 5.2). Some can, in fact, be branches of individual corticospinal neurons. It is likely that some paths operate in parallel, exerting separate cortical controls, while others may be branches ("collaterals") from the main lines. Some of the major descending tracts reaching Ia INs are identified in Fig. 5.2A. The pattern for an opposing pair of muscles is shown in Fig. 5.2B, in which the axon branches of Ia INs are shown to inhibit the Ia IN of the antagonist. Since the coactivationof alpha and gamma MNs is linked by comon descending supraspinal command paths, we have "alpha–gamma linkage in reciprocal inhibition." Ia INs also receive ipsilateral input from "propriospinal" (P) INs, which is a classifying name for INs whose branches reach more than one spinal segment (see Fig. 5.5). Furthermore, Ia INs receive bilateral input from the vestibulospinal tracts, whose locations are indicated diagrammatically in Figs. 5.7 and 5.8. These, and Figs. 5.11 and 5.12, are useful figures to consult whenever new tracts are brought into the story. Finally, Ia INs receive input from flexor reflex afferents (FRA), which we will study in relation to Fig. 5.6.

The basic segmental action of the Ia IN is to inhibit antagonist muscles, which increases the gain (output/input) of the stretch reflex. Figures 5.1 and 5.2 are simplified diagrams suggesting the old view that Ia fibers facilitate (+ in Figs. 3.3 and 5.1) only those MNs that innervate muscles containing the spindles of origin of the Ia fibers ("homonymous" connections).

A

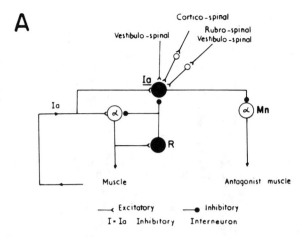

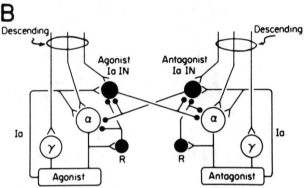

Fig. 5.2. (A) The integrative function of the Ia inhibitory inter-neuron (Ia IN) is revealed by the summing of its various inputs shown in a partial wiring diagram. (B) Diagram of descending paths to alpha (α) and gamma (γ) MNs and Ia INs. Compare to Fig. 5.1 and note that Renshaw (R) cells reach the shortest spinal-reflex paths to Ia INs and alpha MNs. [(A) From Matthews, 1981; (B) from Hult-born, Illert and Santini, 1976; in Schwindt, 1981]

This muscle-limited scheme applies less in higher primates, where Ia fibers converging on a motoneuron pool from functionally cooperating (synergistic) muscles are the important source of excitation. Such "heteronymous" facilitation is important because it adds a fine control over MNs: it can fire them if they are primed, that is, partially depolarized by central commands. Two partial depolarizations *together* can fire the MN, when neither could do so alone. This interdependency offers important opportunities to enact the necessities of motor control as "logical propositions." MNs can function so that they give an output if, and only if, *both* inputs are active. (This kind of connection is called an "and-gate," and is not restricted to MNs.) Another arrangement could be an MN firing with *either* input, in which case it functions as an "or-gate."

As an example, consider the elbow movements discussed in Chaps. 3.4 and 4.1. The biceps and triceps brachii muscles are presented as the antagonistic pair in Figs. 3.6 and 4.6. We know, however, that other muscles are also involved in moving that joint, as illustrated in Fig. 5.3. We recognize triceps as an extensor of the forearm. Biceps flexes the elbow with the palm of the hand upwards; that is, it "supinates" the forearm. Brachioradialis is also a flexor but, unlike biceps, it pulls the forearm into its elbow socket and positions the arm between the supine and prone positions (see Fig. 5.3). When the biceps is stretched as in Fig. 3.6, brachioradialis is a synergist that receives some heteronymous Ia depolarization. *If* the motor task calls for pronation of the hand, then that central command will sum with the peripheral Ia input to activate MNs of brachioradialis. Triceps will be inhibited appropriately. The degree of antagonist co-contraction can be

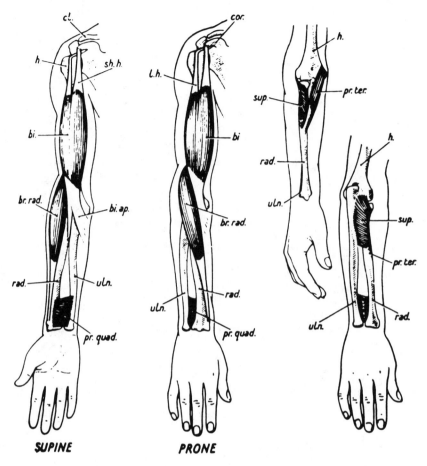

Fig. 5.3. Skeleton and some of the muscles of the human arm used for flexion, supination and pronation. bi., Biceps; br. rad., brachioradialis; h., humerus; pr. quad., pronator quadratus; pr. ter., pronator teres; rad., radius; sup., supinator; uln., ulna. (From Young and Hobbs, 1975: in Alexander, 1981)

controlled with the usual precision because reciprocal inhibition includes alpha–gamma linkage, as shown in Fig. 5.2B.

Figure 5.2A,B shows how "recurrent" inhibition by *Renshaw* (R) *cells* is exerted on alpha MNs as well as on Ia INs; and Fig. 5.4C shows that gamma MNs are reached as well. Renshaw cells, named after their discoverer, are INs innervated by collateral branches of MN axons that run in "recurrent" fashion to other MNs in their own (homonymous) nucleus and to (heteronymous) synergists. R cells inhibit the neurons whose branches drive them, and their synergists. An active "pool" of motoneurons surrounds itself with a shell of recurrent inhibition that depresses the heteronymous "also-rans." In other words, R cells can protect the function of active alpha-MN task groups (Chap. 4.2). Since tonic MN firing predominates over phasic actions (Chap. 4.1, e.g. Fig. 4.5), recurrent inhibition in humans is most important in slow, rather than fast, muscular contractions. R-cell connections can stabilize or change the degree of alpha–gamma coactivation (see above and Figs. 4.7, 4.11 and 4.12), depending on descending influences on R cells. It is difficult, however, to separate supraspinal influences on R cells from those reaching the other, connected, neurons. Such special descending paths may exist, as suggested in Fig. 5.4A. Depending on whether they inhibit or facilitate R cells, the amplification ("gain") of the affected ("target") alpha MNs will rise or fall (see Fig. 5.4B). Since the Renshaw circuit provides negative feedback, facilitation of R cells deepens R inhibition of MN output, which is thus decreased. This is indicated in Fig. 5.4B by the lowered slope of the input–output curve, indicated by the direction of the arrow. Variable gain control is probably of great importance in the adaptation of postures and movements by accommodating small, slow changes of muscle length. R cells can thus function as "variable gain regulators" under central control, because they modulate both alpha and gamma MNs as well as their Ia INs (Figs. 5.2B and 5.4C). R cells inhibit the agonist and disinhibit (reduce the inhibition of) the antagonist. Therefore, R cells promote co-contraction of opposing muscles, while Ia INs promote their alternate actions.

R-cell connections to Ia INs help coordinate the central commands reaching the Ia INs, as drawn in Fig. 5.2. This is another instance where structurally provided, preferred paths can reduce the degrees of freedom needed in the calculation of motor commands. An example of descending control serves to illustrate the integrated use of the Renshaw circuit. R cells are facilitated by a bulbospinal pathway that descends in the dorsolateral reticulospinal tract (the noradrenergic tract is described in Chap. 5.2, and its facilitatory connections to MNs are marked + in Fig. 5.4A and labeled NA in Fig. 5.5). The weaker heteronymous Ia input to muscles is suppressed more than the stronger homonymous input, which survives inhibition better. This restriction enhances the control exerted by the segmental gamma loop over individual muscles. At the same time, the bulbospinal system elevates the control exerted by the corticospinal tract (by another mechanism, to be described in relation to Fig. 5.6). The corticospinal tract has suitable monosynaptic connections to influence individual muscles for the fine control of movements (see Chap. 5.2). The segmental action of R cells in this example is integrated with that of two descending systems, all functioning together to focus control on a particular motor nucleus.

The *Ib INs* mediate messages about active muscle force sensed by Golgi tendon

Fig. 5.4. Renshaw (R) cells can regulate the gain of alpha MNs. (A) Descending facilitation (+) and inhibition (−) of R cells can vary output of MN pool. (B) Input–output relations of MNs, measured as discharge frequencies, ($n \times f_{in}$ and $n \times f_{out}$) are raised and lowered respectively by inhibition and facilitation of R cells (RC). (C) Concept of motor-output stage (framed by *thick lines*). *Broken lines* indicate parallel connections to Ia INs and alpha MNs, as well as to gamma MNs not shown in Fig. 4.8B. (From Hultborn, Lindstrom and Wigstrom, 1979; in Baldissera, Hultborn and Illert, 1981).

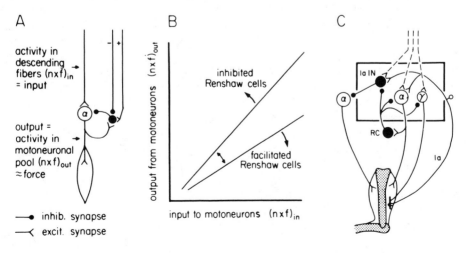

organs to MNs, which they inhibit in proportion to the intensity of the Ib sensory activation. Segmental Ib inhibition of the MNs that generate the sensed force is called "autogenic" (or "autogenetic") inhibition (− in Figs. 3.3 and 5.1). Ib and Ia INs receive the same descending cortical controls, but their subcortical inputs are different (Fig. 5.5A). Instead of vestibulospinal support as for the Ia INs, Ib INs receive dorsolateral reticulospinal inhibition, which, as will be seen in Chap. 5.2, suggests a role in intended movements. For this purpose, the excitatory peripheral inputs to Ib INs from joint and (low-threshold) cutaneous afferents would be useful (see Fig. 5.5A). They would sense, for instance, when a voluntary movement is obstructed by an obstacle, and thereupon would activate the Ib INs, whose autogenic inhibitory signals then would tend to halt the movement and thus avoid forcing the obstacle. This suggested action is directly applicable in "active touch," the exploratory handling of objects discussed briefly in Chap. 3.1. Ib INs also halt muscular exertions before they exceed physiological limits, and may thus prevent muscular fatigue. Inputs from joints or skin (as in Fig. 5.5A) belong to the flexor reflex afferent (FRA) group and thus can make Ib INs part of the chain of INs innervated by the FRA, to be explained below with regard to Fig. 5.6. It will probable turn out that Ib INs are used in as versatile a manner as we are beginning to see for Ia INs. Recently many INs have been found that receive inputs from *both* Ia and Ib afferents.

In the intact animal, Ib INs may have wider scope than this sort of segmental action. Activity in and near the red nucleus, descending in the dorsolateral reticulospinal tract, can alter their activity. When under this influence, they have been found to modulate muscular co-contraction through complex coordination of flexor and extensor MNs. It seems probable that Ib INs in the cat are extensively facilitated by rubrospinal and corticospinal control

that may change according to behavioral needs. It is important to remember, however, that rubrospinal control in *humans* is uncertain. Human cerebellar projection to the red nucleus comes mainly from the lateral cerebellum, not the intermediate one as in the cat. The human lateral cerebellar output projects almost entirely to the parvicellular part of the red nucleus, which in turn communicates with the inferior olive, not the spinal cord (cf. Chap. 14).

All INs with branches reaching more than one spinal segment are classified as *propriospinal neurons* (P INs). They connect with other INs and/or with MNs. "Long" P INs connect cervical and lumbosacral segments, always as *excitatory* connections. (Inspection of Figs. 5.2–5.6 reveals that they share this "long-distance" property of making only facilitatory connections with the corticospinal, rubrospinal, and vestibulospinal tracts. Cortical descending inhibition is probably mediated through reticulospinal tracts). Branches of "short" P INs tend to be restricted to within a few segments at most. Many INs that are classified under other names also have branches outside of one segment, making them also P INs. All P INs may receive cortical descending controls of the types received by Ia and/or Ib INs, as shown for one example in Fig. 5.5B. Peripheral inputs belonging to the FRA group reaching P INs can incorporate them into the polysynaptic chain of FRA INs. (The FRA system is explained below.)

P INs with recurrent axon collaterals reaching, for instance, a cerebellar input nucleus, the lateral reticular nucleus (LRN; see Figs. 5.5B and 5.8), can send "corollary" or "reference" copies about their integrated activities to the cerebrocerebellar circuit. Afferent inputs from the neck and forelimbs are sent to the LRN, through which their information may be used for coordinating rhythmic activities of several limbs such as locomotion (and scratching in some animals; Chap. 10). This instance of FRA function is an example of Lundberg's concept that neurons in ascending

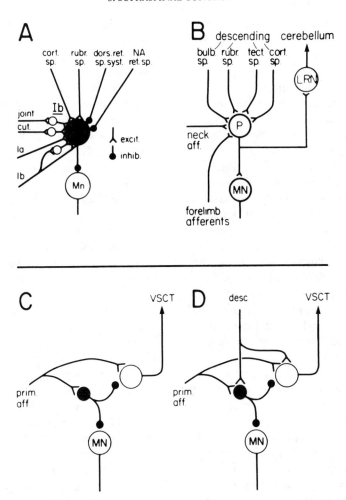

Fig. 5.5. Convergence of peripheral and central inputs on (A) an Ib IN and (B) a propriospinal (P) IN, in the cervical spinal cord. Peripheral afferents include joint, cutaneous, Ia and Ib receptors. Descending central control paths include corticospinal, rubrospinal, dorsal and noradrenergic (NA) reticulospinal, bulbospinal, tectospinal tracts. P IN receives afferents from the neck and forelimb. Note collateral projection from P IN ascending to cerebellar input (lateral reticular, LRN) nucleus. (C) and (D) illustrate how primary afferent and descending inputs [similar to those in (A) and (B)] can excite a spinal inhibitory IN as well as a neuron giving rise to a fiber ascending in the ventral spinocerebellar tract (VSCT). This VSCT neuron also samples the inhibitory output of the inhibitory IN. These successive events could be decoded by recipient cerebellar neurons as a comparison of the inputs and outputs of the spinal inhibitory IN. (Modified from Baldissera, Hultborn and Illert, 1981)

paths monitor the activity of INs in reflex pathways rather than signaling peripheral events. The monitored activity is returned to higher centers as corollary discharges, which are used for updating the movement programs. In fact, ongoing movements can be updated about events that occur during that movement, because the internal loops function swiftly by avoiding the long trip

around the periphery. An example of this concept, which was introduced in Chap. 3.1, could be the participation of cervical P INs in fast updating of visuomotor actions, because the P INs receive input from the optic tectum through a short loop. It has indeed been demonstrated that a cat, when catching moving prey, can redirect the path of its paw within about 50 msec, that is, in less than a quarter of the usual visual reaction time. The tectal loop to P INs is just one of many internal paths available for updating programs.

Activity of INs is monitored by several pathways. Figure 5.5C shows that neurons giving rise to the ventral spinocerebellar tract (VSCT) can be excited by Ia or Ib primary afferent fibers. In fact, some receive input from both. Figure 5.5C illustrates how the VSCT neuron is inhibited by a collateral branch of the Ia IN, whose other branch goes to a MN. The VSCT neuron thus receives first the excitatory input to the Ia IN provided by its primary Ia afferent fiber, followed by the inhibitory output of that IN. The VSCT neuron thus samples first the input and then the output of the Ia IN, which amounts to "comparing" them. As we saw in Fig. 5.2, inputs to the Ia IN include descending facilitatory paths. Figure 5.5D shows that VSCT neurons can also sample those descending inputs and their effects on Ia INs. The information carried by the VSCT reaches the cerebellum, where it is distributed as part of the "mossy" fiber input system, to be described in Chap. 13. This assists the cerebellum in *comparing* descending motor commands reaching lower motor centers with the effectiveness of their execution by those centers.

The acronym FRA stands for *flexor reflex afferents,* that is, the afferents whose action can evoke the well-known polysynaptic flexor reflexes. They consist of fibers with diameters classified as groups II and III (i.e., smaller than Ia or Ib), originating from muscles, joints and skin, that can evoke polysynaptic actions according to the pattern of the ipsilateral flexion reflex and the crossed-extensor reflex, with appropriate reciprocal actions on antagonist MNs. This is the definition given by Lundberg's group, who exclude smaller fibers that mediate noxious stimuli for the withdrawal reflex. Flexor reflexes traverse polysynaptic paths to MNs, but the long chain of FRA INs is not shown in Fig. 5.6. In Fig. 5.6A the spinal INs are lumped together in the circle denoting the "lower motor center," and in Fig. 5.6B they are indicated by a broken line. The FRA INs are not a special group, but are any IN that receives FRA input, be it ever so indirect, through polysynaptic connections. For instance, as mentioned in relation to Fig. 5.5, spinal Ib INs as well as P INs can function in the FRA chain, enabling ascending FRA paths to monitor the effects of descending motor commands on such spinal INs. Figure 5.6B shows how the FRA chain of INs can adjust the balance between different descending motor commands (only one descending path was shown in Fig. 5.6A). Those INs closer to the periphery are reached earlier by incoming neural activity. These "early" INs receive different peripheral input from the more centrally located "late" INs. The peripheral and central inputs of early INs can alter the excitability of late INs and thus can increase or decrease their responses to *descending* commands addressed to them. The differences of innervation of INs in the polysynaptic FRA chain make it a remarkable switching network that can channel the flow of information!

For example, Fig. 5.6B indicates how activation of the dorsolateral reticulospinal tract, drawn on the left, can facilitate inhibitory INs (drawn black) that receive low-threshold cutaneous input. This cutaneous input therefore inhibits the entry of FRA input by early INs, that is, it forestalls (or at least opposes) the flexion reflex. When the activated inhibitory IN silences the early FRA IN, it frees up input opportunities from descending paths to late INs that had previously been kept busy with segmental, interneuronal signals. Late INs can now respond better to descending motor commands (drawn on the right). Thus, by reducing the noisy traffic from early to late INs, the FRA chain has cleared the line (raised the signal/noise ratio) of late INs for signals from the corticospinal, rubrospinal and vestibulospinal tracts. In this consideration we regard the other inputs as unwanted "noise" that interferes with the "wanted" descending commands. In other words, one kind of descending input to the FRA (e.g., the one on the left in Fig. 5.6B) can facilitate the influence of other central inputs (e.g., the ones on the right), using FRA INs as switching devices.

The examples of control exerted by the FRA over descending information (in Figs. 5.5B and 5.6A) suggest uses for particular functions that span "long loops" between the lower and higher levels of the motor hierarchy. For instance, since the FRA can facilitate ascending paths that monitor activity of INs in reflex arcs (Fig. 5.6A), and also can facilitate appropriate descending motor commands (Fig. 5.6B), Lundberg has suggested that the circle between upcoming and downgoing messages may be closed in behaviorally active animals, and

that spinal INs are modulated according to the *needs of active movements* through use of the FRA. These ideas, which rely on activation of preferred paths at the right time, depict the FRA as a system that assists central commands by modulating segmental arcs of the spinal motor servo. The relevant roles of the descending paths are discussed in Chap. 5.2; their use in "long-loop" actions is covered in Chap. 6.2, and in locomotion in Chap. 10.

Peripheral afferent FRA axons have another property worth special mention: they make inhibitory ("presynaptic") connections with some afferent fibers, including Ia afferents. Opposing muscles thus influence each other presynaptically as well through the postsynaptic mechanisms illustrated in Fig. 5.2. "Presynaptic inhibition" selectively depresses *some* inputs to

Fig. 5.6. Interneurons of the flexor reflex afferent (FRA) system can monitor the activity of other spinal interneurons (INs) and can channel their information flow. (A) Ascending paths influenced by the FRA may provide feedback monitoring of activity in lower motor centers, represented by pools of INs that are at the same time reflex arcs and links in descending paths to alpha MNs. (B) The dorsolateral reticulospinal tract can inhibit peripheral FRA input to INs reached "early" by low-threshold cutaneous input. This clears the path to alpha MNs for other descending controls through INs reached "late" in the sequence. Compare to Fig. 5.5. [(A) From Oscarsson, 1973; (B) from Jeneskog and Johansson, 1977; in Schwindt, 1981]

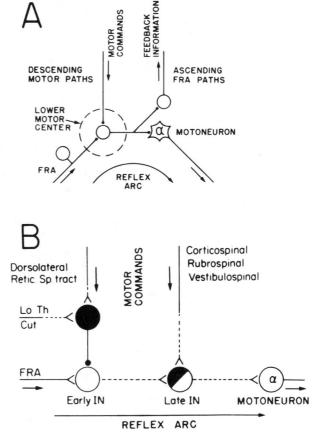

a neuron, while postsynaptic inhibition lowers the response to *all* its inputs. Lundberg views presynaptic inhibition by the FRA as a general mechanism for regulating transmission to first-order INs (early INs in Fig. 5.6). This negative feedback counteracts the positive feedback from peripheral FRA input on descending activation of INs described above. These details are explained mainly to show how hierarchical capabilities reinforce each other. Spinal mechanisms can do a lot of functionally appropriate switching that relieves higher centers from detailed chores. Higher centers can rely on the spinal "smart terminal" to let them get on with their own main job: to give shape to motor commands (Chaps. 2.2 and 3.1).

Fig. 5.7. Diagram of the major brain stem descending pathways concerned with the control of movement in the human (groups **A** and **B**) and their spinal terminations. Corticospinal terminations overlap both **A** and **B**. (From Barr and Kiernan, 1983; modified according to Kuypers, 1981)

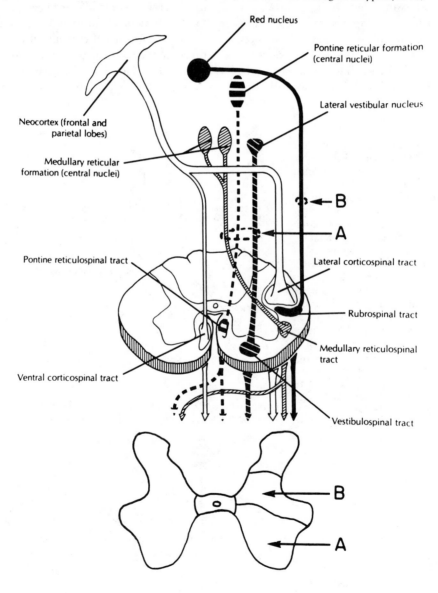

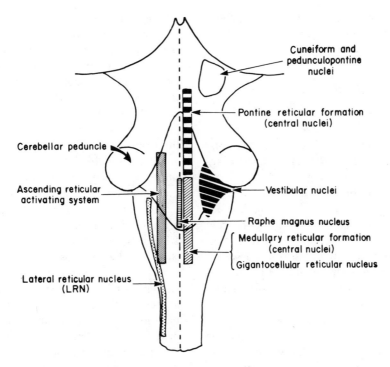

Fig. 5.8. Diagram of some major brain stem nuclei referred to in the text, seen in horizontal section. Nuclei giving rise to descending (type **A**) systems drawn on the *right* side with same conventions as in Fig. 5.7. Nuclei giving rise to ascending systems drawn on *left*. (Modified from Barr and Kiernan, 1983).

Synaptic Neurotransmitters

Figures 5.2–5.6 provide the opportunity for a brief summary of the neuro-transmitters involved. Knowing *which* neurotransmitters are active *where* is of great importance, because this knowledge offers therapeutic opportunities as pharmacological interventions in neurotransmission become increasingly feasible. Primary afferents, such as Ia and Ib probably excite alpha MNs through release of glutamate or aspartate. Excitatory spinal INs probably release aspartate. Renshaw cells are driven by acetylcholine (ACh) released from recurrent MN collaterals. Descending corticofugal paths release glutamate as the excitatory neurotransmitter. Inhibitory spinal INs are also driven by glutamate and aspartate, and release glycine for postsynaptic inhibition. Presynaptic inhibition operates through release of gamma-aminobutyric acid (GABA). Reticulospinal

cells are probably excited by glutamate or aspartate and are inhibited by glycine. Vestibulospinal cells are inhibited postsynaptically by GABA.

2. Descending Control Paths

Possibilities for complex instructions abound for spinal interneurons but instructions toward what end? The most global answer, introduced in Chap. 2.2, would be "to fulfill the intent of the individual." The hierarchical system substitutes more limited, specific tasks that can be carried out at different levels. The example of the FRA, taken up in the preceding unit, illuminates Bernstein's concept of these capabilites that simplify the function of the brain. A practical goal is to acquire a good understanding of the anatomy and functional relations of the descending systems. This unit is divided into three related subtopics: anatomical organization, postural actions, and control of ascending information.

Anatomical Organization

It is helpful to remember that *motor tracts originate in the brain stem with the exception of the pyramidal (or corticospinal) tract.* The most important descending tracts are shown in Figs. 5.7, 5.10, 5.11, and 5.12. The brain stem is indicated as medulla oblongata and pons in Fig. 2B and C and the nuclei corresponding to the tracts are shown and labeled in Fig. 5.8. The phylogenetically oldest tracts descend more medially in the medulla; they are labeled group **A** in Fig. 5.7, following Kuyper's classification.

Figure 5.9 indicates that the brain steers "fractionated" limb movements by means of the corticospinal tract (drawn as a heavy line on the right) as well as the corticorubrospinal and some corticoreticulospinal pathways (brain stem group **B**.) Group **A** paths, which coordinate posture and locomotion, include four reticulospinal tracts and the two vestibulospinal tracts

(cf. Fig. 9.2). They receive input from cerebral areas rostral to, but not from, the primary motor cortex (precentral area 4). They continue in the ventral and ventrolateral spinal funiculi, terminating in the intermediate zone of the spinal cord (Figs. 5.7 and 5.9), where they connect with long propriospinal INs and MNs of proximal limb muscles as well as of eye, ear, neck and back muscles. These are essential postural components, whose integration into movements will be taken up in Chap. 9.

The terminal regions in the spinal cord are simplified in Fig. 5.7 to those marked **A** and **B**; the detailed laminae are not shown. The regions, and the laminae within them, indicate where afferent and efferent paths have their endings, but to appreciate the capabilities of spinal integration we must remember that the dendrites of MNs, and of some INs, extend through many laminae and thus provide functional choices for activation of alternate anatomical connections. The vestibular pathway terminates in the same region as other fibers of pontine origin, while the rubrospinal and corticospinal fibers overlap with others of medullary ori-

Fig. 5.9. Summary of the muscle groups controlled by corticoreticulospinal, corticorubrospinal and corticospinal paths. Note the overlapping control of arm–hand muscles, but the nearly exclusive control of one or two digits by the corticospinal tracts, drawn in *heavy lines.* (From Humphrey, 1979; in Humphrey, 1983)

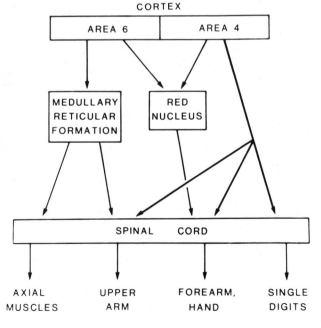

gin (Fig. 5.7). The pontine systems facilitate physiological extensors and the medullary systems physiological flexors. Throughout their downward course these tracts give off many collateral branches. Group **A** clearly is well suited for the synergistic activation of many muscles and not for fine control of fractionated movements. This is borne out by the consequences of sectioning group **A** pathways in subhuman primates, described below. They constitute the basic movement system that ensures erect posture, integration of body and limb movements, orientation movements of body and head, and direction of locomotion.

The *rubrospinal tract* is the main member of group **B** in subhuman primates. It is less important in the human. It receives a projection from precentral cortex and descends through the ventrolateral part of the medulla and continues into the dorsolateral funiculus. It terminates in the dorsal and lateral parts of the spinal intermediate zone (Fig. 5.7), from which short propriospinal INs originate. It also connects with MNs of the distal extremities. Throughout its descent the group **B** rubrospinal tract gives off very few collaterals. This organization suggests use for movement fractionation. Group **B** provides the capacity for independent, flexion-biased movements of the extremities and shoulders, particularly the elbow and hand, but not of the fingers (see Fig. 5.9)

Figure 5.7 shows the course of the *corticospinal tract*, labeled neither **A** nor **B** because it is not a brain stem tract but instead originates in the sensorimotor cortex. This cortex consists of several areas that all contain cells of origin of the corticospinal tract. The cortical areas are marked in Fig. 2.1A as the "premotor association area" and the "motor area," the "sensory area" and also include part of the "sensory association area." The first two, comprising areas 6 and 4, which appear in Fig. 5.9, are part of the frontal lobe, which is located rostral to the central sulcus. The numbers of the cortical areas are marked

in Fig. 11.1. The sensory areas and their association cortex are part of the postcentral, parietal lobe. They are areas 2, 1 (together, SI) and 5, as well as the "second somatic sensory area" (SII, buried in the dorsal wall of the lateral sulcus). Areas 2 and 1 are the "primary somatosensory areas," and area 5 is the rostral part of the "somesthetic association cortex" located in the superior parietal lobule. Area 3, which also belongs in this group, occupies the walls of the central sulcus, and being thus buried is not visible on the surface of the cerebral mantle. Area 4 is the "primary motor cortex" or "primary motor area" (PMA). The lateral part of area 6 is called the "premotor area," and the medial part, buried from view in the longitudinal fissure, is called the "supplementary motor area" (SMA). All these areas together make up the "motor cortex" (see Figs. 2.7, 5.10 and 11.1).

A little less than one-half of the neurons giving rise to axons that traverse the medullary pyramid (pyramidal tract) are located in the precentral, primary and supplementary motor areas, and the rest are postcentral. Our anatomical orientation requires us to understand which ("corticofugal") tracts leaving the cortex function primarily in the motor realm, and which act more on sensory information. How motor acts are served by sensory adjustments was touched on in Chap. 3.1 and is taken up below under the heading, "Control of Ascending Information." Figures 5.10 and 5.11 provide anatomical orientation. The postcentral origins (in the sensory, somesthetic areas) of the input-adjusting components of the pyramidal tract are indicated, together with some of the afferent paths affected. Figure 5.11 is a diagram of the main components of the descending fiber systems. Corticothalamic and the corticoreticular fibers (the most medial sets) end in the ipsilateral thalamus and bilaterally in the pontine and medullary reticular formation, whose responsiveness they adjust. The corticobulbar fibers end in the contralateral dorsal column nuclei (gracilis and cuneatus), where they adjust afferent input to the medial lemniscal system going to the primary sensory cortex. Also indicated are the tracts descending from the reticular and the raphe nuclei (cf. Figs. 5.7 and 5.8). These "extrapyramidal" projections, derived from postcentral cortex, have, of course, motor influences besides their control of ascending sensory input, as judged by the enhanced spasticity caused by postcentral lesions when added to precentral ones, and by their compensatory actions during dysfunction of the motor cortex (in monkeys).

The motor cortex on each side of the human brain sends about one million pyramidal tract axons to the medulla, of which more than three-quarters continue further down to the spinal cord as corticospinal (CS) axons in the lateral and ventral corticospinal tracts. The motor fibers of the CS systems are traced in more detail in Fig. 5.12. More than three-quarters of the corticospinal neurons cross ("decussate") as part of the lateral CS tract; the rest continue ipsilaterally as the ventral CS tract. These tracts terminate in the spinal cord in the areas of the brain stem **A** and **B** groups deep in the intermediate zone, and in the ventral horn, mostly in the cervical and lumbar enlargements.

The corticospinal system serves exploratory manipulatory activity. Axons of corticospinal neurons (CSNs) in the precentral cortex predominantly modulate the activity of alpha MNs as well as of static and dynamic gamma MNs. Denny-Brown has pointed out that "the pyramidal system is concerned not so much with discrete movements of individual muscles or individual joints as with those spatial adjustments that accurately adapt the movement to the spatial attributes of the stimulus. Thus grasping is adapted to the shape of the thing to be grasped, whether a particle of food, a pen or a surface, only in the presence of the pyramidal tract." Accordingly, CSNs are organized to coordinate related motor nuclei even if they are located in separate spinal segments, because

individual axon branches innervate several MN nuclei. An instance is illustrated in Fig. 5.13A. We must remember, however, that not all of the connections shown are active at the same time; they are under the sway of a number of converging influences. This pattern also applies to other descending tracts, such as the rubrospinal, vestibulospinal and reticulospinal ones. Postcentral CS axons, in contrast, probably modulate interneurons in the dorsal horn of the spinal cord (see Fig. 5.10). In lower mammals the corticospinal tract is as much a sensory as a motor control system, connecting predominantly with spinal interneurons. Corticospinal fibers of monkeys make monosynaptic connections with MNs of hand and finger muscles (see Fig. 5.9), and in the chimpanzee and human these connections reach even the MNs of proximal muscles. The extent of monosynaptic corticomotoneuronal (CM) connections relates to how well limb movements can be fractionated. Alpha MNs with many CM synapses also receive many Ia connections. Phillips has pointed out that this makes the CM drive highly responsive to changes of load on muscles and sets the stage for muscular adjustments through a "long loop" traversing the sensorimotor cortex. Use of long loops is discussed in Chap. 6.2.

CSNs have a unimodal distribution of sizes in the monkey, and presumably in humans as well. Less than one-quarter of the monkey's CS axons are >5 μm—that is, conduct faster than 25 m/sec. The small-fibered, slow-conducting majority is more easily modulated by synaptic inputs than the fast-conducting minority. Similar rules operate in the cerebral cortex as do in the spinal cord: slow CSNs tend to be recruited first because synaptic currents produce bigger voltage drops across their membranes, since their input resistance is two to three times higher than that of fast CSNs (see Henneman's size principle in Chap. 4.1). In the alert monkey, the activity of slow cells is related to resting limb postures and to finely graded movements.

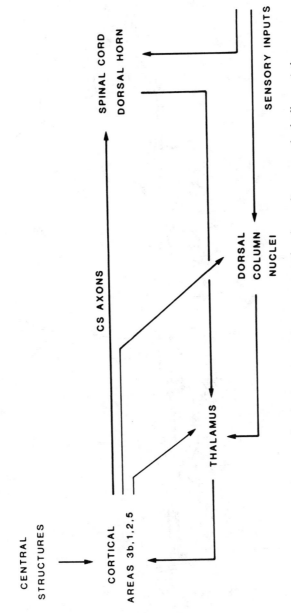

Fig. 5.10. Summary of paths from sensorimotor cortex for descending control of afferent information. Corticospinal (CS) neurons in these areas act principally to modulate reflex and somatosensory transmission during movement, and are affected by both central and peripheral inputs. (From Humphrey, 1983)

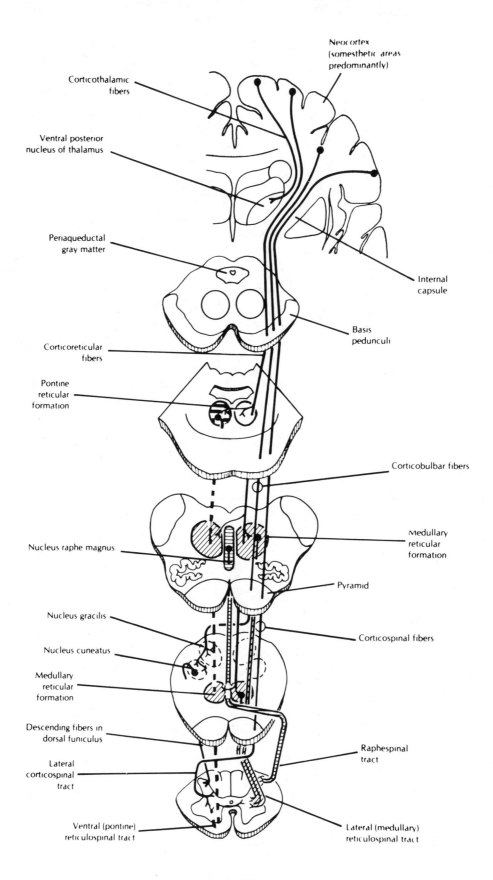

Neocortex
(somesthetic areas
predominantly)

Corticothalamic
fibers

Ventral posterior
nucleus of thalamus

Internal
capsule

Periaqueductal
gray matter

Basis
pedunculi

Corticoreticular
fibers

Pontine
reticular
formation

Corticobulbar fibers

Medullary
reticular
formation

Nucleus raphe magnus

Pyramid

Nucleus gracilis

Corticospinal fibers

Nucleus cuneatus

Medullary
reticular
formation

Descending fibers in
dorsal funiculus

Raphespinal
tract

Lateral
corticospinal
tract

Ventral (pontine)
reticulospinal tract

Lateral (medullary)
reticulospinal tract

Fast CSNs, in contrast, probably discharge during movement onset when inertia of the limb needs to be overcome to change from one posture to another. These actions depend on the great synaptic security of transmission across CM synapses, which is assisted by presynaptic facilitation of transmitter release when impulses follow one another at about 5 msec, their natural frequency. This is illustrated by the lowermost trace in Fig. 5.13B, which presents responses of a spinal MN when driven at that rate by precentral stimulation. The intracellular records show the buildup of the synaptic responses to CM activation at 200 stimuli/sec (i.e. 5 msec intervals). This buildup is specific to the CM input, because no such potentiation is produced by activation of Ia fibers to that MN at the same rate (upper traces). The neocortical connection here functions as a local amplifier that speeds up the summation of tension in selected muscles and hence their ability to accelerate a joint quickly. This selectivity is a great addition to the ability of the ancient motor system, the basal ganglia, to regulate acceleration through speed of recruitment on an overall basis.

At this point it is well to remember that CSNs, because of their branches, can discharge spinal MNs monosynaptically as well as polysynaptically (with after-discharge) through INs in the intermediate zone of the spinal cord. In addition, CSN branches also promote the inhibition of antagonist muscles by reaching Ia INs related to the agonist MN (see Fig. 5.2). Finally, it should be mentioned that descending corticospinal fibers also control local cholinergic muscle vasodilatation in preparation for muscular activity.

The main *extrapyramidal* paths originating in the cerebral cortex are the corticostriate, corticoreticular, and cortico-

rubral systems. Their parts and functions are summarized here, to be followed by more detail in Chaps. 11–14. The striatum is the input to the basal ganglia, innervated partly from area 4. The corticoreticulospinal system originates mostly in the medial and lateral area 6 (Fig. 5.9). These systems serve postural control with axial orienting movements and limb projections. The reticulospinal systems deal mostly with central inputs and also with some somatosensory feedback from truck and axial muscles (Fig. 5.11). Impulses in this large-fibered system reach the spinal cord earlier than those of the pyramidal tract. The corticorubrospinal system (Fig. 5.9) consists of two parts. The smaller one originates from the arm and leg regions of area 4 and projects to the magnocellular part of the red nucleus, which gives rise to the rubrospinal tract, a component whose importance in humans is uncertain. The larger corticorubral part projects from areas 4, 6 and 5 to the parvocellular part of the red nucleus, which, in turn, connects to the cerebellar circuit through its inferior olivary input nucleus. (This is taken up in Chap. 13.1.)

The third system descending from the brain stem, not shown in Fig. 5.7 but in Figs. 5.8 and 5.11, was mentioned in Chap. 2 in connection with walking: the monoaminergic fibers descending from the brain stem nuclei subcoeruleus and raphe (see Figs. 5.8 and 5.11), mostly to terminations in the dorsal horn. They include two reticulospinal tracts, and will be taken up again with regard to descending control of afferent input below and to locomotion in Chap. 9.

Kuypers' view of the group **A** and **B** systems is based on the different motor defects following selective interruption of these paths in the rhesus monkey. Pyramidal lesions cause grave loss of initiative to

Fig. 5.11. Descending pathways that modulate transmission of sensory information from the spinal cord to the cerebral cortex. Compare to Figs. 5.8 and 5.10 where the same codes of hatching are used. (From Barr and Kiernan, 1983)

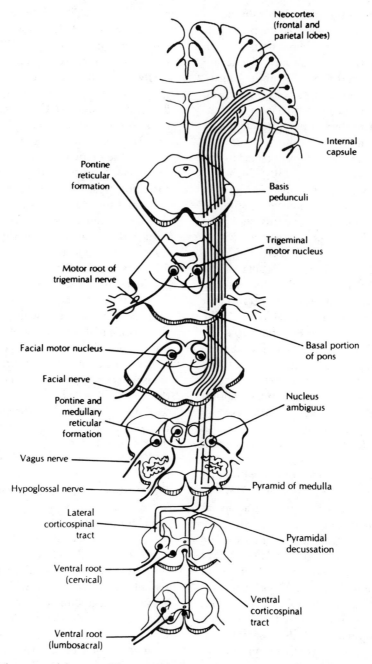

Fig. 5.12.   The pyramidal system. The corticobulbar and corticospinal neurons are shown as well as the "lower motoneurons," which are drawn as *heavier lines*. (From Barr and Kiernan, 1983)

use the opposite extremities, but not complete loss of their use. They can be brought to act if the normal side is restrained. The following is an instuctive summary made from Kuypers' description.

Bilateral pyramidotomy mainly interferes with steering of the extremities, a mixture of **A** and **B** properties. Immediately after the operation, the animals can sit with their heads up. There is no forward slumping of the head and

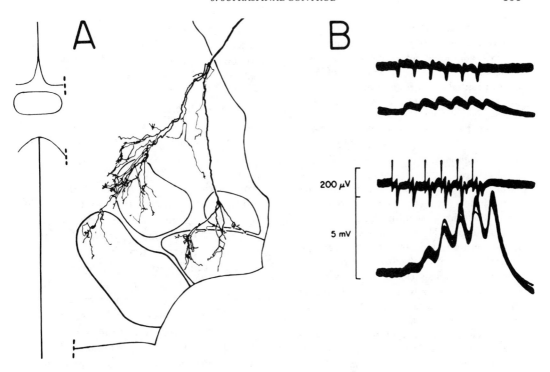

Fig. 5.13. Anatomical and physiological properties of corticospinal (CS) endings. (A) Axon branches of a CS neuron (located in the hand area of a monkey's motor cortex) reaching four groups of spinal MNs. The upper and lower pairs of MN nuclei shown in this transverse reconstruction give rise to the ulnar and radial nerves, respectively. (B) Presynaptic facilitation is evoked by repetitive activation of corticomotoneuronal (CM) monosynaptic synapses of CSNs on a spinal MN (lower traces), but not of Ia monosynaptic synapses on the same MN (upper traces). Each pair of traces presents extracellular and intracellular records of excitatory postsynaptic potentials (EPSPs) evoked by stimulation at 200/second (Hz, i.e., 5-msec intervals), at strengths for equally sized first EPSPs. [(A) from Shinoda, 1981; (B) from Phillips and Porter, 1964]

body, which happens only if lesions extend into the medullary tegmentum, damaging group **A** pathways. The animals can walk, run and climb immediately postoperatively, but they cannot pick up pieces of food with their hands, which they limply place on the food without grasping it. Yet they can use their hands and feet in clinging to the cage bars.

During recovery the animals regain the capacity to pick up food with their hands. Initially, reaching consists of a hooking, circular adduction ("circumduction") of the whole arm, and the closure of the hand forms part of this whole-arm movement. As recovery proceeds, closure of the hand, which consists of flexion of all fingers together, becomes progressively independent of the arm movements, so that ultimately the animals can reach out and open and close the hand with a stable, outstretched

arm. Yet, even 4–5 years postoperatively, individual finger movements such as the thumb and index finger precision grip do not return. (This loss of fine or discrete control is called "paresis.") *Unilateral* pyramidotomy produces roughly the same sequence, but restricted to the contralateral limb. This suggests that the corticospinal tract serves independent finger movements. If sectioned soon after birth, this capacity never develops. Ablation of precentral cortex in different species is followed by flaccid paralysis of a severity that is related to the extent that those species have developed corticomotoneuronal (monosynaptic) connections.

The specific deficiencies caused by section of group **A** or **B** are best revealed after recovery from bilateral pyramidotomy, which we saw causes loss of independent finger control. *Brain stem motor control* returns after bilateral pyramidal transection, but it is different for groups **A** and **B** as demonstrated by the consequences of their additional respective sections in the same animals. Bilateral interruption of **A** produces postural changes of trunk and limbs, a prolonged inability of the animal to right itself, and a severe deficit in the steering of axial and proximal limb movements. Distal dexterity is less imparied. Flexion of trunk and limbs persists throughout the recovery period. Shoulders are elevated and arms adducted, especially when sitting or when supine. The animals cannot right to a sitting position until some weeks later, when they are still unsteady and tend to slump forward. They learn to walk again but remain unsteady and have difficulty in avoiding obstacles. In contrast, hands and distal parts are very active: animals can hold pieces of food very soon postoperatively, and can manipulate as well as they did just after bilateral pyramidotomy. There is a difference however, in how they reach for food. If only pyramidotomized, they will turn toward it and reach for it with an outstretched arm and an open hand. Animals with *additional group* **A** *damage*, however, follow food only with the eyes while body and arms remain relatively stationary. They bring arm and hand to the food by flexing the elbow, but only when it is close to the hand.

Animals with *additional group* **B** *transection* are able to right themselves immediately. They sit up in their cages, walk, climb and do not have the axial and proximal limb flexion posture that occurs after **A**-transection. The **B**-group shows striking changes, however, in the use of the ipsilateral limbs, particularly the affected arm, which hangs loosely from the shoulder with the elbow slightly flexed and the fingers extended. Finger and wrists are limp postoperatively. In reaching for food the elbow is held semiflexed and the hand is brought to the food by circumduction of the arm in the shoulder. The food is grasped by flexion of the fingers, but this is part of the total arm movement. The affected limb shows less defect however, when used in walking or climbing.

Postural Actions

Working from this overview of the descending systems, we can now ask: which descending tracts *promote antigravity reflex patterns that are used for standing* and which ones *oppose* them to liberate limbs for use in *intended movements?* The cerebral cortex of the monkey gives rise to the corticospinal (*pyramidal*) and the corticorubrospinal tracts (Fig. 5.7). The role of the (group **B**) rubrospinal tract in the human is uncertain, however, because its size has dwindled in evolution. From what we have learned so far, it comes as no surprise that both tracts *liberate muscles and joints from postural roles imposed by gravity* through their tendency to inhibit "antigravity" muscles (that hold the body up against gravity) and to facilitate their opposites. In humans, pyramidal activation for voluntary action takes the form of inhibition of flexors and facilitation of extensors of the upper limbs, and conversely, inhibition of extensors and facilitation of flexors of the lower limbs. Corticospinal and rubrospinal connections are mostly through INs except for control of the fingers, where finesse is needed most. Fine control is brought about by use of MNs receiving matched densities of monosynaptic pyramidal connections with those from muscle spindles. This exemplifies the usual mode of operation in motor control: provision for striking a *fine balance between two mechanisms.* In this instance they happen to be central feedforward and peripheral feedback controls.

Movements require preparations well before the implementation of muscular action, in fact before the central commands for action are issued. These preparatory aspects of motor control are carried out largely by the paths originating in the brain stem: the four reticulospinal and two vestibulospinal tracts. They function as parts of more complex control systems, including other extrapyramidal structures as well as the pyramidal tract.

The *antigravity reflexes for standing are promoted* by the (group **A**) rostrolateral *pontine reticular formation* (cf. Figs. 5.7 and 5.8). In humans, this is achieved without direct cortical control by tonic facilitation of flexors in the upper limbs and extensors in the lower limbs—that is, just the opposite of pyramidal action. As would be expected from Fig. 5.2, Ia INs are influenced in the same direction as alpha MNs. The fibers descend in the *pontine reticular tract*, also known as the *medial reticulospinal tract* because it runs (at least partly) through the medial longitudinal fasciculus (MLF) together with vestibulospinal fibers. In the human, it passes through the sulcomarginal edge of the anterior spinal columns, near the vestibulospinal tract, which also promotes reflex standing.

Mobilizaion of the spinal-output stages from antigravity functions by the pyramidal system is preceded and accompanied by equivalent actions emanating from the *ventromedial reticular formation*, which is part of group **A** but has some spinal lateral (**B**) terminations and properties. This part of the reticular formation is a site of convergence of pyramidal branches from precentral cortex and of dentate projections from lateral cerebellum. (Specifically, it is the caudal part of the gigantocellular reticular nuclei located in the bulbar region near the inferior olive: see Figs. 5.8 and 5.11.) Preparations for movement include effects from several structures on MNs and on segmental reflex patterns, that is, on INs. The *medullary reticular formation* (corresponding to part of Magoun's original "inhibitory" area) tends to inhibit segmental stretch-reflex patterns for standing. It causes this "release" from segmental reflex function by postsynaptic inhibition of (primarily) extensor MNs as well as of Ia INs, and to a lesser extent of some other inputs to MNs. Medullary reticulospinal fibers descend bilaterally in the *lateral (medullary) reticulospinal tract* in the *ventral* half of the cat's cord and (possibly in the lateral spinal columns in the human).

A second medullary reticulospinal inhibitory path, the *dorsolateral* one, also activates circuits, particularly for coordinated stepping movements, by releasing them from segmental reflex function. The dorsolateral tract tonically inhibits segmentally active FRA and Ib polysynaptic paths. This path is another A-part with some B-terminations and properties. Its fibers descend in the *dorsolateral funiculus* of the spinal cord. Figure 5.6 shows how activation of the dorsolateral reticulospinal tract can inhibit FRA peripheral input, making the INs closer to alpha MNs (late INs) in the FRA polysynaptic chain more readily available for descending control messages from the corticospinal, rubrospinal and vestibulospinal systems. Branches of the dorsolateral path facilitate dynamic gamma MNs (Chap. 13.1).

Preparations for locomotion that liberate spinal circuits from segmental duty are aided by two more reticulospinal inhibitory paths that are distinguished by containing *monoaminergic reticulospinal fibers* (the third group of Kuypers). They "release" long-latency FRA paths from previous inactivity so that they may be used for coordinated stepping movements. This release is brought on by tonic inhibition of segmental FRA and Ib polysynaptic paths, without affecting Ia disynaptic inhibition (compare Fig. 5.2 with Figs 5.5 and 5.6). The monoaminergic system, which is activated by the midbrain locomotor center, consists of serotonergic fibers originating in and near the raphe nuclei located close to the midline of the pontomedullary brain stem, and of noradrenergic fibers originating near the locus coeruleus (see Fig. 5.8). The fibers descend in the lateral and ventral funiculi.

The *vestibular system* is primarily organized to stabilize the head in space by action on neck muscles, and to stabilize the eyes in space during head movements by action of the vestibulocular reflex on the external eye muscles. It is *not* a general system for impressing vestibular input directly on limb posture or movements except to counter changes applied to the position of the head, which will be considered in Chap. 9.1. The lateral vestibular tract, however, does reach limb MNs. Interactions between head and body are the topic of Chap. 9.2. The vestibular nuclei (located in the brain stem: cf. Figs. 5.7 and

5.8) receive vestibular input from the labyrinthine and spinal somatic peripheral inputs, as well as more integrated information relayed from the reticular formation and the cerebellum. The vestibulospinal tracts (see Fig. 9.2) are part of group **A** and, like the pontine reticular formation, promote standing reflexes. Actions on alpha and gamma MNs and on Ia INs (cf. Fig. 5.2) follow these rules, always with regard to the starting positions of head, trunk and limbs in relation to intended posture or movements. The balancing function of the vestibulospinal system uses converging bilateral descent to spinal MNs. Since alpha MNs thus receive synergistic inputs from either side of the midline, vestibulospinal integration affects the contralateral FRA, as we have already seen in Fig. 5.6. This stands in contrast to the unilateral actions on MNs by the corticospinal, rubrospinal, and reticulospinal tracts that only involve ipsilateral peripheral afferents.

The *lateral vestibulospinal tract* (LVST) is part of group **A**, but like some others mentioned, has some **B**-terminations and properties. It conveys integrated cortical and cerebellar commands, as is suggested by its pattern of branching to cervical as well as lumbar segments. It descends ipsilaterally from the lateral vestibular (Deiters') nucleus, which receives peripheral vestibular as well as central cerebellar and reticular inputs. [The *medial vestibulospinal tract* (MVST) projection is mostly restricted to neck muscles, converging with LVST, through the medial longitudinal fasciculus MLF together with some fibers from the rostroponal reticular formation.] Since the most intense action of the LVST is on the cervical cord, the neck, rostral trunk and forelimb muscles receive more influences from labyrinthine reflexes than the hindlimbs. Vestibulospinal output facilitates extensor muscles and inhibits flexors. The tract excites static gamma MNs monsynaptically, which tightly couples alpha–gamma coactivation. This neural action is probably used for isometric con-

tractions of human hand and finger muscles. Release of Deiter's nucleus is partly responsible for the pathological extensor tone in the decerebrate cat (see Chap. 7.2).

The cerebellum provides the largest central input to the vestibular nuclei with direct Purkinje cell projections from the vestibulocerebellum (vestibular input) and from the spinocerebellum, as well as indirect projections of spinal input via the fastigial nucleus. The connections of the cerebellar nuclei are illustrated in Fig. 13.2. The second largest projection to the vestibular nuclei comes from the reticular formation, mostly from the gigantocellular nucleus and the caudal reticular pontine nucleus (see Fig. 5.8), which are under direct control from the cerebral cortex, cerebellum and superior colliculus.

One last descending system should be mentioned, because it is important for rotary movements of the head and truck in response to visual signals. That is the *tectospinal tract,* which originates in the superior colliculus (as part of group **A**), and after crossing descends in the anterior columns of the spinal cord, mixed with vestibulospinal fibers. Its "orienting" actions, which assist subjects to examine ("foveate") visual targets, are analogous to those of the vestibulospinal tract to labyrinthine input. It is possible that eye position may be signaled to the superior colliculus from spindle-like receptors in extraocular muscles (see Chap. 9.2). The tectospinal system is under the influence of the basal ganglia through the nigrotectal fibers to the superior colliculus.

Control of Ascending Information

The foregoing has made it clear that the CNS operates through looped circuits that can influence one another. Descending controls affect the information flow for sensory and motor events together; the two are inextricably entwined (Chaps. 2.2, 3.1, and see Figs. 5.2–5.6 as examples). Eccles has been using the term "evolving movement" for that reason. Only a few examples will be given here to illustrate the main points about descending control of ascending information.

Sensorimotor cortical areas 1, 2 and 3B project to pools of INs in the dorsal horn of the spinal cord, and areas 3a and 4 to INs and MNs in the dorsal horn base, intermediate (gray) zone, and lateral ventral horn (see the lower part of Fig. 5.7, and Fig. 5.9). There they modulate sensory afferent endings and interneurons, partly by presynaptic inhibition. Corticofugal activity also presynaptically inhibits primary afferent fibers from rapidly adapting mechanoreceptors (in the cat). This control is input-specific and may be related to the somatomotor functions of the cortical areas. Areas 1 and 2, for instance, receive short-latency somatic inputs from skin and joints, respectively, which they modulate, but they do not inhibit noxious inputs to spinothalamic cells. (The descending inhibition may be mediated by reticulospinal projections after they have been activated by pyramidal fibers.) Figures 5.2–5.6 show that all INs can receive corticospinal input, which is always excitatory. Some of these INs are neurons giving rise to axons ascending in the spinocerebellar and spinoreticular tracts. Cortical descending input can generally be found where there is FRA input, which led to Lundberg's formulation of FRA function, explained with respect to Fig. 5.6. In the dorsal column nuclei of the medial lemniscal system— that is, in the first synaptic nucleus of the main specific somatosensory input—postcentral sensorimotor cortex excites interneurons, which in turn can inhibit output cells from the nuclei. In contrast to the above pyramidal action, rubrospinal and vestibulospinal tracts mostly influence spinal cord tract cells.

The pyramidal tract also modulates afferent input above the spinal cord, in "relay" nuclei where the ascending information in the medial lemniscal system is processed. For instance, corticobulbar fibers (from the caudal part of the primary motor area and from postcentral areas) can facilitate and inhibit activity in the dorsal columns and more rostral somatosensory nuclei during voluntary movement. These effects are modality-specific, in that they can enhance some and suppress others in a task-related manner. The facilitation of inputs from joints and muscles by skin contact may be an example. Connections for these effects are drawn diagrammatically in Fig. 5.12.

Why do higher centers govern their own inputs and those of related brain parts? The example cited above, for instance, would be a useful device in "active touch," the interplay of sensory and motor events during tactile exploration of a surface or of an object. More generally, higher centers can change the gain or the composition of inputs. They may change how elective a receiving center is for different input modalities, and they may switch channels of information flow. Figure 5.6 illustrates an example of a cellular mechanism for that point, and also how the signal/noise ratio on a particular line can be changed. When this occurs, it could be experienced by the individual as a change of sensations or it might occur subconsciously. Experimenters observing events in the nervous system would record changed responsiveness of neurons to afferent inputs. Figure 5.14 illustrates such a change for three neurons in the dorsal horn of a lumbar segment in a decerebrate cat with intact brain stem and when the animal was spinalized by cold block of the thoracolumbar border. Removal of descending influences changed which natural stimuli were "adequate" and altered the boundaries of their "peripheral receptive fields." In the decerebrate, but not in the spinal state, the effects of passive movement of the ankle and claws were prominent. In the spinal state without descending controls, however, the cells were dominated by input from the skin. This type of change could have come about through influence of the pyramidal tract, perhaps by interactions in the FRA chain, referred to in relation to Fig. 5.6.

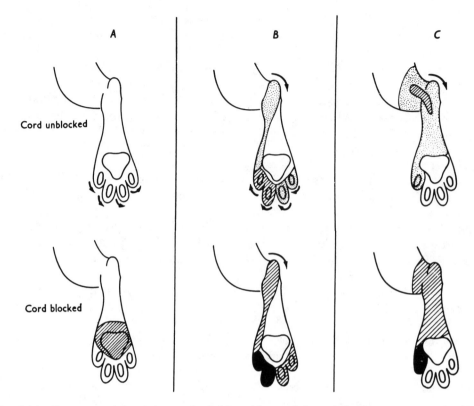

Fig. 5.14. Responses of three neurons in the dorsal horn of the cat's lumbar spinal cord (A–C) to natural stimulation are under tonic descending control from the brain stem. In the decerebrate animal with intact brain stem (top row: cord unblocked), there was predominance of input from joint movement *(arrows)* and "deep" cutaneous inputs (touch, *hatched*; pressure, *stippled*). Interruption of descending controls by making the animal spinal through thoracic cord block (bottom row: cord blocked) decreased the efficacy of these inputs and released "superficial" skin input (e.g., from brushing, *black*). (From Wall, 1967)

Another way to look at descending inhibition would be that internal descending discharge from sensorimotor areas could be programmed to inhibit certain inputs that would otherwise occur as the result of the movement-to-come. Perhaps some inhibitions are meant to prevent interference with (i.e., facilitate) the operation of movement programs. An example would be "predictive programming" of neurons in motor cortex and spinal cord according "motor set," which suppresses responses to muscle stretch when they are not wanted in the task context (Chap. 12.3).

Descending inhibition can be targeted on painful, potentially injurious (nociceptive) stimuli that generate impulses that are relayed centrally through the spinothalamic system. They receive a number of controlling projections from the brain stem and midbrain. A powerful pain-suppressing projection originates in the *midbrain reticular formation* and the adjoining *periaqueductual gray matter*. It projects indirectly, polysynaptically to the tonically active medullary raphe nuclei, mainly the *raphe magnus nucleus* (see Fig. 5.8), whose output descends in the dorsolateral funiculus of the spinal cord to terminations mostly in the dorsal horn. Stimulation of the gray matter produces analgesia by means of the raphe serotonergic pathway, which is effective on cells in the primate spinothalamic and ventral spinocerebellar tracts.

Figure 5.15 illustrates the selective nature of this descending inhibition by comparing its effectiveness before and during local anesthesia of the descending tract (by cold block) in a cat under general anesthesia. When the tonic inhibition was active (upper graphs), gentle stimuli such as hairbending (H) excited the spinocervical neurons about as much as noxious, intense heating of the skin, graphed below the histograms of cellular discharge frequency. However, when the descending inhibition was blocked from reaching the neurons (lower graphs), they responded disproportionately more to noxious inputs such as

Fig. 5.15. Pain is under tonic descending control from the brain stem. Response of a neuron in the dorsal horn of the lumbar spinal cord of an anesthetized cat with intact brain stem (top row: cord unblocked) and after thoracic cord block (bottom row: cord blocked). Block of descending inhibition released greater responses to pain-producing inputs (P, pinprick and heating the skin to 40 to 50°C). Superficial input, as from hairbending (H), increased far less. (From Cervero, Iggo and Moloney, 1977; in Willis and Coggeshall, 1978; and in Brooks, 1983)

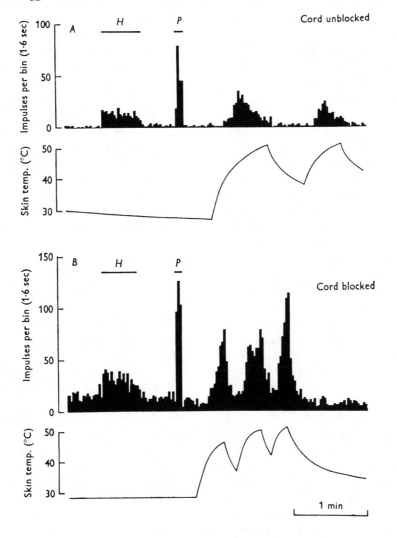

heat or pinprick (P) than to gentle hair-bending (H).

3. Summary

Spinal-output stages include alpha and gamma MNs and all spinal INs. Together with the controlled muscle and its sense organs, this functional assembly constitutes the motor servo, which is self-adjusting but can still be controlled by descending commands. Supraspinal control is mediated mostly through descending input converging on INs, which, in turn, influence alpha and gamma MNs. Ia INs receive the same descending inputs as their connected alpha or gamma MNs. Coordination of antagonist muscles is preserved at the segmental level through reciprocal inhibition by Ia branches of the Ia IN of the antagonist. In addition, Renshaw (R) cells, responsible for recurrent inhibition, innervate alpha MNs and their Ia INs as well as their gamma MNs. R-cell action can be useful in adjusting the gain of the motor servo and in focusing segmental control on a particular muscle. Ib INs can assist exploratory manipulation by autogenic inhibition of MNs that would otherwise force a sensed obstacle. Ib INs receive the same corticospinal and rubrospinal facilitation as Ia INs, but instead of vestibulospinal facilitation they are inhibited by the dorsolateral reticulospinal tract. All INs with branches reaching more than one spinal segment are called propriospinal (P) INs. Some send corollary messages back to higher centers about their integrated efferent activity. All INs, including Ib and P INs, which receive group II afferents from muscles, joints or skin—that is, flexor reflex afferents (FRA)—can then function as part of the polysynaptic FRA input chain in INs. Their diverse central inputs can strengthen or weaken inputs to other INs in the FRA chain. Such segmental actions can raise the effectiveness of central commands directed at INs in the chain. Thus, all INs do their segmental work in coordination with su-

praspinal commands. It is likely that studies of intact animals will reveal the roles of all spinal INs to be wider than is presently realized.

Supraspinal motor control is directed toward two major goals. The first deals with keeping the body in an erect posture, integrating body and head movements, and the direction of locomotion. This postural goal is achieved by the reticulospinal and vestibulospinal tracts (group **A**) originating in the brain stem, which promote segmental reflex activity that opposes gravity. These tracts activate synergistic muscles of the neck, back, eyes, ears and proximal limbs. The second goal deals with the capacity for independent, flexion-biased movements of the extremities and shoulders. The rubrospinal tract (group **B**) provides these mostly for the elbow and hand, while the corticospinal tract is particularly responsible for independent finger movements. These two tracts promote voluntary movements, and liberate muscles and joints from postural roles imposed by gravity. These functions are assisted by some group **A** tracts. The lateral reticulospinal tract receives projections from motor cortex and the lateral cerebellum. Locomotion is facilitated by the dorsolateral reticulospinal tract and by two monoaminergic reticulospinal paths. The corticospinal tract is the only descending control tract that descends without interruption from the cerebral cortex (and hence it is additional to groups **A** and **B**). It coordinates finger and hand–arm movements and is essential for the fine control of independent finger movements.

Supraspinal control includes, as part of the motor programs, descending effects on afferent, ascending inputs. There are differential mechanisms for governing kinesthetic and somatosensory information as opposed to the central control of pain. Controls descending to the spinal cord can alter sensory as well as motor patterns. Motor systems govern their own sensory inputs to avoid the sensory consequences of intended movements that might interfere with their execution. The pyramidal tract, for example, alters ascending information flow in the medial lemniscal system, while the rubrospinal and vestibulospinal tracts mostly influence spinal cord tract cells. Pain can be suppressed by a midbrain reticular system, mediated by the serotonergic outflow from the raphe nuclei to inhibit spinothalamic neurons.

References

Alexander, R. McN. 1981. Mechanics of skeleton and tendons. In *Motor control*. Sect. 1, Vol. 2. *Handbook of physiology*, ed. V. B. Brooks, pp. 17–42. Bethesda, Md.: American Physiological Society. [Fig. 5.3]

Alstermark, B., Eide, E., Lundberg, A., Gorska, T., Lundberg, A., and Petterson, L.-G. 1984. Visually guided switching of forelimb target reaching in cats. *Acta Physiol. Scand.* 120:151–153.

Baldissera, F., Hultborn, H., and Illert, M., 1981. Integration in spinal neuronal systems. In *Motor control*. Sect.1, Vol. 2. *Handbook of physiology*, ed. V. B. Brooks, pp. 509–595. Bethesda, Md.: American Physiological Society. [Figs. 5.4 and 5.5]

Barr, M. L., and Kiernan, J. A. 1983. *The human nervous system*. 4th ed. Philadelphia: Harper & Row. [Figs. 5.7, 5.8, 5.11 and 5.12]

Brooks, V. B. 1984. The cerebellum and adaptive tuning of movements. In *Motor integration in the nervous system*, eds. O. Creutzfeldt, R. F. Schmidt, and W. D. Willis. *Exp. Brain Res.* Suppl. 7, pp. 170–183.

Brooks, V. B. 1959. Contrast and stability in the nervous system, *Trans. N.Y. Acad. Sci.* 21:387–394.

Brooks, V.B. 1983. Study of brain function by local, reversible cooling. *Rev. Physiol. Biochem. Pharmacol.* 95:1–109. [Fig. 5.15]

Cervero, F., Iggo, A., and Moloney, V. 1977. Responses of spinocervical tract neurones to noxious stimulation of the skin. *J. Physiol. (Lond.)* 267:537–558. [Fig. 5.15]

Denny-Brown, D. 1966. *The cerebral control of movement* (The Sherrington Lectures VIII). Springfield, Ill.: Charles C Thomas.

Denny-Brown, D. 1960. Motor mechanisms—introduction: the general principles of motor integration. In *Neurophysiology*. Sect. 1, vol. 2. *Handbook of physiology*, ed. H. W. Magoun, pp. 781–796. Washington, D.C.: American Physiological Society.

Eccles, J. C. 1969. The dynamic loop hypothesis of movement control. In *Information processing in the nervous system* ed. K. N. Leibovic pp. 245–268. Heidelberg: Springer.

Houk, J. C. 1974. Feedback control of muscle: a synthesis of the peripheral mechanisms. In *Medical Physiology*, ed. V. B. Mountcastle. 13th ed. St. Louis: Mosby. [Fig. 5.1]

Houk, J. C., and Rymer, W. Z. 1981. Neural control of muscle length and tension. In *Motor control* Sect. 1, vol. 2. *Handbood of physiology*, ed. V. B. Brooks, pp. 257–323. Bethesda, Md.: American Physiological Society.

Hultborn, H. M., Illert, M., and Santini, M. 1976. Convergence on interneurones mediating the reciprocal Ia inhibition of motoneurones. I. Disynaptic Ia inhibition of Ia inhibitory interneurones. *Acta Physiol. Scand.* 96:193–201. [Fig. 5.2B]

Hultborn, H. M., Lindstrom, S., and Wigstrom, H. 1979. On the function of recurrent inhibition in the spinal cord. *Exp. Brain Res.* 37:399–403. [Fig. 5.4]

Humphrey, D. R. 1983. Corticospinal systems and their control by premotor cortex, basal ganglia and cerebellum. In *The clinical neurosciences*. vol. 5. *Neurobiology*, eds. W. D. Willis, Jr. and R. N. Rosenberg, pp. 547–587. New York: Churchill Livingstone. [Figs. 5.9 and 5.10]

Humphrey, D. R. 1979. On the cortical control of visually directed reaching: contributions by nonprecentral areas. In *Posture and movement*, eds. R. E. Talbot and D. R. Humphrey, pp. 51–112. New York: Raven Press. [Figs. 5.9]

Jeneskog, T., and Johansson, H. 1977. The rubrospinal path. A descending system known to influence dynamic fusimotor neurones and its interaction with distal cutaneous afferents in the control of flexor reflex afferent pathways. *Exp. Brain Res.* 27:161–179. [Fig. 5.6B]

Krnjevic, K. 1981. Transmitters in motor systems. In *Motor control*. Sect. 1, vol. 2. *Handbook of physiology*, ed. V. B. Brooks, pp. 107–154. Bethesda, Md.: American Physiological Society.

Kuypers, H. G. J. M. 1981. Anatomy of the descending pathways. In *Motor control*. Sect. 1, vol. 2. *Handbood of physiology*, ed. V. B. Brooks, pp. 597–666. Bethesda, Md.: American Physiological Society. [Fig. 5.7]

Magoun, H. W. 1950. Caudal and cephalic

influences of brain stem reticular formation. *Physiol. Rev.* 30:459–474.

Matthews, P. B. C. 1981. Proprioceptors and the regulation of movement. In *Motor coordination*. Vol. 5. *Handbook of behavioral neurobiology*, eds. A. L. Towe and E. S. Luschei, pp. 93–137. New York: Plenum Press. [Fig. 5.2A]

Oscarsson, O. 1973. Functional organization of spinocerebellar paths. In *Somatosensory system*. Vol. 2. *Handbook of sensory physiology*, ed. A. Iggo, pp. 339–380. Berlin: Springer, Verlag. [Fig. 5.6A]

Phillips, C. G. 1969. Motor apparatus of the baboon's hand. The Ferrier Lecture. *Proc. R. Soc. Lond. (Biol.)* 173:141–174.

Phillips, C. G. and Porter, R. 1964. The pyramidal projection to motoneurones of some muscle groups in the baboon's forelimb. In *Physiology of spinal neurones*, eds. J. C. Eccles and J. P. Schade. *Prog. Brain Res.* 12:222–242. [Fig. 5.13B]

Pierrot-Deseilligny, E., Katz, R., and Hultborn, H., 1983. Functional organization of recurrent inhibition in man: changes preceding and accompanying voluntary movements. In *Motor control mechanisms in health and disease*, ed. J. E. Desmedt. *Adv. Neurol.* 39:443–457.

Proske, U. 1981. The Golgi tendon organ: properties of the receptor and reflex actions of impulses arising from tendon organs. In *Neurophysiology IV*, ed. R. Porter. *Int. Rev. Physiol.* 25:127–171.

Sasaki, K., and Gemba, H. 1984. Compensatory motor function of the somatosensory cortex for dysfunction of the motor cortex following cerebellar hemispherectomy in the monkey. *Exp. Brain Res.* 56:532–538.

Schwindt, P. C. 1981. Control of motoneuron output by pathways descending from the brainstem. In *Motor coordination*. vol. 5. *Handbook of behavioral neurobiology*, eds. A. L. Towe and E. S. Luschei, pp. 139–230. New York: Plenum Press. [Figs. 5.2B and 5.6B]

Shinoda, Y. 1978. Intraspinal mutliple projections of single corticospinal neurons in the cat and monkey. In *Integrative control functions of the brain*, eds. M. Ito, N. Tsukahara, K, Kubota, and K. Yagi, vol. 1, pp. 137–151, New York: Elsevier/North-Holland.

Shinoda, Y. 1981. Divergent projection of individual corticospinal axons to motoneurons of multiple muscles in the monkey. *Neurosci. Lett.* 23:7-12. [Fig. 5.13A]

Sjolund, B. H., and Bjorklund, A., eds. 1983. *Brainstem control of spinal mechanisns*. Amsterdam: Elsevier Biomedical.

Smith, O. A. Jr., Nathan, M. A., and Clarke, N. P. 1976. Central nervous system pathways mediating blood pressure changes. In *Hypertension*, ed. J. E. Wood, vol. 16, pp. 9–22. New York: American Heart Association.

Tanaka, R. 1983. Reciprocal Ia inhibitory pathways in normal man and in patients with motor disorders. In *Motor control mechanisms in health and disease*, ed. J. E. Desmedt. *Adv. Neurol* 39:433–441.

Wall, P. D. 1967. The laminar organization of dorsal horn and effects of descending impulses. *J. Physiol. (Lond.)* 188:403–423. [Fig. 5.14]

Wiesendanger, M. 1984. Pyramidal tract function and the clinical "pyramidal sydrome." *Hum. Neurobiol.* 2:227–234.

Willis, W. D. 1979. Supraspinal control of ascending pathways. In *Reflex control of posture and movement*, eds. R. Granit and O. Pompeiano. *Prog. Brain Res.* 50:163–174.

Willis, W. D., and Coggeshall, R. E. 1978. *Sensory mechanisms of the spinal cord*. New York: Plenum Press. [Fig. 5.15]

Wilson, V. J., and Peterson, B. W. 1981. Vestibulospinal and reticulospinal systems. In *Motor control*. Sect. 1. vol. 2. *Handbook of physiology*, ed. V. B. Brooks, pp. 667–702. Bethesda, Md.: American Physiological Society.

Young, J. Z., and Hobbs, M. J. 1975. *The life of mammals: their anatomy and physiology*. 2nd ed. Oxford: Clarendon Press. [Fig. 5.3]

6
Motor Set

When we "get set" to carry out a planned motor task, we rely on our past experience and act according ot our present mood and attention to the task. The term "motor set" indicates that the CNS is ready to carry out a planned motor action, that preparations have been made to implement the intention. Procedures have been started to make the motor plan become reality by putting the various programs and many subprograms into place, ready to enable them upon command. It resembles the countdown toward a rocket launch: a hierarchical command sequence is followed step by step while making sure that all systems are operational, those already engaged and those to be engaged later. Motor set implies that (1) high-level planning is conveyed to the middle level of the motor hierarchy where the framework of the external world is transformed into coordinates of the internal world; and (2) middle-level programs are transformed into subprograms of the lowest level, specifying muscular actions.

This chapter examines two major aspects of motor set, beginning with a brief survey of the timetable of brain activation to define the cadence of preparation for a voluntary motor act. The second aspect is how the middle level of the motor hierarchy controls the lowest level; one important means identified is called "long-loop

actions" between the cerebrum and the spinal cord. Here we stress their function during ongoing movements, while Chap. 7 concentrates on their use in beginning movements. Students might well be surprised at how quickly our investigation reaches the limits of current knowledge in motor control and will take note of the intense ongoing search for unifying concepts.

Motor set for motor execution is created only with the integrated guidance of experience, mood and attention. What are the neural task systems for these psychological entities? We learned in the introductory survey (Chap. 2.1) that memory traces of past experience are stored in a distributed manner in the brain, rather than being confined to any one location. Yet, moving them into and out of storage requires the activity of the hippocampus and temporal lobe, structures that are part of, or closely linked to, the limbic system. Limbic functions are also essential for the formation of mood and attention, which depend as well as on the reticular (ascending) arousal system and high-order association areas of the cerebral cortex (Figs. 2.2–2.5 and 2.7). Getting set for motor action thus involves many successive translations between different parts of the brain. Instructions for components of motor plans are passed between association areas and are converted into premotor commands for the middle level where, after further internal interactions, they become specifications for spinal implementation. This was portrayed earlier in the cartoon of Fig. 2.4, which indicates that the neural task systems for these integrations are huge and all-embracing. The systems can perform their functions only if all components are ready to do their part; high-level plans, middle-level programs and their many subprograms, and the routines of the lowest level. To cite once more a familiar example, postural supports have to be coordinated early to steady the body, head and limbs for the expected movements. Throughout the "countdown to launch," external and internal ("corollary") feedback ensures that all the functions enumerated above proceed correctly and in a manner appropriate to the circumstances of the moment. Ongoing feedback makes it possible to amend commands, which is a ubiquitous occurrence. Once more we should remind ourselves that none of the parts of the brain "comprehend" the overall meaning of the purposeful messages handled by them. Comprehension is the product of the entire nervous system, the result of many actions occurring in many places: it is a distributed property.

1. Timetable

To start a voluntary motor act, we get ready and get set to go in just under 1 second. The first general process of getting ready is reflected in a "readiness potential" that can be recorded from the scalp over anterior parietal and precentral cerebral cortex on either side of normal human subjects. Figure 6.1 shows that it begins 0.8 second before onset of EMG activity for self-initiated finger movements. The potential probably originates from the premotor association area of the cerebral cortex (Fig. 2.1A)—more precisely, the medially located supplemental motor area (SMA, Chap. 11.1). This is suggested by in-

creased regional blood flow in the SMA earlier than that in other areas before an *imagined* sequence of finger movements. The potential is also generated by activity in other closely linked areas, such as the parietal sensory association area and the precentral and postcentral motor and sensory areas (Fig. 2.1A). The frontal lobes (prefrontal cortex) are also involved if the movements are made in response to a known warning signal, rather than being entirely self-initiated. (With prefrontal involvement, the potential is called the "contingent negative variation"—CNV—not illustrated). The negative-going readiness potential is succeeded by a premotor positivity originating from the active precentral motor cortex when it begins to issue motor commands about 0.1 second before muscle action (Fig. 6.1).

The preparatory timing sequence measured by scalp potentials has been confirmed by recording the discharge of neurons in these cortical areas of monkeys in equivalent behavioral situations. Instructions to get ready for a motor act trigger a certain class of neurons in prefrontal cortex. Within 0.3 second, tonic activity in motor cortex contralateral to the operant limb changes from previous unattentive, uninstructed levels to a level that is preparatory for action. This state can be maintained for seconds or minutes if necessary, until the subject receives the final signal for action. Neural activity in other connected structures now begins to increase by stages. The supplementary motor area (as we noted before) comes to life well before movement onset, about several hundred milliseconds for task-related neural firing changes. Certain groups of neurons in the lateral premotor cortex change together with those in the two assisting circuits to which they are connected: the putamen circuit of the basal ganglia (whose output is through the globus pallidus or "pallidum"), and the lateral cerebellum (whose output is the dentate nucleus). The thalamic nuclei linking these circuits to the cerebral cortex also contain

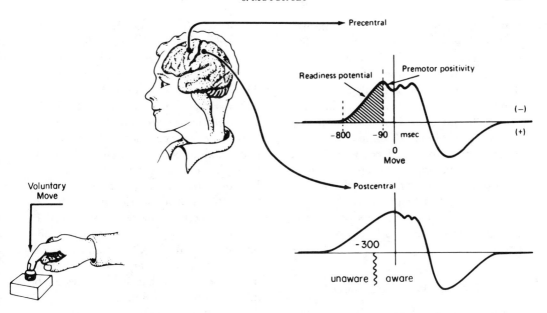

Fig. 6.1. Human premotor potentials, recorded from the scalp over the sensorimotor cortex, begin about 0.8 second before a voluntary movement. Conscious awareness of having wished to initiate movement, however, begins about 0.5 second after onset of potentials, that is, about 0.3 second before movement (EMG) onset. (Modified from Deecke and Kornhuber, 1971; in Ghez, 1981; with addition after Libet et al., 1983, and McCloskey et al., 1983)

neurons whose activity changes shortly before that of the motor cortex. This precentral output stage of the middle level projects its calls for action to the spinal cord, about 0.1 second prior to EMG onset. During the time of cortical and subcortical activity prior to motor cortex involvement, the stiffness of joints is adjusted from maintaining premovement postures to those appropriate for the impending movement (premovement "tuning," Fig. 1.3 and Chaps. 2.2 and 5.2). Finally, after the adjustment of tonic levels, phasic cortical movement commands activate phasic muscular changes.

Figure 6.1 directs us to yet another aspect of "getting set"; it also indicates the timing of our attention and awareness of what we are doing. What happens in the brain when we are "paying attention"? It is an altered state, made evident by widespread desynchronization of the alpha rhythm of the electroencephalogram (the 8- to 12-Hz component of the EEG). These

signs indicate the opening of thalamic gates from the prefrontal association cortex to the sensorimotor cortex. The alerting stimulus is screened for its meaning, and if it is perceived as significant for the impending motor action, it evokes especially large potentials over the frontal cortex.

Finally, there is a surprise hidden in the apparently routine analysis of self-initiated movements when we want to get started on a motor act, such a ringing someone's doorbell as in Fig. 6.1 (without outside "alert" and "go" signals). We make the wish to move and indeed start the brain working on it, as witnessed by the readiness potential, but, surprisingly, we are not conscious of having made the wish (i.e., the "decision," having given an internal "command") until about 0.5 second later! This approximate timing, indicated in Fig. 6.1 by a wavy line, has been confirmed in several ways. For instance, subjects can compare the time when they consciously realize that they have made the (internal) wish to begin with some external reference signal, such as a mild touch on the skin given by the observer, or some visual display. The subjects have only to compare which occurred first; the actual timing is done by the observer. The wavy line in Fig. 6.1 reveals that internal commands for voluntary action are perceived within about 0.3 second before EMG onset, that is, mostly during the time that the middle level of the motor hierarchy is active. We have no conscious awareness of the preceding work of the high-level association cortex.

2. Long-Loop Responses

In previous chapters we have touched several times on the interactions of volitional acts and reflexes. Since supraspinal participation in both types of actions is inevitable, we realize that the two processes are always blended to varying degrees. The routes for interaction between the middle level of the hierarchy and the spinal cord were taken up in Chaps. 5.1 and 5.2. Now, we can refocus our enquiry on the *relative* importance of spinal and supraspinal contributions. Long-loop responses to perturbations of a limb during intended motor acts serve a significant purpose: they restore the limb to the intended state as originally decreed by commands from the middle level; that is, they implement motor set. Long loops connect that level to deal with muscle stretches imposed by the environment that are beyond the range of control of the spinal motor servo (Chaps. 3.2 and 4.2).

Long-loop responses can be recognized by their latencies, because it takes longer for nerve impulses to traverse a long loop than a short, spinal one. A typical test setup is illustrated in Fig. 6.3A. When a subject maintains an intended limb posture and that limb is perturbed (pushed or pulled), stretched muscles react with a spinal stretch reflex of short latency and an amplitude that depends on the subject's

motor set. If the subject had been instructed to resist the perturbation, the stretch reflex is larger than if the instruction had been to yield (i.e., not to resist). The initial spinal reflex is followed by a voluntary movement according to the instruction, but in the time between them, long-loop "reflexes" occur that are under considerable voluntary control. The voluntary component is larger for those with later onset times. Thus, there is a gradation without sharp boundaries from reflex to voluntary action. The best way to think of a reflex is as a tightly coupled input–output relation in the CNS that can occur without conscious participation. Yet we need to remember that such reflexes can be influenced by motor set.

The time ranges for the successive muscular responses, named M1, M2 and M3 by Tatton and Lee, are illustrated in Fig.6.2A. M1, the spinal stretch reflex, begins 25–35 msec after a wrist perturbation and peaks before 50 msec. M2 (the medium-latency response, hatched for identification) begins after 50 msec and peaks before 80 msec, followed by and sometimes commingled with M3 (the long-latency response), which begins near 85 msec and peaks before 100 msec. Activity thereafter is called "intended" or "voluntary" (Vol. in Fig. 6.2A). The EMG records have been processed for clarity. "Raw" records, as in Figs. 6.5, 6.7 and 6.8, are averaged after their positive- and negative-going phases have been "rectified," that is, made to deflect all in the same direction. The distinctions between M2 and M3 are not always as clear as in Fig. 6.2, nor are those between M3 and the following voluntary activity. The latencies of long-loop responses depend on the length of the conduction pathway, being longer for the legs than for the hands. (Compare the approximate M2 latencies for the thumb: 40 msec in Fig. 6.9, 60 msec for the wrist in Fig. 6.2, 80 msec for the elbow in Fig. 6.7, and 100 msec for the leg in Figs. 6.5 and 6.8.)

These latencies of responses to limb perturbations delay the mechanical limb reactions sufficiently to make them useless for corrective ("servo") feedback. They would always arrive too late and would thus make the limb oscillate instead of steadying it. Since such oscillations do not occur normally, long-loop responses are probably feedforward, instead of feedback, controllers, which is suggested by their cortical connections anyway. Segmental afferent inputs do participate in their generation, however, because M2–M3 bursts occur *only* if perturbations displace a joint long enough to give peripheral information time to reach the spinal cord for interaction. The CNS can then calculate ahead to provide long-loop responses. (In Fig. 6.2 the perturbations had to last for at least 40 msec leaving 15 msec of neural "calculation" time until the appearance of the M2 response at 55 msec.)

The most outstanding properties of long-loop responses are their susceptibility to prior instructions given to the subject, and their task-related adaptiveness (which occurs unconsciously). Instructions have more influence on M3 and later components than on M2. [Extra force is provided when called for: in fact, the gain (output/input) can increase 10-fold for what appears to be the voluntary component according to its timing. Adaptive gain changes of this magnitude are brought about most likely by supraspinal effects on alpha MNs; Fig. 4.11.] Prior instructions have different impact on early, middle and late stretch responses because the later responses are more accessible to supraspinal influences. M1 is a tightly coupled, segmental stretch reflex, while M2 is less dependent on segmental connections, and M3 least.

How are we to distinguish the relative contributions made to their generation by spinal and supraspinal control, discussed in the previous two chapters? Melvill Jones, and Houk have both pointed out some indicators by which to distinguish reflex "servo" actions (using negative feedback), which are generated by the spinal motor servo drawn in Fig. 5.1, from "vol-

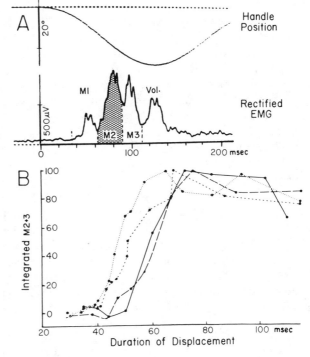

Fig. 6.2. Successive muscular responses of a normal subject who resists a perturbation from an intended posture. (A) Average of 20 rectified EMGs from wrist extensor following sudden flexor displacement of the wrist (*hatched area, M2*). Downward deflection of *upper trace* represents wrist flexion by torque, which starts at *vertical line.* (B) Long-loop components occur only when perturbations create displacements of at least 40–50 msec duration, as in (A). Normalized, integrated averages of 20 EMGs of M2 + M3 from four normal subjects. There was no change of M1. [(A) From Tatton and Lee, 1975, in Houk and Rymer, 1981; (B) from Lee, Murphy and Tatton, 1983]

untary" actions. Latencies of muscular responses are poor criteria because they depend on the nature and strength of the signal as well as on the experience and attention of the subject. A better way is to compare the shapes and directions of responses to perturbations in either direction when the subject has been given different instructions, such as to resist (i.e., to "compensate") in contrast to not intervene (i.e., to "yield"). Reflex (servo) responses, made without conscious intent to resist, have springlike properties and magnitudes that vary in proportion to the perturbations that they oppose (Fig. 6.3B,C). Servo responses thus can vary in *amplitude* but not in direction. Errors in *direction* do occur, however, with voluntary movements (Fig. 6.3C).

Long-loop responses change in a task-related manner. This may come from explicit instructions to a subject, as in Fig. 6.3, or from unconscious adjustments made in response to changing environmental conditions. For example, most people preserve their postural body balance on shifting surfaces by long-loop responses in their leg muscles. Figure 6.4A and B demonstrates how the motor hierarchy adjusts the posture of the individual by changing responses of synergic groups of leg muscles according to prevailing circumstances. Muscle tensions change in relation to each other in useful *patterns* (Fig. 6.4A: ratios of active muscles). These ratios are preserved when making small or large movements; that is, there is an overall scaling that is probably carried out by the basal ganglia (Chap. 2.2). Another important change appears in Fig. 6.4B: the *adaptation* of response amplitudes in just a few successive trials, according to their postural usefulness.

The observations by Nashner show that responses of particular muscles are enhanced when they are useful and are diminished when they are counterproductive. Those of gastrocnemius, for instance, remain about the same during forward sway (Fig. 6.4A), but fade during backward sway (Fig. 6.4B) from high to low levels in successive trials. Thus, the motor hierarchy implements the intent of the subject by changing long-loop responses according to the needs of the moment. When these needs are met, the reaction to induced sway is based on the *expectation* of now-known circumstances, and muscle actions differ little from those used in the equivalent *intentional* motor act. Leaning forward is accomplished by programming the activation of wanted muscle synergies and suppression of unwanted participants (e.g., gastrocnemius). The cerebellar deficits depicted in the right column (Fig. 6.4C,D) will be taken up, together with those in Fig. 6.9, in Chap. 13.

Long-loop and voluntary movements are the products of motor programs that are "triggered" by the middle level of the hierarchy. They are also called *reaction-time movements*, because their latencies can vary greatly in comparision to those of servo responses. This is illustrated in Fig. 6.5, where the records on the left represent muscle responses that were evoked from gastrocnemius by sudden and sustained dorsiflexion of the foot. The records on the right, in contrast, were obtained from the same muscle, but are of a voluntary contraction made upon a signal that consisted of application of a similar force to the heel, but without dorsiflexing the ankle and hence avoiding stretch of the gastrocnemius. The latencies of the resulting "voluntary" responses were longer and more varied than those of the "functional stretch" reflexes or responses, as the medium-latency muscle bursts were named by Melvill Jones. Latencies become particularly variable if there is uncertainty about the direction of an impending perturbation, but they shorten with experience if there is no uncertainty. By these criteria, intended actions begin as early as 70 msec (or even less) after a perturbation; that is, they include M2 and M3, reflecting the voluntary components in their makeup. This mix of tightly coupled reactions with those looping through "volition" makes

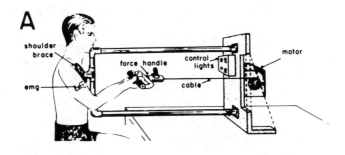

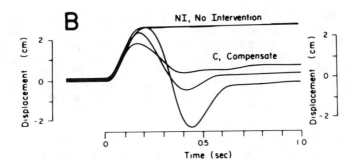

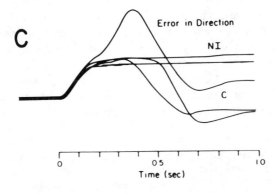

Fig. 6.3. Directional errors occur only with intended (reaction-time) movements. (A) Arrangement in which subjects react according to instructions, given by control lights, to changes of loads on the handle imposed by a motor. (B,C) Position traces (displacement) of two different subjects responding to load changes (at time 0) when instructed to resist (compensate) or to yield (no intervention). Attempts to compensate can cause an error in direction (C). [From Crago, Houk and Hasan, 1976; (A) in Houk, 1978; (B,C) in Houk and Rymer, 1981]

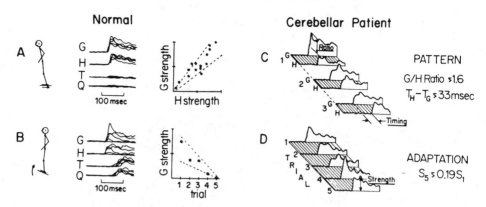

Fig. 6.4. Stabilization of human stance requires cerebellar guidance. (A,B) Figurines indicate normal stabilization by means of (long-loop) functional stretch responses in leg muscles when subjects sway forward in response to backward movement (A) or upward tilt (B) of platform on which they stand. (C,D) Cerebellar deficit occurs as functional stretch responses of muscles are activated neither in functional *pattern (upper row)*, nor in *adapting* sequence *(lower row)*. EMGs are from gastrocnemius (G), hamstrings (H), tibialis anterior (T) and quadriceps (Q). At *right,* minimum criteria for classifying response as abnormal. (From Nashner and Grimm, 1978; also in Brooks, 1985)

the term long-loop "responses" preferable to "reflexes." The terms indicate differences in the *degree* of tight, seemingly automatic, input–output coupling. There is no longer an all-or-none distinction between reflexes and voluntary actions.

What are the functions of the long-loop responses? We recognize them now as largely "triggered reactions" with at least two relations to motor tasks. The most important may be that their phasic actions help match appropriate movement veloci-

ties to the intended path; that is, they adjust movement "trajectories." After perturbations, for instance, they restore the programmed relation between velocity and movement path ("trajectory compensation"). Chapter 7.1 will show that this function of long loops in largely isotonic movements is only a particular application of a more general function, which is to impress the program for phasic change of a controlled variable in relation to the background level of that variable. Figure 7.5

Fig. 6.5. Intended movements have longer and more variable latencies than those of long-loop responses. EMGs from gastrocnemius of a normal subject. *(Left)* Long-loop responses (functional stretch reflex) to sudden dorsiflexion of the foot evoking gastrocnemius stretch; *(right)* intended (voluntary) responses to a signal consisting of a jolt that is of same force but does not stretch gastrocnemius. (Chan, Melvill Jones and Catchglove, 1979)

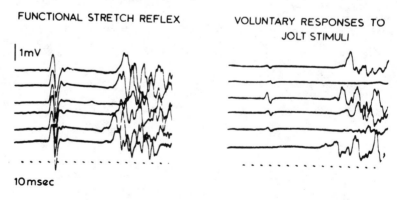

shows that the same rules apply to changes of force in isometric movements as apply here to changes of velocity in isotonic movements. Both are based on the programming by the middle hierarchical level of the spinal cord, which already operates this kind of relation by virtue of Henneman's size principle of spinal recruitment (cf. Chap. 4.1).

Long-loop responses are phasic; that is, they are synchronized muscular contractions, for phasic aspects of movements: acceleration and velocity. Their participation in restoring appropriate movement speeds to intended displacements was first recognized by Cooke and is illustrated for human elbow movements in Fig. 6.6. Unperturbed flexions and EMGs are shown on the left and their perturbed counterparts on the right. (The spinal M1 component is missing in this instance because the perturbation rose too slowly to evoke it.) The lowermost, convex traces plot the trajectory (i.e., the path and its rate of change); with velocity plotted along the ordinate and limb position along the abscissa (as a "phase-plane" plot, rather than against time, as in the traces above). Excellent trajectory compensation is demonstrated by the match of the normal and perturbed plots on the bottom right. Trajectory compensation and bracing the limb for assumption of another posture (a form of load compensation) are parts of the same planning process to match move and hold programs introduced in Chap. 1.2 (Fig. 1.5). We have used the analogy of controlled rocket flight before. Here it evokes the image of an automatic, corrective "burn" in order to fly at the right speed at a particular stage of the journey. This is necessary because the physical properties of the craft and its environment form part of the basis of the flight plan (or program).

Long-loop responses of opposing muscles help to stabilize the limb not only *after* unexpected perturbations (as in Figs. 6.3–6.6), but also for intended resistance to *expected* perturbations. Figure 6.7 illustrates an instance where a subject resists a persisting perturbation, whose progress

Fig. 6.6. Long-loop responses assist in "trajectory compensation" of a limb when subjects resist perturbations of an intended movement, made as rapidly as possible. Records of 20 averaged *normal* and *perturbed* elbow flexions made by a normal subject. Position traces are enclosed by standard deviations *(dots)*. Movement onset at *filled triangles,* perturbation at vertical *broken line* (which is also shown for reference in the normal record on the left). Trajectory compensation is indicated by *arrows* in position, velocity, and trajectory traces. Rectified EMGs of biceps and triceps. Trajectory records are averaged ("phase-plane") plots of velocity against limb position. (Calibrations are 30 deg, 50 deg/second, and also apply to position and velocity traces.) (From Cooke, 1980; also in Brooks, 1985)

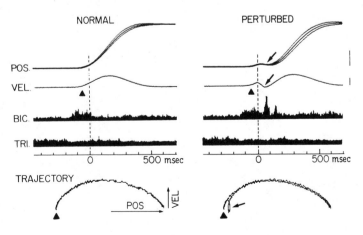

can therefore be calculated ahead by the brain. The order to "resist" calls forth a muscular response that is an appropriately timed "load compensation" bracing the limb, and is equivalent to providing a postural base for the next intended posture or movement. (If a movement follows, then load compensation is a part of trajectory compensation, as in Fig. 6.6.) Muscular co-contraction stiffens the joint before the (medium-latency, M2) long-loop response. This stiffening is illustrated in Fig. 6.7 by the stippled area. The instruction "Resist" sets the agonist phasic medium-latency EMG component (M2 of triceps brachii, not illustrated) and generates co-contrac-

Fig. 6.7. Long-loop responses precede "load compensation" of the arm when subjects resist a persisting perturbation of an intended posture. The traces in the upper part of the figure indicate rising ramp torque, starting at the *vertical broken line* at time 0, which alters intended angular displacement *(solid trace)* of the elbow. Agonist EMG medium-latency component (M2, starting at *vertical arrow*) helps to stabilize limb stiffness, which is plotted in the lower part of the figure. Stabilization precedes intended correction of perturbation in order to resist *(solid line)*. When subject yields, there is neither EMG medium-latency component nor stiffness stabilization *(broken line at bottom of dotted area)*. (From Kwan, Murphy and Repeck, 1979; in Lee, Murphy and Tatton, 1983; also in Brooks, 1985)

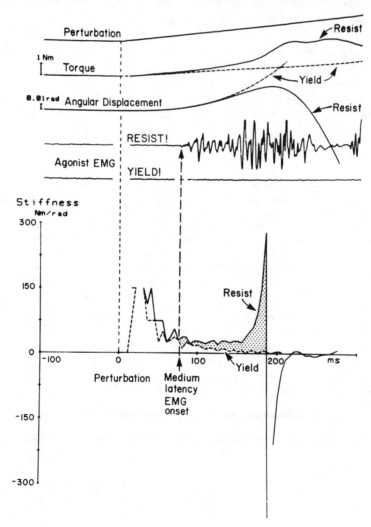

tion to maintain a steady elbow stiffness (solid trace). This contrasts with the decay of muscle stiffness when the subject has been instructed to "Yield" (broken trace at the bottom of the dotted area). Long-loop responses stabilize limbs also because they are dispersed over some time, rather than synchronous like a spinal stretch reflex to a sudden perturbation (shown in Fig. 6.8). This asynchronous application of muscular force acts as a damper against oscillations (clonus) that could follow perturbations. It seems reasonable to assume that the stiffening action operated through long-loop paths applies as much to the *tonic* maintenance of intended postures as to their *phasic* corrections. The paths of long loops are presumably also available for relaying the responses to internal commands, rather than only those to external perturbations. Thus, long-loop paths may be functional components in the control and regulation of normal postures and movements.

Long-loop responses are a highly visible form of postural adjustment that are usually triggered by muscle stretches lasting longer than 40–50 msec (Fig. 6.1B). This minimal duration presumably arises from the time needed to integrate peripheral and supraspinal signals. Building upon the steady stiffness plateau (the horizontal stippled area in Fig. 6.7), the medium-latency M2 EMG component precedes the generation of a large stiffness increase that contributes to the effective opposition against the imposed ramp displacement (a persistently rising perturbation). Large changes of stiffness are likely caused by supraspinal, voluntary efforts, rather than by adaptive gain changes (Chap. 4.2).

The idea that long loops restore the trajectory against external perturbatons fits with the original suggestion by Melvill Jones that these largely programmed "functional stretch responses" help to maintain normal, intended movements and postures. In natural circumstances the brain often "knows" when a limb is expected to encounter a resistance. In Fig.

1.1, for instance, the arm is braced before the end of the golfer's swing for the impact of the club on the ball, just as it is for the ramp displacement of the horizontal elbow movement in Fig. 6.7. Long-loop (functional stretch) responses are the first predictively generated force for damped landings when a person is falling or stepping. In these instances, signals about changes of gravity from the otoliths in the vestibular system are part of the response trigger mechanism (Chap. 9). This will be considered also for stopping of head and limb movements in Chap. 9.2 and for locomotion in Chap. 10. The reader will have realized by now from the many considerations about programs that bracing at an expected time is a prerequisite for matching subprograms for limb movements and for limb postures. Each is the end of one and the beginning of another. The smoothness of their transition reflects how well move and hold subprograms are fused into overall programs for movements with continuous velocity profiles (Figs. 1.3 and 1.5).

Trajectory control may be most significant as a means to make *patterned* movements by fitting simple paths into compound movements. This typically human activity demands scaling of abstract patterns in time or space (to be taken up in the next chapter). While patterns may be the product of the brain's highest level, scaling is done by the middle level of the motor hierarchy. Trajectory control simplifies the scaling process by combining direction, rate, and range of movements into one functional entity: the relation of the directional path to its rate of change. As pointed out above, the same arguments apply to any program for patterned application of force, no matter what displacement of the limb occurs as a result. Scaling of handwriting patterns are considered in relation to Figs. 7.1 and 7.2, and scaling of walking patterns in relation to Figs. 10.2 and 10.3.

Long-loop responses require intact connections between the sensorimotor cortex and the spinal segmental apparatus (i.e., the "motor servo"). Figure 6.8A contrasts electromyographic responses to sudden and maintained stretch of a normal human subject and a patient with spastic paraplegia. Their responses are similar when tested for their arms (biceps, above the spinal lesion), but very different for their legs (gastrocnemius, below the lesion). The spinal cord below the lesion cannot generate functional stretch responses, but there is an indication of the beginning of a prolonged spinal response. Figure 6.8B shows that the missing supraspinal structure is in the cerebral hemisphere, because late responses are absent in the arm and leg on the affected side of a hemiplegic patient, while they are normal on the unaffected side.

Further evidence for involvement of the sensorimotor cortex in human long-loop responses is provided by their absence in patients with lesions in the dorsal columns, disconnecting the sensorimotor cortex. Such a case is illustrated in the upper part of Fig. 6.9, showing loss of the medium- and long-latency responses on the affected side. Stretch of the long thumb flexors was followed only by the spinal (M1) reflex in this patient who had a unilateral lesion in the brain stem, leading to sensory losses but no apparent motor deficits. Marsden commented that "this evidence is consistent with the hypothesis that the long-latency stretch reflex [on which servo responses are based] uses a supraspinal, possibly a transcortical, reflex arc...." Neurons in the sensorimotor cortex (of monkeys) have indeed been shown to participate in a transcortical loop that facilitates M2 muscular responses to stretch. Precentral signals for generation of M3 and voluntary contractions begin later, well after the cortical arrival of sensory stretch information (Fig. 12.11, later).

The motor cortex influences the final common path under the guidance of the cerebellum, whose dysfunction therefore also depresses long-loop responses. The lower part of Fig. 6.9 shows loss of the me-

dium-latency response after cerebellar disconnection, on the affected side. (The patient, who suffered from a unilateral acoustic neuroma, had ataxia on that side without other motor or sensory deficits.) Stretch of the long thumb flexors caused the appearance of another response 40–50 msec later (i.e., at about 80 msec). This later response is not linked as strongly to the stimulus as the earlier, lost one (see Fig. 6.4 for loss of posture-related patterns and adaptation of long-loop responses of leg muscles). Figures 6.8 and 6.9 indicate that motor set is implemented through the middle level, particularly the cerebellocerebral circuit. Cortical and cerebellar contributions to posture and motion will be considered further in Chaps. 11–13.

3. Regulation and Control

We have learned in this chapter that long-loop responses are a means whereby the motor cortex helps to specify the actions necessary to maintain intended trajectories, that is, the direction and speed of intended movements (an idea introduced in Chap. 2.3) as well as intended postures. How are the supraspinal commands actually impressed upon the muscles? The answer involves their length–tension curves (whose spinal adjustments were introduced in Chap. 3.2). The spinal motor servo can regulate the stretch reflex sufficiently well to adjust muscle lengths to perturbations caused by self-generated muscular changes, but not by imposed, external perturbations. Small muscular changes shift the equilibrium points of muscles along particular length–tension curves without change of stiffness (e.g., as in Fig. 3.4, when the antagonist shifts from the filled square to the open circle). *Regulation* means preservation of a property near a constant value, while *control* means adjustment or variation of that property. Distinguishing the meaning of these terms is a helpful tool that is not used, however, by all workers in this field.

Up to now control has been considered

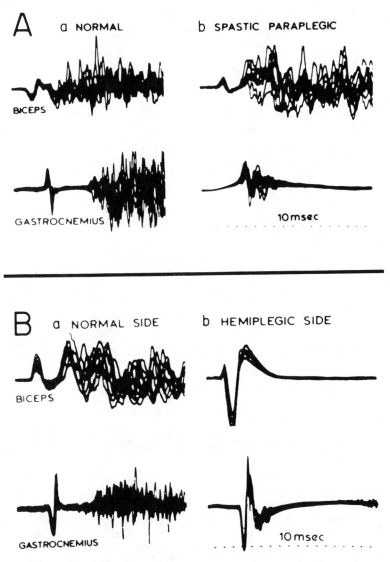

Fig. 6.8. Long-loop (functional stretch, M2) responses depend on intact supraspinal connections (A), specifically between the spinal cord and the motor cortex (B). (A) Superimposed EMG responses in a spastic paraplegic patient *(right column)* show lack, below the level of cord transection, of functional stretch responses (M2 at about 100 msec) to sudden and maintained stretch, starting at beginning of traces. (B) Lack of functional stretch responses on the affected side of a hemiplegic patient. (From Chan, Melvill Jones, Kearney, and Watt, 1979; in Evarts, 1981a; also in Chan, 1983; Brooks, 1985)

as the exclusive province of supraspinal commands. Yet, we must remember that a property which is regulated at one level of the motor hierarchy may be controlled by another. The motor servo not only regulates, for instance, but it can also exert control by adaptive *gain* changes of the stretch reflex (which is expressed by the slope of the length–tension curve). This mechanism operates well, however, only below 10% of the maximal torque that can be generated at the joint (Chap. 4.2). Most experiments suggest that supraspinal participation is required to change the reflex *threshold* by shifting the muscle action from one length–tension curve to another

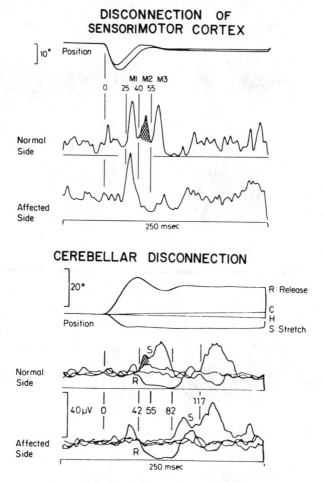

Fig. 6.9. Long-loop responses depend on intact connections of the spinal cord with the sensori-motor cortex (upper set of traces) and the cerebellum (lower set). *(Upper set of traces)* Displacements of the right and left thumbs from an intended position in a patient with a unilateral brain stem lesion. Below, comparison is made for the normal and affected sides of muscular responses to a fast, brief stretch of the long thumb flexor (at time 0; averages of rectified EMG records, M2 *hatched*). *(Lower set of traces)* Responses to sustained stretch or release of the long thumb flexor in a patient with a unilateral cerebellar disconnection. The upper traces show the position of the thumb on the affected side (also shown: C, control; H, halted; all at time 0). Below, comparison is made of the muscular responses on the normal and affected sides. On the normal side, M2 *(hatched)* merges with M3 and is followed by a voluntary response (at 117 msec). On the affected side, M2–M3 are absent but an-other response occurs instead at 82 msec. (From Marsden, Merton, Morton and Adam, 1978; in Houk and Rymer, 1981; also both in Brooks, 1985)

(see Figs. 3.4 and 4.6). Figure 6.7 implies that long-loop responses of medium la-tency are an expression of supraspinal commands calling for muscular co-con-traction to reset (control) the joint stiff-ness. Since long-loop responses can adjust large changes of joint angle, their predom-inant action is far more likely to be on alpha than on gamma MNs (Chap. 4.2).

The two types of influence—regulation and control—are drawn in Fig. 6.10A, sep-arating muscle regulation *along* a length-tension curve at constant stiffness, from the control transit *between* two such curves, which changes stiffness. (The threshold changes, but the slope—or reflex gain—remains the same.) The equilibrium points of the motor servo at the initial and final loads are marked by filled and open circles, which indicate how this process stretches the muscle along the constant upward slope of the solid line, **a**. In the mechanical analog, shown in Fig. 6.10B, this servo regulation is drawn as a spring that can be pulled on, but that has constant stiffness (force change/length change) as a property of how it is made. If the final load is to be supported at the *initial* length, however, supraspinal control is brought to bear and a reaction-time shift occurs to the dashed length–tension curve with a different threshold. In the hypothetical diagram (Fig. 6.10A), that shift is drawn as an isotonic shortening of length along the horizontal arrow, **b**. In the mechanical analog (Fig. 6.10B), this is indicated by a change of spring slack, or threshold, represented by the rack-and-pinion control that would alter how tightly the spring is wound to support a particular load. Houk thus posits that reflex actions *regulate* (i.e., tend to keep constant) the equilibrium stretch of the spring like muscles for a particular

load. The "regulated compliance" in Fig. 6.10B is the inverse of stiffness, and is kept constant by the motor servo. [See Fig. 5.1 and also refer back to Figs. 4.6B and 4.9A, to see how the stretch reflex tends to preserve (i.e., regulate) muscle stiffness linearly against various loads despite the nonlinear properties of muscle tissue.] The motor servo thus damps oscillations, which improves smooth matching of move and hold programs. As stated above, however, supraspinal motor commands are needed to *control* (i.e., to reset) muscle stiffness for a particular load, which is accomplished by adjusting reflex thresholds. Transcortical loops of co-contracting muscles help to steady the joint against expected load changes.

The foregoing text has outlined some means whereby motor set can use motor programs to operate long-loop pathways and mechanisms for generation and maintenance of *intended trajectories and postures*. Thus, spinal alpha MNs can be programmed by the middle level. These processes are based on the assumption that the brain has internal knowledge of the joint stiffness that obtains at an intended end point, a conclusion reached by Fel'd-

Fig. 6.10. (A) Diagram to illustrate length–tension changes produced by spinal reflex (**a**, along *heavy line* in direction of *upward-sloped arrow* toward the right), and by voluntary, intended component of response to a load perturbation (**b**, along *horizontal arrow* toward the *broken line* on the left). Compare to Fig. 3.4. (B) A mechanical analog of the motor servo drawn in Fig. 5.1, explained in text. [(A) From Houk and Rymer, 1981; (B) from Houk, 1978)]

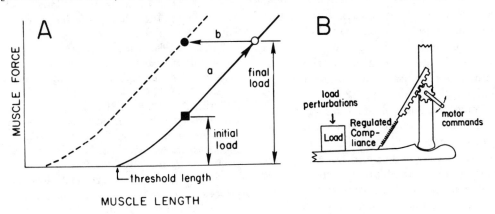

man (Chap. 4.2) and by Bizzi (Chaps. 7.1 and 9.2.)

4. Summary

Motor set indicates that the CNS is ready for a particular motor act. One way to test intent and set is to perturb an intended position or movement and observe the muscular corrections. Such perturbations evoke successive muscular responses. All can be brought under voluntary control, depending on the instructions and the circumstances. The first (M1, 25–50 msec) is the spinal stretch reflex. The second (M2, 50–85 msec) also has some spinal servo properties but is under stronger voluntary control than M1. The third (M3, 85–100 msec) is almost entirely voluntary. Servo responses are characterized by oscillatory response intensities that are proportional to that of the perturbation and oppose it. Only voluntary responses ever err in the direction of the response.

Long-loop (or functional stretch) responses can control and regulate intended limb trajectories and postures by adjusting joint stiffness. They restore perturbed velocities of intended movements to appropriate values (trajectory compensation). They occur before joints are stabilized against perturbations (load or unload) by co-contraction of opposing muscles (load compensation). Stiffness is probably adjusted in response to large perturbations by shifting the equilibrium point of muscles to new length–tension relations, which permit generation of greater force at the original length. Stiffness may also be adjusted in part by altered gain of the stretch reflex through adaptation of the servo gain, a mechanism suitable for dealing with small perturbations.

Long-loop and voluntary responses are mediated through the motor cortex and depend on cerebellar guidance for their adaptive task relationship. Long-loop responses are emitted predictively in programmed postural adjustments, for instance in leg muscles, when an individual runs or hops on, or falls toward, a surface. They occur too late to brace the leg for landing, but their use might well be for the *following* rhythmical movement. (In this case they are triggered also with the assistance of vestibular gravity receptors, acting through the vestibulospinal tract.) It is suggested that responses generated by supraspinal commands, and routed through the descending limb of long-loop paths, participate in normal movements as part of the motor program, and thus of motor set. They are important in the overriding function of matching the move and hold programs, which together create smooth, programmed motor acts. It seems reasonable to assume that long loops function in the steady maintenance as well as in the corrections of intended postures (isometric versus isotonic muscular contractions). The outstanding properties of long-loop responses are their susceptibility to instructions given to a subject, and their task-related adaptations to changing circumstances. Long-loop responses to imposed perturbations probably function through their influence on alpha MNs, because gamma MNs produce inadequate changes of gain.

References

Abrahams, V. C. 1981. Unresolved questions concerning muscle afferents. *Can. J. Physiol. Pharmacol.* 59:656–659.

Brooks, V. B. 1985. How are "move" and "hold" programs matched? In *Cerebellar functions*, eds. H. J. Dichgans, W. J. Bloedel, and W. Precht. pp. 1–23. *Proc Life Sciences*. Berlin: Springer Verlag. [Figs. 6.4, 6.6–6.9]

Burke, D. 1980. The activity of human muscle spindle endings in normal motor behavior. In *Neurophysiology IV*, ed. R. Porter. *Int. Rev. Physiol.* 25:91–126.

Burke, D. 1983. Critical examination of the case for or against fusimotor involvement in disorders of muscle tone. In *Motor control mechanisms in health and disease*, ed. J. E. Desmedt. *Adv. Neurol.* 39:133–150.

Chan, C. W. Y. 1983. Segmental versus suprasegmental contributions to long-latency stretch responses in man. In *Motor control mechanisms in health and disease*, ed. J. E. Desmedt. *Adv. Neurol.* 39:467–508. [Fig. 6.8]

Chan, C. W. Y., Melvill Jones, G., and Catchglove, R. F. H. 1979. The "late" electromyographic response to limb displacement in man. II. Sensory origin. *Electroencephalogr. Clin. Neurophysiol.* 46:182–188. [Fig. 6.5]

Chan, C. W. Y., Melvill Jones, G., Kearney, R. E., and Watt, D. G. D. 1979. The "late" electromyographic response to limb displacement in man. I. Evidence for supraspinal contribution. *Electroencephalogr. Clin. Neurophysiol.* 46:173–181. [Fig. 6.8]

Cooke, J. D. 1980. The organization of simple, skilled movements. In *Tutorials in motor behavior*, eds. G. E. Stelmach and J. Requin. *Adv. Psychol.* 1:199–212. [Fig. 6.6]

Crago, P. E., Houk, J. C., and Hasan, Z. 1976. Regulatory actions of human stretch reflex. *J. Neurophysiol.* 39:925–935. [Fig. 6.3]

Deecke, L., and Kornhuber, H. H. 1971. Cerebral potentials and the initiation of voluntary movement. In *Attention, voluntary contraction and event-related potentials*, ed. J. E. Desmedt, *Prog. Clin. Neurophysiol.* 1:132–150. [Fig. 6.1]

Evarts, E. V. 1981. Role of motor cortex in voluntary movements in primates. In *Motor control.* Sect. 1, vol. 2. *Handbook of physiology*, ed. V. B. Brooks, pp. 1083–1120. Bethesda, Md.: American Physological Society. [Fig. 6.8]

Evarts, E. V. 1981. Sherrington's concepts of proprioception. *Trends Neurosci.* 4:44–46.

Evarts, E. V., Shinoda, Y., and Wise, S. P. 1984. *Neurophysiological approaches to higher brain functions.* New York: John Wiley & Sons.

Ghez, C. 1981. Cortical control of voluntary movement. In *Principles of neural science*, eds. E. R. Kandell and J. H. Schwartz, pp. 323–333. New York: Elsevier/North-Holland. [Fig. 6.1]

Houk, J. C. 1978. Participation of reflex mechanisms and reaction-time processes in the compensatory adjustments to mechanical disturbances. In *Cerebral motor control in man: long-loop mechanisms*, ed. J. E. Desmedt. *Prog. Clin. Neurophysiol.* 4:193–215. [Figs. 6.3A and 6.10B]

Houk, J. C., and Rymer, W. Z. 1981. Neural control of muscle length and tension. In *Motor control.* Sect. 1, vol. 2. *Handbook of physiology*, ed. V. B. Brooks, pp. 257–323. Bethesda, Md.:American Physiological Society. [Figs. 6.2A, 6.3B,C, 6.9 and 6.10A]

Kwan, H. C., Murphy, J. T., and Repeck, M. W. 1979. Control of stiffness by the medium-latency electromyographic response to limb perturbation. *Can. J. Physiol. Pharmacol.* 57:277–285. [Fig. 6.7]

Lee, R. G., Murphy, J. T., and Tatton, W. G. 1983. Long-latency myotatic reflexes in man: mechanisms, functional significance, and changes is patients with Parkinson's disease or hemiplegia. In *Motor control mechanisms in health and disease*, ed. J. Desmedt. *Adv. Neurol.* 39:489–508. [Figs. 6.2B and 6.7]

Libet, B., Gleason, C. A., Wright, E. W., and Pearl, D. K. 1983. Time of conscious intention to act in relation to onset of cerebral activity (readiness-potential). *Brain* 106:623–642. [Fig. 6.1]

Marsden, C. D., Merton, P. A., Morton, H. B., Adam, J. E. R., and Hallett, M. 1978. Automatic and voluntary responses to muscle stretch in man. In *Cerebral motor control in man: long-loop mechanisms*, ed. J. E. Desmedt. *Prog. Clin. Neurophysiol.* 4:167–177. [Fig. 6.9]

Marsden, C. D., Rothwell, J. C., and Day, B. L. 1983. Long-latency automatic responses to muscle stretch in man: origin and function. In *Motor control mechanisms in health and disease*, ed. J. Desmedt. *Adv. Neurol.* 39:509–539.

Matthews, P. B. C. 1981. Proprioceptors and the regulation of movement. In *Motor coordination.* Vol. 5. *Handbook of behavioral neurobiology*, eds. A. L. Towe and E. S. Luschei, pp. 93–127. New York: Plenum Press.

McCloskey, D. I., Colebatch, J. G., Potter, E. K., and Burke, D. 1983. Judgements about onset of rapid voluntary movements in man. *J. Neurophysiol.* 49:851–863. [Fig. 6.1]

Mortimer, J. A., and Webster, D. D. 1983. Dissociated changes of short- and long-latency myotatic responses prior to a brisk voluntary movement in normals, in karate experts, and in Parkinsonian patients. In *Cerebral motor control in man: long-loop mechanisms*, ed. J. E. Desmedt. *Prog. Clin. Neurophysiol.* 4:541–554.

Nashner, L. M., and Grimm, R. J. 1978. Analysis of multiloop dyscontrols in standing cerebellar patients. In *Cerebral motor control in man: long-loop mechanisms*, ed. J. E. Desmedt. *Prog. Clin. Neurophysiol.* 4:300–319. [Fig. 6.4]

Prochazka, A., and Hulliger, M. 1983. Muscle afferent function and its significance for motor control mechanisms during voluntary movements in cat, monkey, and man. In *Motor control mechanisms in health and disease*, ed. J. Desmedt. *Adv. Neurol.* 39: 93–132.

Skinner, J. E., and Yingling, C. D. 1977. Central gating mechanisms that regulate event-related potentials and behavior. In *Attention, voluntary contraction and event-related cerebral potentials*, ed. J. E. Desmedt. *Prog. Clin. Neurophysiol.* 1:30–69.

Tatton, W. G., and Lee, R. G. 1975. Evidence for abnormal long-loop reflexes in rigid Parkinsonian patients. *Brain Res.* 100:671–676. [Fig. 6.2A]

Tatton, W. G., North, A. G. E., Bruce, I. E., and Bedingham, W. 1983. Electromyographic and motor cortical responses to imposed displacements of the cat elbow: disparities and homologies with those of the primate wrist. *J. Neurosci.* 3:1807–1817.

Thach, W. T., Perry, J. G., and Schieber, M. H. 1982. Cerebellar output: body maps and muscle spindles. In *The cerebellum: new vistas*, eds. S. L. Palay and V. Chan-Palay. *Exp. Brain Res.* Suppl. 6, pp. 440–454.

Vallbo, A. B., Hagbarth, K. E., Torebjork, H. E., and Walling, B. G. 1979. Somatosensory, proprioceptive, and sympathetic activity in human peripheral nerves. *Physiol. Rev.* 59:919–957.

Vallbo, A. B., and Hulliger, M. 1981. Independence of skeletomotor and fusimotor activity in man? *Brain Res.* 223:176–180.

Wallin, G., and Hagbarth, K. E. 1978. Muscle spindle activity in man during voluntary alternating movements, Parkinsonian tremor and clonus. In *Physiological tremor, pathological tremors and clonus*, ed. J. E. Desmedt. *Prog. Clin. Neurophysiol.* 5:150–159.

7

Controlled Variables

This chapter asks what properties ("variables" or "parameters") are controlled in postures and movements. The answer depends on what instructions have been given to the subject or are perceived implicitly by the subject from the surrounding circumstances. Instructions, however received, direct our attention, control our sensory awareness and set our motor readiness. The answer also depends on the level of task control that we wish to describe; for instance, all that occurs in Fig. 1.1, or only in one of the figurines, or in just part of one?

We first compare the control of variables in simple and in compound movements. This comparison permits us to identify some common, basic rules and an important control principle: that the brain singles out the body part requiring the greatest attention and simplifies the guidance of its trajectory by subordinating those of other parts of the body. Second, we consider some mechanical limb properties that enter into the control process. The chapter goes on to the neural control of the hierarchical levels, and concludes with demonstrations of the importance of our perceptions, in particular our "sense of effort."

1. Simple and Compound Movements

Everyday experience tells us that we can do almost anything if we put our minds to it. To quote from an article by Stein: "We can put the right *spring* in our step, control the *position* of our limbs with the required precision ..., control the patterns of *force* generated by our vocal cords and our fingers to sing a song while playing the accompaniment on the piano at speeds at which detailed feedback must be impossible, and control the *velocity* of a golf club so that it strikes the ball optimally ..." How is it done? To understand the control of variables, we need to consider motor tasks of different complexities. Let us start with a difficult task in which many joints are used, such as writing, and then work our way down to simple movements.

Overall plans for well-learned movement sequences, such as handwriting, encode the temporal relationships, the relative instead of the actual time intervals, between movements that may vary in size and speed. With this kind of "phasing" we can produce the same recognizable handwriting even when we use different joints to do so (see Fig. 2.6). Individual writing patterns are preserved because we always use the same *proportions of space and time,* no matter whether we write large or small, slowly or in haste. This analysis (by Terzuolo, illustrated in Figs. 7.1 and 7.2), shows that we control the *patterns* of successive muscular activities. For example, when a person is instructed to write with different amplitudes, writing duration often remains unchanged despite large differences in letter size. Writing speed is increased automatically and in proportion to the change of size. Figure 7.1 demonstrates how the same motion patterns are repeated for three different sizes of writing, although the actual velocities are largest for large writing and smallest for small ones. The brain here controls the amplitudes of the well-practiced movement patterns

while preserving the proportions of space and time. Actual velocities are therefore not a controlled variable in this case. Pattern regulation emerges just as clearly when the speed, instead of the amplitude, of writing is controlled. Figure 7.2 shows that as the total movement duration decreases, instantaneous velocity values increase proportionally, which regulates (i.e., keeps invariant) the ratios of the times of occurrence of the major features of the pattern. They all line up in Fig. 7.2. (The inset in the top left-hand corner explains how tangential velocities are established for the curved writing paths that constitute individual parts of the pattern.) Naturally, these velocities decrease as the pen goes around sharp bends, that is, at points of maximal curvature. As before, the ac-

Fig. 7.1. Learned movement patterns are preserved when writing in different sizes. The pattern records describe the time course (abscissa) of tangential velocities (*V*, left ordinates) reached in writing the signatures shown. The *upward-sloping lines* represent the lengths of the trajectory (right ordinate; note that trajectory lengths of upper two traces reset, that is, they traverse the 10-cm calibrated distance several times). Abscissa represents time (seconds). How tangential velocities are measured is shown in Fig. 7.2. (From Viviani and Terzuolo, 1980)

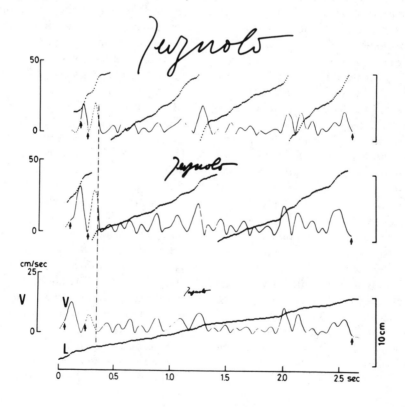

tual velocities of the constituent movements are not controlled, but they vary here as the consequence of the controlled writing speed.

We encountered an example of scaling when we considered the muscle synergies used in balancing the body in the upright posture (cf. Fig. 6.4). Overall scaling of pat-terned movements is accomplished with the aid of the basal ganglia, which simplifies supraspinal control along the lines suggested by Bernstein (Chap. 2.2). We note in this connection a well-known property of unconscious movement planning: speed is traded for accuracy. Large and small movements can be made equally accurately

Fig. 7.2.   Learned movement patterns are preserved when writing at different speeds, while keeping size constant. *Inset* at top left shows how tangential velocity (*V*) is computed by fitting circles *(dotted line)* to segments (1–6) of the handwritten letter *a*. The resulting velocity segments are numbered (1–6) on the lowermost velocity trace, plotted against time (abscissa). The *dotted lines* interpolating the times of occurrence of the major features of the velocity profiles all have a common origin. (From Viviani and Terzuolo, 1980)

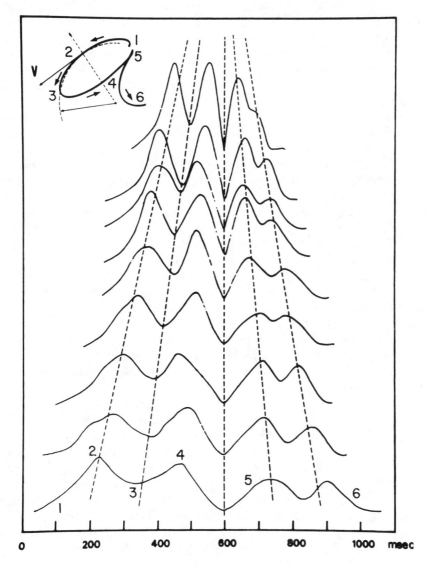

if given enough time, larger ones taking longer to execute than small ones. But if large and small movements have to be made in the same amount of time, then movement accuracy and errors increase roughly in proportion to movement size. This is referred to as Craik's ratio rule, which becomes a precise, semilogarithmic relation for fast and fairly large intended movements (Fitt's ratio rule). Thus, human strategies depend on the task requirements. If absolute accuracy is required, then movement time varies with amplitude. If rapid movements are required, however, absolute accuracy suffers, although we preserve relative accuracy between sizes of movement and those of their errors. The errors seem to be scaled along with the movement patterns; they presumably represent the limit of useful programming.

The same rules as those for writing apply to other patterned movements, such as typing (not illustrated). The patterns of how the fingers are used are reflected, although not displayed, in the constant ratios of the times taken to strike particular keys, regardless of actual typing speeds. This example is mentioned here because it offers a useful way in which to assess motor tasks that can be timed, or sampled, only intermittently. Patterns of leg use during walking are discussed in Chap. 10.1.

We learned early in this study that intended (programmed) movements can be recognized by their distinctive "continuous" velocity profile with only one peak (Figs. 1.3 and 1.5). This property not only serves as a useful guide but tells us much more, because such velocity profiles apply not only to single-joint (simple) movements, but also to the *path of the object of greatest attention* of the central nervous system for intended multi-joint (compound) movements. For arm movements, this is usually the path of the hand. (For head movements it is usually the direction of gaze of the eyes; see Chap. 9.) Figure 7.3 illustrates the hand path for a multi-joint,

free reaching movement of a human subject using shoulder, elbow and wrist to grasp a pin stuck in the table. The hand path is mostly straight. The velocity profile of the hand path (broken line) is continuous except for a few deviations (marked by arrows). The cause of the deviations becomes apparent by comparison of the plots on the left (with time as the abscissa) with the pictorial representation on the right (with distance as the linear abscissa and 20-msec time markers shown as dots along the flight path). The first deviation occurs about 150 msec after lift-off, when the movement slows during redirection toward a more horizontal flight path. The second and third deviations may be the result of changing the object of attention from the hand to the fingers, which open for the grasp about 100 msec after peak velocity and begin to close about 200 msec before landing. The fourth deviation is caused by the combined final slowing for landing and by the completion of finger closure for the grasp. Although the velocity profile of the hand path is mostly continuous, the profiles of the limb paths for the joints that transport the hand are not necessarily continuous, because their actions are fitted to support the intended hand path (not illustrated). We do know, however, that the relations between their paths are programmed together as a pattern. An example of this is given for leg movements during walking in Figs. 10.1 and 10.2.

Analysis of three-dimensional movements is difficult, which makes it more profitable to study two-dimensional ones that are carried out on a flat surface (i.e., in one plane). Writing has already been presented as an example (Figs. 7.1 and 7.2), but it is complicated by the use of many joints: those of the fingers, the wrist, and even the elbow and shoulder. Less complicated movements in one plane can be studied more conveniently, for example arm movements that are restricted to the shoulder and elbow. More informative descriptions can be obtained from movements

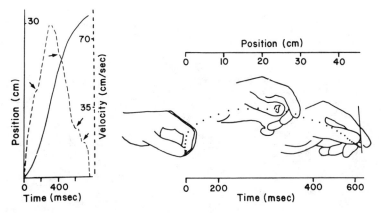

Fig. 7.3. The hand path of a free reaching movement made with the shoulder, elbow and wrist moves in a straight line and has a bell-shaped, "continuous" velocity profile. Graphs on *left* have two ordinates: position (*solid line*, cm) and velocity (*broken line*, cm/second). Abscissa is time (msec). Side view of hand path on *right* has two abscissas: position (cm) above, and time (msec) below. Time is also indicated by 20-msec dots along hand path. For details see text. (From Jeannerod and Prablanc, 1983; also in Brooks, 1985)

that are restricted to two joints operating in the same plane (two degrees of freedom).

This has been studied for elbow and shoulder movements by Bizzi's group, who had subjects move a jointed lever in the horizontal plane (Fig. 7.4A,B). Positions of the upper arm and forearm can be followed by sensors located in the lever joints, the angles of which relate to those of the shoulder and elbow. Traces 1–5 of Fig. 7.4C represent the hand paths of a subject who moves the lever handle either from one target to another in a straight line (**1**), or follows around several targets in increasingly curved paths (**2–5**). The velocity profiles, in Fig. 7.4D, grade from single-peaked (**1**, continuous) to multiple-peaked (**5**, discontinuous) as the hand paths become more curved and are traversed increasingly in successive, short segments.

Figure 7.4C,**1** shows that the hand tends to move in almost straight paths, that the velocity profiles of hand movements are continuous, and that they are independent of where they occur in the work space, which can be any part of the horizontal surface shown. Moreover, the same hand paths are obtained when the subject moves

the handle while standing with the surface at waist height, in which case shoulder and elbow movements differ greatly from those used in the sitting position (not illustrated). The paths of the "supporting players," the shoulder and elbow, do vary with the work space and are not necessarily as straight as the hand paths. Subjects can move the hand around obstacles or follow prescribed nonlinear hand paths by making successive, minimally curved, short segments. The points of greatest curvature are indicated by arrowheads in Fig. 7.4C and by vertical lines in Fig. 7.4D. The velocity profiles grade from nearly continuous (Fig. 7.4C,**1**, on the left) to discontinuous (or "segmented," Fig. 7.4C,**2–5**). The segments, which are analogous to the successive "steps" in single-joint discontinuous movements (Figs. 1.3 and 1.5), are probably controlled by successive subprograms for limited, nearly straight movements. They call for muscular net forces in slightly different directions ("force vectors").

Force vectors are the common denominator of segments of multijoint movements and of whole single-joint movements: they traverse near-straight paths. Thus, *force vectors are an output speci-*

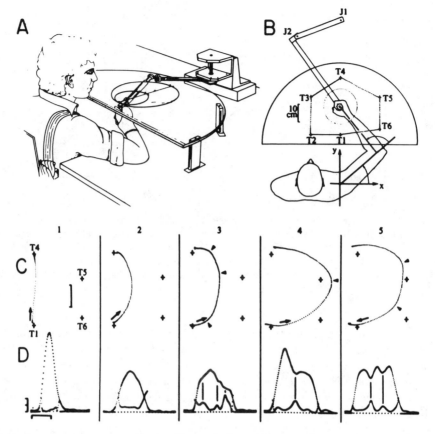

Fig. 7.4. Arm movements use the shoulder and elbow joints to optimize transport of the hand. (A,B) A subject holds a handle with two joints (J1, J2). T1–T6 mark visual targets on the horizontal work space. (C,D) Rapid aiming movements yield continuous velocity profiles (e.g., **1,2**), while nonlinear movements are discontinuous (**3–5**). *Arrows* indicate directions from T1 to T4 (**1–4**) and from T4 to T1 (**5**). Calibration in **1** is 10 cm. *Arrowheads* indicate greatest path curvatures. (D) Velocity profiles of movements **1–5**, whose minima are aligned by vertical lines to maxima of path curvatures, plotted below. Time calibration: 500 msec. (From Abend, Bizzi and Morasso, 1982; partly also in Bizzi and Abend, 1983; also in Brooks, 1985)

fied by simple motor programs. For multi-joint movements this is a matter of control, while for single-joint movement is merely the consequence of their anatomical range. Two-joint movements, with two degrees of freedom, can control direction and force, whereas one-joint movements can only control the degree of force; the direction is fixed by the arc described by the limb about the joint. Control of force yields control of velocity, which appears to be scaled in relation to the path or trajectory (Fig. 6.6). The speed–path relations in Fig. 7.4C suggest that when subjects

move the handle from one point in the horizontal workspace to another without special instructions how to do it, the arm movements are programmed in terms of the trajectory of the most important object (body part), the hand. All other matters seem to be subject to this overriding objective.

The paths of nonlinear movements made with multiple (more than two) joints, as in handwriting, also reflect patterns of successive segments oriented along different directions. As in two-joint movements, their junctions are traversed at minimal velocities (which are marked in Fig. 7.4D,3–5 by the vertical alignments of the greatest path curvatures and the smallest velocities). As Bizzi points out, the simplicity of the hand path is another example of Bernstein's theory in action: overall, high-level plans are assisted by the availability of low-level programs. The move program for the hand makes it easier (reduces the degreees of freedom) to plan the overall move of the two-jointed limb. The overall hold program of the limb also resembles that for one joint: steady hand postures are determined by the summed joint stiffnesses in the work plane.

The foregoing considerations of overall trajectories still do not reveal the secrets of their creation. The brain has to translate the coordinates of real space ("Cartesian" coordinates) into those of the joints and into the torques required to achieve them. This translation from sensory to motor representation probably occurs in the middle level of the motor hierarchy for voluntary movements, but we do not know how it is achieved (see Fig. 2.4). That is the subject of a major quest in current neuroscience, because it helps to decipher the system "language" for much of the basic logic of the brain. No matter how the "inverse" kinematics and dynamics are arrived at (from the brain to the outside world), it is plain that the trajectory of the most important object, in this case the hand, determines the actions of those parts of the limb that serve to transport the hand.

It is useful at this point to illustrate the variety of ways in which single-joint movements can be made at different speeds. Continuous movements of moderate speed were illustrated in Fig. 1.3 as being propelled and braked by a triphasic sequence of bursts of muscle activity. There are many gradations of slow speeds, however, that can still retain a single-peaked velocity profile. Figure 7.5 provides an instructive example. A seated human subject (sketched in Fig. 7.5C) performs a step-tracking task with the right arm,

which is held in a splint and cannot be seen by him. The trunk and shoulders are stabilized with belts and a padded block. For relatively fast isotonic movements (of a freely moving, unloaded handle), a triphasic pattern of muscle bursts is used (Figs. 1.3 and 7.5B), which optimizes efficiency with respect to one of the factors listed in Fig. 7.9. When only low speeds are required (Fig. 7.5A), a different movement tactic is used that optimizes energy expenditure. What matters most seems to be the preservation of the continuous trajectory. Note when the biceps (antagonist) ceases to hold the arm in flexion and when the triceps (agonist) begins to discharge. What is driving this movement in which biceps ceases well before movement onset, and triceps begins only after peak velocity has already been reached? The answer lies in the physical properties of muscle tissue as expressed in the length–tension relations of the two opposing muscles (Figs. 3.4, 3.6 and 4.6). When the triceps brake is released, the joint rotates until equilibrium is reached with biceps, which then commences its holding action at an intensity proportional to the load it opposes. Muscle action in slow, simple movements can grade from a mixture of "pulses" and "steps" (as in Figs. 1.3 and 7.5B) to pure steps, as in Fig. 7.5A. If very slow velocities suffice for the task, such movements can have shallow-peaked continuous profiles, fashioned entirely from use of elastic energy stored in the muscles. Metabolically supported muscle bursts are then not needed. The "neutral" joint positions are cheapest because they are maintained without any muscular effort by the balance of agonist and antagonist tissue properties (see Chaps. 3.2 and 4.1).

An important general rule is revealed by comparison of the isotonic movements (Fig. 7.5A–C) studied by Bizzi's group with the isometric movements studies by Ghez and associates (Fig. 7.5D). The records are obtained in the same way as those in Fig. 7.5A,B, except that the subject presses against a fixed bar. The instruction in the

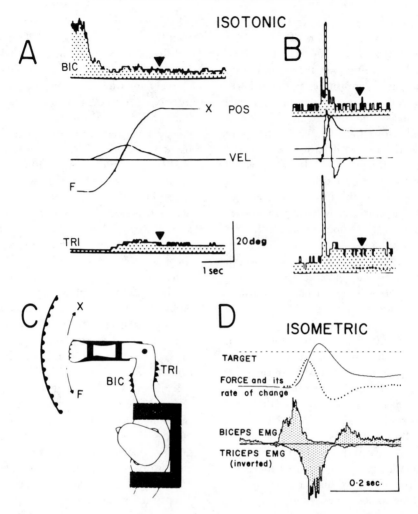

Fig. 7.5. Human subjects display the same tactics of muscle use for isotonic and isometric efforts when step-tracking positions of target lights by flexing (F) and extending (X) the forearm in the horizontal plane (A–C); or force targets by flexing against the stationary handle (D). Position and velocity are monitored by a potentiometer *(black dot)* under the elbow (C), force by transducer (not shown) on handle. EMG leads on skin over triceps and biceps. (A) Slow extension starts by release of tonic biceps (braking) action, which holds the arm in flexion, and then by a late triceps step grading over into tonic holding of the arm in extension *(dotted areas:* integrated, rectified EMG; *arrowheads* mark holding postures). (B) Triphasic pattern of muscle force pulses for smooth take-off and landing at faster speed. Triceps step holds the arm in extension posture. (D) Triphasic EMG pattern caused force trace *(solid line)* to reach, overshoot, and then fall away from force target *(horizontal broken line).* Relation of EMG to rate of force change *(dotted trace)* is the same as that to velocity in (C). Calibrations: 58 Newton (N) (a measure of force); 1575 N/second. [(A–C) Adapted from Lestienne, Polit and Bizzi, 1981; also in Brooks, 1985; (D) adapted from Gordon and Ghez, 1984]

step-tracking task is similar to that in Fig. 7.5B, namely to match the target as rapidly as possible. The target is a visual representation of a required force level (indicated in Fig. 7.5D by the horizontal broken line). The subject has to attain the prescribed

force—after which it may relax, which can be seen by following the force trace toward the target—surpass it and then decline (F, solid line). The rate of force change (*dF/dT*, dotted line) has a continuous profile, equivalent to those of the velocity traces in Fig. 7.5B,C. The relation between the controlled parameter and its rate of change (i.e., the force trajectory) has the same appearance (not illustrated) as that for position and velocity (Fig. 6.6.). The force trajectory is produced by the familiar triphasic EMG pattern. Various force levels are always reached in the same length of time in this task; that is, the rise time is held constant (regulated), while the rate of rise is the controlled variable. This relation, producing pulses of constant duration but variable amplitudes, is already known for human finger movements from the study of Freund, illustrated in Fig. 7.6. (As an aside we take notice that eye movements are controlled differently, in that both the amplitudes and durations can be varied for saccades.)

Studies of human subjects moving and holding their arms against various loads, in a manner much like that in Fig. 7.5, convinced Fel'dman that we aim single-joint movements according to the length-tension characteristics of the muscles involved, in fact that we program according to the joint stiffness at the desired final position (Figs. 3.4 and 4.6). This hypothesis has received experimental verification by Bizzi through the use of monkeys in a task situation illustrated in Fig. 7.7D. The animals were trained to point the handle to targets that were designated by lights. In this task (as in similar tests illustrated in Figs. 1.5 and 7.5) the subjects had to use proprioceptive feedback about their arm positions, because their operant arm was covered from their view by an opague surface. No particular movement speeds were called for. The animals pointed correctly to previously learned target positions (Fig. 7.7A), even when their arms had been pushed away from or toward the target at the beginning of the movement (Fig. 7.7B,C). The most remarkable finding was that the animals could perform just about normally after the operant arm had been deafferented (Fig. 7.8). This indicates that the brain had acquired internal knowledge of the lengths and tensions of the participating muscles when they balanced each others' efforts at the intended end point. As we saw in Fig. 3.4, these values obtain at the intersection of their length-tension curves. This idea is expressed in Fig. 7.7E. In other words, the brain seems to have learned the required joint stiffness for the desired end point, presumably through corollary discharge during motor learning. One criterion, however, betrays a relative lack of skill in the (feedforward) performance of the deafferented animals. They found it easier to perform the task with a stiffer arm than preoperatively (i.e., co-contracted more postoperatively). We know that co-contraction of opposing muscles is governed by descending supraspinal paths, particularly to the Ia IN (Fig. 5.2), and Chap. 13 will show that this is under cerebellar control.

Timing of the electrical and mechanical events of the muscles when the arm is moved passively (with the torque motor, unknown to the deafferented monkey) reveals operation of the learned motor program, made visible by the intended muscle excitation, which can, however, get out of step with the actual positions imposed on the limb. The most telling demonstration of how remembered length-tension properties are used comes from trials in which the animal was tricked by having its arm moved passively into the desired target position at a time when it expected to make that movement actively (Fig. 7.8A). Upon

Fig. 7.6. Pulse durations of voluntary isometric contractions are constant when a human subject contracts m. extensor digicis as fast as possible to reach several prescribed force targets. Compare to Fig. 7.5. (From Freund and Büdingen, 1978)

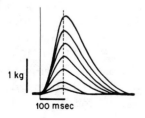

1 kg

100 msec

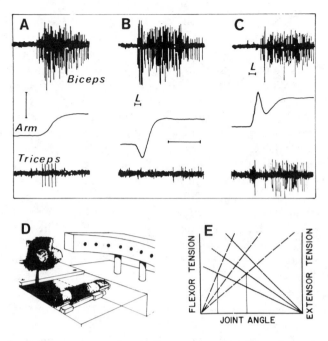

Fig. 7.7. Learned movements are aimed according to remembered length–tension curves of participating muscles. Flexion movements made by a monkey to visual targets without sight of its limbs, using the setup in (D). (A) Normal, unloaded movement and biceps, triceps EMGs. (B,C) Movements in which the torque motor has displaced the arm away from, and toward, the target. In both cases, the forearm reached the correct final position; note increased activity of stretched muscles. Calibrations: time, 1 second; vertical bar, 15 deg; *L*, timing and duration of load application. Target light is on during actual pointing. (E) Schematic representation of flexor and extensor length–tension curves. [(A–D) From Polit and Bizzi, 1979; (E) from Bizzi et al., 1982; partly in Bizzi and Abend, 1983]

appearance of the command (the target light) to move actively into that target, the trained monkey activated the neural process to make the learned movement from its beginning to its end, as evidenced by appropriate EMG activation after the usual reaction time (Fig. 7.8A). Although the arm was in fact in the correct position to gain a reward for the animal, it was not kept there but instead returned to the base position where it would have been had it not been displaced, and *then* it returned to the indicated target. During this to-and-fro movement the agonist discharged as it would do normally, when undisturbed.

As Bizzi put it,

Thus, in the presence of flexor muscle activity, we observed movement in the extensor direction. This remarkable finding cannot be explained if muscles are regarded purely as force

generators, but is readily explained if the length dependence of muscle force is taken into account. . . . If alpha MN activity evoked by the target light had *rapidly* achieved levels appropriate for the new final position, then no return movement should have taken place [see Fig. 7.7E]. The fact that a return movement did occur indicates that the control signal shifted *slowly* towards the final position [italics mine].

If the trajectory depended on a simple, rapid shift to a final equilibrium position, the displaced arm should have moved late but not in a to-and-fro motion. That this did occur suggests that the animals learn not only the end points and their stiffness, but also a series of intermediate equilibrium positions. In other words, they learn an internal "reference" trajectory that determines the path to be followed and generates torques appropriately to reduce mismatch between the intended and actual events. The control signal for moving the arm from one position to another is thus a gradual shifting, instead of sudden jumping, from one length–tension curve to another. These signals are timed in advance to accommodate the slowdown from electrical to mechanical events in muscle, a necessity with which we are familiar from Fig. 1.3. *Thus, reference trajectories are a sequence of length–tension relations that define the move programs. The initial and final relations are the hold programs.*

The same rules apply to the intended components of pursuit-tracking movements made to match the position of a moving target (c.f. Chap. 1.2). Tanaka has shown that they consist of three phases: an initial catch-up, the pursuit, and the termination. The initial catch-up phase is an intended small movement whose peak velocity is scaled to overcome the delay inherent in the visuo-motor reaction time, so as to reach the target which is already advancing at the moment of movement onset. The middle phase is stepped by smaller corrections, and the termination is a final, intended step.

2. Some Mechanical Factors

Why do human subjects and animals tend to make continuous movements, even if they are not required to do so (Fig. 1.5)? The answer may be that continuous movements offer the greated choice of economical trajectories. What is being economized? It can be a number of items, depending on what is most called for. Figure 7.9 shows calculated velocity profiles of hypothetical continuous movements of the same amplitude. They can optimize one of several minima without much change of shape, that is, without much change of programming: that for peak acceleration, jerk (rate of change of acceleration), energy, or alternately the constancy of stiffness. Changes from one type to another actually occur in jaw movements during speech. Which one is most useful at

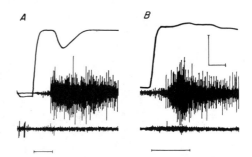

Fig. 7.8. The brain forms "reference trajectories" for learned single-joint movements, based on remembered length–tension curves of participating muscles. (A) Movements of deafferented forearm of a monkey in the absence of visual feedback. Same task situation as in Fig. 7.7D. Displacement of the forearm to a flexion position at which a target light was displayed. At the termination of the servo motor action *(horizontal bar),* note the movement of the arm toward extension and subsequent return to the position specified by the target. Flexor activity (upper EMG) evoked by the target light is similar to that which was observed during undisturbed movements of same amplitude. Lower EMG is of extensors. (B) Same animal. Displacement of the forearm to a flexion position at which a target light was displayed. No movement of the forearm at the termination of servo motor action. Flexor EMG was triggered by appearance of target light, and is similar to that during undisturbed movements. Calibrations: time, 550 msec; vertical bar, joint angle of 20 deg. (From Bizzi, Accornero, Chapple and Hogan, 1982)

any given time depends on the circumstances; trade-offs between particular goals is a familiar theme in motor control. The velocity profile with minimal peak velocity (V, Fig. 7.9) approaches that of a segment, or step, of a discontinuous movement, which makes sense for dipping economically into the recurring "velocity valleys" between force vectors in that type of movement. (Examples for single-, double-, and multiple-joint movements appear in Figs. 1.5A, 7.2 and 7.3D.) Minimization of acceleratory transients (jerk) is likely to be very important for the path of the object of greatest attention for the CNS.

Discussions about motor performance often pose the question just how move-

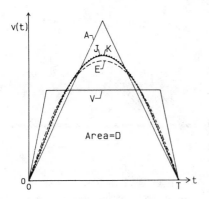

Fig. 7.9. Continuous movement profiles can optimize one of several variables without much adjustment. Comparison of velocity profiles, calculated for the same movement time and distance which are optimum with respect to five different objectives. Ordinate: V(t), velocity at time t, plotted on abscissa. **A,** Minimum peak acceleration *(solid line);* **E,** minimum energy *(dashed);* **J,** minimum jerk *(solid);* **K,** constant stiffness *(dotted).* **V,** which is not a continuous profile, minimizes peak velocity *(solid).* (From Nelson, 1983; also in Brooks, 1985)

ments are improved. Are they changed so as to require less work, have they become more efficient, or what other aspects are controlled toward optimal values? Work is the product of the average force and the distance over which it acts. Efficiency relates muscular input to a kinematic output; it is proportional to the work divided by the sum of the integrated EMGs of all muscles acting on a joint. Power is the rate of change of efficiency (i.e., work/time, which equals force × velocity) divided by the summed EMGs. Which factors are favored depends on the task situation; there are no uniform answers except that the CNS seeks the simplest methods of programming.

Interactions between joints are important factors for the execution of all naturally occurring movements because they influence motor programs. Several points concern us most. First, gravity dictates that the torque required to move a joint depends on the positions of the other joints. For instance, wrist extension from the horizontal forearm is harder work in the

pronated position (palm down) from where it has to lift against gravity, rather than in the supinated position (palm up) when it falls with gravity (see Fig. 5.3). Limb position also affects which muscles are active and the economy of their efforts, depending on whether they are stretched while contracting or lengthening. (Figure 4.6C reminds us of the asymmetrical properties in the interaction of two opposing muscles.) For instance, biceps brachii is the main flexor for the elbow in the horizontal plane if the hand is held halfway between pronation and supination (thumb on top, Fig. 6.3A), but not if the hand is pronated, when brachioradialis becomes more active. Biceps brachii, like many other muscles, produces another interaction because it *spans two joints* (Fig. 5.3). Third, mechanical cross-coupling effects cause reactions in all joints linked to one that is rotating. These effects are of great physiological importance because they influence active muscle groups that maintain body posture ("synergies," Fig. 6.4; also see Fig. 9.9).

What are the interactions when a joint moves? Three kinds of torques occur, which are illustrated in Fig. 7.10, taken from the discussion of these problems by Bizzi and Abend. The left-hand diagram indicates how rotation of joint J1 causes a reactional force (or "torque," since we are considering angular motions) that is proportional to acceleration, in the opposite direction at J2 (and vice versa, not illustrated). The right-hand diagram illustrates centripetal interaction torque (toward the rotating joint) caused by the reaction (force) to the centripetal force acting on the mass at the end of line 2. The centripetal force, which is proportional to the square of the angular velocity of joint 2, acts on J1 trhough the arm L. Thus, a movement at J1 induces a centripetal torque at J2. A third kind, called Coriolis torque, which is proportional to the product of the two angular velocities, acts about joint 1. All these interaction forces need to be balanced by appropriate mus-

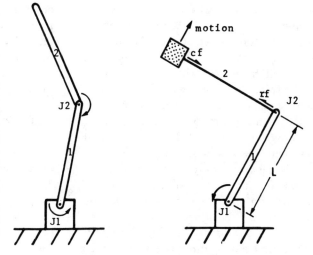

Fig. 7.10. Schematic illustration of interaction torques. *(Left)* Horizontal two-link arm is fixed at one end to a wall with a joint (J1). Second degree of freedom is provided by joint J2. If J1 is rotated as indicated by *arrow*, a reaction torque will move J2 as indicated by arrow. *(Right)* Motion at J1 caused by centripetal interaction torque. *rf*, Reaction force; *cf*, centripetal force. Explanation in text. (From Bizzi and Abend, 1983)

cular actions in order to achieve smooth and accurate movements. A comprehensive scheme that takes all these interactions into account is presented in Chap. 9.6.

3. Synopsis of Neural Control Levels

Movement patterns are specified by overall motor plans. Why are patterns preserved, rather than some other aspect? Presumably the brain can formulate and remember complex tasks best by storing the generalized sequence, the *cadence of successive movement directions in relation to movement amplitudes.* This would enable the CNS to coordinate the action of several joints, including the most human activity: creation of symbolic patterns. Such generalized functions are carried out by high levels of the motor hierarchy, "headquarters" that select what is important, make it the object of attention, and then issue general commands to deal with the important matters in such a way that they can apply in diverse circumstances (see Figs. 2.4 and 2.5). Neurons in high-order association cortex discharge in relation to some aspect of the task, but these cortical areas are not organized to represent the details of sensory or motor maps of the body.

Somatotopy is first encountered in the spinal cord and continues in the transition to the middle level of the hierarchy (Fig. 2.5). The middle (staff) level scales motor execution for the required amplitudes and directions, fitting them into real time. Neurons in motor cortex are, among other things, directionally tuned; each activates the spinal cord most intensely for a particular direction of movement. As a group, they can thus specify directional force in terms of the activity of appropriate muscle groups. The middle-level task system is assembled through activation of appropriate sensorimotor cell assemblies at suitable times and intensities for the desired *trajectory* (i.e., the speed in relation to the path). When that is disturbed, it is restored by the motor cortex with cerebellar guidance (Fig. 6.4). That guidance is also essential for the performance of normal, unperturbed movements, when it provides predictive timing based on the motor programs in use. This smooths performance (and holds tremor in abeyance) by accurately matching move and hold programs (Chap. 6.2). Unless prescribed by higher commands, movement velocities are determined finally at the lowest (work force) level, which "knows" how the selected muscles can best manage within the constraints of their length–tension relations (refer again to Figs. 3.6 and 4.6 and remember our previous analogy of the skiers coming down the hill). We learned about the work force level of the CNS in previous chapters. For instance, in Chap. 4.2 we noted that parametric control is limited at the spinal level, but that it is assisted by supraspinal control of the balance of static and dynamic gamma MNs. How the work is apportioned to CNS headquarters and staff will be taken up in Chaps. 11–14.

It is important to reiterate that the way in which a subject controls a motor action depends on the *instructions* received by the subject. (Recall from Chap. 2.1 the equivalent dependence of motor action on the relevance of a stimulus with reference to drive-motivation.) Instructions govern even the simplest circuits, such as the spinal motor servo. For instance, the tonic stretch reflex used in simple arm movements can vary either with an externally applied force or with the angle of the elbow, depending on whether the instruction was to regulate (keep constant) the exertion of muscular force or, alternately, the angular position of the elbow. How many levels of the motor hierarchy participate in such simple controls is still a matter of remarkably vigorous debate! The hierarchical arrangement follows the lines postulated by Bernstein. Each level of command relies on the capabilities of the one beneath it (Fig. 2.4) and equally relies on interaction with those above and below (Chap. 2.2).

The investigation of brain functions would be a hopeless task, were it not for our ability to obtain experimental data from animal models. This research, which leads to relief of human suffering, is warranted because the brains, and the sensorimotor integration that they create, follow many of the same rules in monkeys and human subjects.

4. Sense of Effort

When we estimate how much effort has to be spent on a task, we reach back to previous experience for the answer because our perceptions of the present are rooted in the past. This also applies to motor programs, whose subroutines have to estimate how much force to apply where and when, "how much is enough." Movement parameters are thus determined centrally until the program is adapted by peripheral feedback to suit the current circumstances (Fig. 4.11). Memory is converted into muscular effort by motor commands from the middle level of the hierarchy (Figs. 2.2 and 2.3). These motor commands are updated by peripheral feedback, even for skilled ballistic movements. Pure feedforward control is rarely used, and probably only for maximal, uncontrolled, all-out efforts. These points were discussed in Chap. 1.1, and so was the fact that ascending sensory feedback is adjusted ("edited") by the brain according to the needs of the task (Chaps. 1.2 and 3.1). How does this sensorimotor integration affect the variables of motor performance?

Integration of control over sensory input and motor output is most conspicuous for the muscle spindles. Their sensitivities are governed by the brain through supraspinal steering of gamma MNs. We saw in Chap. 4.2 that this fusimotor control is run as a corollary to the commands sent to alpha MNs. We also learned that corollary discharges provide opportunities for the CNS to enact subprograms for holding and moving, which might involve gamma MNs if it benefits spindle function within the task context (Fig. 4.12). Corollary discharges of motor commands were discussed in Chap. 2.2, where we learned that they either cancel the sensory consequences of intended movements or modify the reaction of the sensory systems to them. Corollary discharges affect sensations as a consequence of the distribution within the CNS of *motor* commands addressed to spinal to alpha MNs. This definition by McCloskey (whose views we generally follow here) excludes the internal consequences of sensory information ("reafference"). The latter are often included in these discussions, however, since they serve a similar function for the comparison of the expected and the actual course of events (see Chap. 5.1; Fig. 5.5B). Corollary discharge of motor commands *is* involved in sensations of static muscular force (or "effort") and in extracting useful kinesthetic information from the discharges of muscular receptors, but it is *not* involved in sensations of movement or altered limb position. These conclusions, which are based on illusions created by muscle vibration or anesthesia of nonmuscular receptors (Chap. 3.1; Figs. 3.1 and 3.2), mark the importance of corollary discharge for the determination of the variables in a motor task.

Vibration creates the illusion of movement only when the spindle responses can be modulated, when there is an extra fraction of spindle discharge that can be ascribed to something other than the *expected,* actual sensory events, that is, when the spindle response range is not saturated. The illusion of joint rotation (and of its speed) fails during strong contractions of the vibrated muscle, because alpha–gamma coactivation makes the intrafusal muscle fibers contract as well, saturating spindle responsiveness (see Chap. 4.2). A linear relation between muscle load and illusory speed of the human forearm is illustrated in Fig. 7.11. That figure also happens to rule out the participation of tendon organs in the illusion (created by loading the muscle), because the sensitivity of tendon organs to active muscle tension would increase, rather than decrease, the illusion when the muscle is fatigued.

Figure 7.11 has the interesting implication that alpha and gamma MNs are coactivated over the entire range of the expected muscular effort *without normally causing illusions.* We conclude that the internal corollaries of motor commands relate movement variables to external realities, and that at the same time they instill in us perceptions of what we are doing. Muscle vibration, and the tonic vibration reflex set up by it, cause illusions (Figs. 3.1 and 3.2). Vibration was found to be a useful clinical tool by Hagbarth soon after the discovery of its effects. Vibration of weak muscles can evoke spinal reflexes larger than those that could be evoked by stretch of those muscles. Vibration of weak muscles in hemiplegic patients can restore the balance between conflicting tonic stretch reflexes of antagonistic muscles, and thus inhibit unwanted postures. Why the tonic vibration reflex is especially useful with weak muscles will become apparent below.

The amount of force that we apply to lift, move or oppose an object depends on our perception of how heavy the object is. This can be tested objectively by having a subject match the perceived weight handled by the limb on one side with various weights on the other, control side. What creates the sensation of heaviness, the perception of force? The clinic teaches us that this sensation is associated with weakness. The sensation is unlikely to arise from peripheral sense organs, because they would continue to signal the actual pressures and tensions. Even muscle spindles are exempt because, as reported by Hagbarth, subjects feel a decrease of tension (instead of an increase) when muscles contract involuntarily during vibration. Similarly, subjects perceive themselves to be exerting less (isometric) force during a tonic vibration reflex. By exclusion, it appears that *the sensation of heaviness (or "effort") is caused by awareness of the descending motor command.* This conclusion of McCloskey's fits the important observation that weakness can be overcome by encouragement. A summary of the factors affecting perceived heaviness (or muscular force) is presented in Fig. 7.12. It includes lesions at the middle level of the motor hierarchy (motor cortex, cerebellum) or abnormal changes of input from peripheral receptors (e. g., vibration), as well as neuromuscular block and fatigue. McCloskey points out that the simplest explanation for the associations in Fig. 7.12 is that motor commands irradiate sensory centers, which is supported by known anatomical connec-

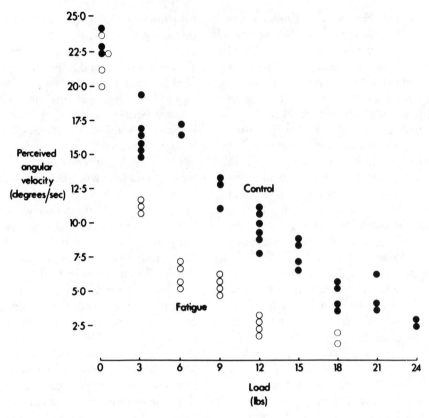

Fig. 7.11. Perceived velocity of illusory movements declines when muscle contracts. Angular velocity of elbow extension induced by vibration of biceps brachii at 100 Hz (ordinate) plotted against load borne by tensing vibrated biceps. *Filled circles* are points obtained when biceps carried its loads only briefly and was not fatigued. *Open circles* are equivalents when biceps was fatigued by prolonged weight bearing. (From McCloskey, 1973, in McCloskey, 1981)

tions and also by the timing of our conscious awareness of motor commands (Fig. 6.1).

Another glance at Figs. 2.2 and 2.5 suggests that the motor commands responsible for the sense of heaviness (which are never accompanied by any sense of movement) may be communications between the highest and the middle levels of the motor hierarchy, as well as between the middle and lowest levels. Both are likely in view of clinical findings concerning one-sided motor strokes. Two detailed accounts exist by neurologically knowledgable patients who suffered pure motor strokes (without sensory loss) that rendered them weak but not paralyzed. Both

felt an increased sense of heaviness when attempting to move the affected limbs. Brodal described his awareness of the "force of innervation" required to make muscles contract, and Mach commented on the "effort" needed to "move the arm or leg which seemed an enormous burden." The sense of heaviness is capable of crossing from the limbs on one side of the body to those on the other (as tested by matching weights), *below* the level of the corpus callosum, as established with tests in patients where it was divided for cerebral excisions (see Fig. 2.1C).

A similar phenomenon to a changed sense of heaviness occurs when we lower or raise our bodies by muscular effort in

SENSE OF EFFORT (HEAVINESS)

INCREASED   DECREASED

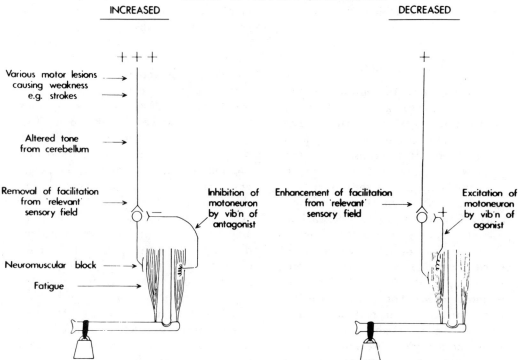

Fig. 7.12. Summary of factors affecting perceived muscular force or heaviness (i.e., "sense of effort"). (From McCloskey, 1981)

abnormal gravitational fields. When we *are* heavier (as in a diving aircraft), lowering ourselves during a kneebend creates the illusion of making us float off the ground, while raising ourselves with the antigravity leg muscles creates the illusion of pushing the ground down (Chap. 1.3). The phenomenon is best explained by the assumption of having fooled the inexperienced brain about the expected consequences of alpha–gamma coactivation, calibrated for normal gravity. The neural task system for sense of effort includes long loops between sensorimotor cortex and the spinal cord, that is, the middle level of the hierarchy (Chap. 6.2).

Access to motor commands at relatively low levels is also suggested by another finding listed in Fig. 7.12, namely that anesthesia of nonmuscular receptors of the

thumb increases the sense of heaviness, that is, that it is normally facilitated by skin input (Chap. 5.2). The neural connections shown in Fig. 5.6B could produce this sensitization because greater skin input raises the effectiveness of corticospinal commands. The sense of heaviness is related to motor cortex once more by Marsden's report that the gain of the long-loop response of the thumb (which is known to emanate from the motor cortex, see Fig. 6.9) is changed by skin anesthesia produced with a pressure cuff. The gain changes in relation to the "effort made by the subject rather than the actual presure exerted by the thumb." We conclude that commands from the motor cortex reach our awareness as a sense of effort (or heaviness) that crudely compares the intended force with that actually exerted. This sense of effort influences the intensity, and other variables, of our voluntary muscular actions.

5. Summary

At the highest level of control, the brain concentrates its guidance on the object that requires its greatest attention. This converts motor set into motor execution. Motor set depends on the instructions that are given explicitly to a subject or are gained implicitly through the subject's perception from the surrounding circumstances. Control can be exerted on limb position, or on the stiffness with which it is maintained, or on the acceleration and velocity, or its braking to adjust the force of impact, and other factors. In the case of arm movements, the brain usually pays the greatest attention to the path of the hand.

The controlled variables in sequential, multi-joint movements are movement *patterns* (proportions of space and time), especially if the task has been well learned (e.g., handwriting, which has many degrees of freedom). These patterns of constituent movements in different directions are scaled into real time and space at the middle hierarchical level according to the instructions received by the subject. The middle level also transforms the scales of the external world into motor commands for the internal world of the body. The lowest level translates them into activity of particular muscles.

For simpler tasks, carried out with two joints in one plane (two degrees of freedom), the overall program controls the *trajectory* (directional path at suitable speeds) of the most important object, for example the hand in the case of arm movements. When a subject makes such a movement without special instructions how to do it, the handpath tends to be straight and the trajectory is that of a continuous movement, with a single velocity peak just like that described for single-joint movements. The hand path is the outcome of a generalized, overall program that can be scaled to fit the particulars of any work space. Nonlinear paths for two-joint movements have segmented (discontinuous) velocity profiles. They are composed of successive segments formed by force bursts tuned to a sequence of directions (force vectors).

Single-joint movement programs control the *force* with which they move along the path prescribed by the joint. The changes of force determine the speed along the path, and hence the trajectory of isotonic movements. Typically, the initial rate of rise of force is a programmed variable. Transition from the start to the end position is determined by a gradual shift along equilibrium positions determined by the length–tension properties of the muscles moving the joint. The brain has internal knowledge of this sequence, constituting a "reference trajectory" on the basis of which torques are generated to minimize mismatch between actual intended positions. Continuous movements can optimize several variables, such as acceleration, or its rate of change, constancy of stiffness, or energy. The first three apply mostly to moderate speeds, generated by muscle force pulses delivered in the well-known triphasic pattern. The last one seems to be the most desirable factor when movements are made as changes between alternate postures as steps of muscle force. Reference trajectories (i.e., move programs) are a series of length–tension relations, of which the initial and final ones are the hold programs.

The same programming rules hold for isometric applications of force as for isotonic movements. They are both carried out with the same patterns of muscle use. Fast use of isometric tension at single joints is programmed as a pulse of force, with the rate of rise of force as the controlled variable, following a reference force trajectory. Programming of patterns of force vectors are the common denominator for movements of all kinds.

Several mechanical factors have to be taken into account because they influence the subsidiary guidance of movements.

These factors are (1) position of the limb (which alters the relative use of muscles), (2) use of muscles that span two joints, and (3) purely mechanical interactions between joints. The last group derives from reactive forces that cause equal and opposite torques in adjacent limb joints. These forces, in turn, cause centripetal interactions that affect the most proximal joint. The latter also has impinging on it a (Coriolis) torque caused by the velocities of the moving parts of the limb.

The variables of task execution are also under the influence of our perception of how much effort we need to put into carrying out the task. The *sense of effort* reflects our awareness of motor commands. We probably sense it as the consequence of events involving the middle level of the motor hierarchy. It is influenced by such simple factors as peripheral sensations or neuromuscular fatigue. The sense of effort can adjust movements properly only with a normally functioning central nervous system. This would be expected, because it involves comparisons of what is wanted with what is actually achieved.

References

Abend, W., Bizzi, E., and Morasso, P. 1982. Human arm trajectory formation. *Brain* 105:331–348. [Fig. 7.4]

Alexander, McN. 1982. *Animal mechanics.* 2nd ed. Oxford: Blackwell Scientific Publications.

Alexander, McN. 1981. Mechanics of skeleton and tendons. In *Motor Control. Handbook of physiology,* ed. V. B. Brooks, Sect. 1, vol. 2. pp. 17–42. Bethesda, Md.: American Physiological Society.

Beppu, H., Suda, M., and Tanaka, R. 1983. Slow visuomotor tracking in normal man and in patients with cerebellar ataxia. In *Motor control mechanisms in health and disease,* ed. J. E. Desmedt, *Adv. Neurol.* 39:889–895.

Bizzi, E., and Abend, W. 1983. Posture control and trajectory formation in single- and multi-joint arm movements. In *Motor control mechanisms in health and disease,* ed. J. E. Des-

medt. *Adv. Neurol.* 39:31–45. [Figs. 7.4, 7.7E and 7.10]

Bizzi, E., Accornero, N., Chapple, W., and Hogan, N. 1982. Arm trajectory formation in monkeys. *Exp. Brain Res.* 46:139–143. [Figs. 7.7E and 7.8]

Brodal, A. 1973. Self-obervations and neuro-anatomical considerations after a stroke. *Brain* 96:675–694.

Brooks, V. B. 1985. How are "move" and "hold" programs matched? In *Cerebellar functions,* eds. W. J. Bloedel, J. Dichgans, and W. Precht, pp. 1–23 *Proc. Life Sciences.* Berlin: Springer Verlag. [Figs. 7.3, 7.4, 7.5A–C, and 7.9]

Brooks, V. B. 1979. Motor programs revisited. In *Posture and movement,* eds. R. E. Talbott and D. R. Humphrey, pp. 13–49. New York: Raven Press.

Freund, H. J., and Büdingen, H. J. 1978. The relationship between speed and amplitude of the fastest voluntary contractions of human arm muscles. *Exp. Brain Res.* 31:1–12. [Fig. 7.6]

Gordon, J., and Ghez, C. 1984. EMG patterns in antagonist muscles during isometric contraction in man: relations to response dynamics. *Exp. Brain Res.* 55:167–171. [Fig. 7.5D]

Granit, R. 1972 Constant errors in the execution and appreciation of movement. *Brain* 95:649–660.

Hagbarth, K.-E., and Eklund, G. 1966. Motor effects of vibratory stimuli in man. In *Muscular afferents and motor control,* ed. R. Granit. 1st ed., pp. 177–186. New York: John Wiley & Sons.

Hagbarth, K.-E, and Eklund, G. 1969. The muscle vibrator–a useful tool in neurological therapeutic work. *Scand. J. Rehabil. Med.* 1:26–34.

Hollerbach, J. M. 1982. Computers, brains and the control of movement. *Trends Neurosci.* 5:189–192.

Jeannerod, M., and Prablanc, C. 1983. Visual control of reaching movements. In *Motor control mechanisms in health and disease,* ed. J. E. Desmedt. *Adv. Neurol.* 39:12–29. [Fig. 7.3]

Kelso, J. A., ed. 1982. *Human motor behavior: An introduction.* Hillsdale, N.J.: Lawrence Erlbaum Assoc.

Lackner, J. R., and Graybiel, A. 1984. Perceptions of body weight and body mass at twice earth-gravity acceleration levels. *Brain* 107:133–144.

Lestienne, F., Polit, A., and Bizzi, E. 1981.

Functional organization of the motor process underlying the transition from movement to posture. *Brain Res.* 230:121–131. [Fig. 7.5A–C]

Marsden, D. C., Merton, P. A., and Morton, H. B. 1976. Servo action in the human thumb. *J. Physiol. (Lond.)* 257:1–44.

McClockey, D. I. 1981. Corollary discharges: motor commands and perception. In *Motor control.* Sect. 1, vol. 2. *Handbook of physiology,* ed. V. B. Brooks, pp. 1415–1447. Bethesda, Md.: American Physiological Society. [Figs. 7.11 and 7.12]

McCloskey, D. I. 1978. Kinesthetic sensibility. *Physiol. Rev.* 58:763–820.

Nelson, W. L. 1983. Physical principles for economics of skilled movements. *Biol. Cybern.* 46:135–147. [Fig. 7.9]

Partridge, L. D., and Benton L. A. 1981. Muscle, the motor. In *Motor control.* Sect. 1, vol. 2. *Handbook of physiology,*ed. V. B. Brooks, pp. 43–106. Bethesda, Md.: American Physiological Society.

Polit, A. and Bizzi, E. 1979. Characteristics of motor programs underlying arm movements in monkey. *J. Neurophysiol.* 42:183–194. [Fig. 7.7.A–D]

Schmidt, R. A. 1982. *Motor control and learning. A behavioral emphasis.* Champaign, Ill.: Human Kinetics Publishers.

Soechting, J. F., and Lacquaniti, F. 1981. Invariant characteristics of a pointing movement in man. *J. Neurosci.* 1:710–720.

Stein, R. B. 1982. What muscle variable(s) does the nervous system control in limb movements? *Behav. Brain Scis.* 5:535–577.

Viviani, P., and Terzuolo, C. 1980. Space-time invariance in learned motor skills. In *Tutorials in motor behavior,* eds. G. E. Stelmach and J. Requin. *Adv. Psychol.* 1:525–533. [Figs. 7.1 and 7.2]

III

Posture and Locomotion

The brain links willed and unwilled actions in the control of motor performance. This part (Chaps. 8–10) explores the control of two aspects of this performance: posture and locomotion. Postural control is brought about by plans and programs that assemble task-related automatic adjustments of movements and postures. Intended and automatic actions are blended by the CNS to create the intended results by letting planned programs "exit" appropriately into reflex (servo) adjustments. The adjustments are executed largely by interactive stretch reflexes that can be triggered by a number of sensory inputs, ensuring activation if not by one means, then by another. This is a system with many backups. Postural reactions are integrated swiftly to help us keep our balance even during such complex acts as the golf swing in Fig. 1.1, or to keep our eyes trained on objects of interest. The predictive actions of postural programs utilize the brainstem, cerebellum, basal ganglia and cerebrum, whose influence is brought to bear through the descending systems (Figs. 5.7–5.12). This complex task system supports our upright posture through facilitation of postural, antigravity, segmental stretch reflexes and through other postural reactions.

This part begins with a consideration of muscle tone—already introduced in Chap. 3.2—and then progresses to postural control. Brodal made the following eloquent statement about postural reactions.

> *Postural reflexes* is a collective name for a large number of reflexes which tend to preserve the body's posture. The Postural Reflexes ... are of great importance because they are present in the normal human being and are essential for normal motor performances. In lesions of the brainstem the tonic neck and labyrinthine reflexes may appear in exaggerated form.... Furthermore they may be influencing other reflexes.... *They are, therefore, of clinical interest, the more so since some use may be made of these and other postural reflexes in physiotherapeutic exercises in some instances* [italics mine].

Review of the postural reactions is followed by a second, more detailed look at postural programs, to reassess how the brain uses the mass-spring properties of muscle, a concept first introduced in Chaps. 3.2 and 4.2. The chapter concludes with some applications of Nashner's theoretical framework for the control of posture. From the consideration of posture we proceed in Chap. 9 to an analysis of locomotion. Going from stance to step and from step to stance is governed by rhythmic spinal programs that are under tonic control descending from the brain stem, as well as under ascending afferent control from the limbs. Sensory information is evaluated and used for motor adjustments by the middle level of the motor hierarchy for locomotion as it is for posture (and for breathing). Here we deal once more with a well-defined interplay between voluntary and automatic reactions, and as for posture, with a system of great clinical importance.

8
Muscle Tone

1. Normal Tone

Tone is the resistance offered by muscles
to continuous stretch, such as that produced by passive flexion or extension of a
joint. Tone was formerly judged by the examiner's subjective perception of the resistance offered to passive joint rotations, or
sometimes also by the feel of firmness or
other observable activities such as the
EMG. Any measure can be used only,
however, during imposed ("passive")
stretch of the muscles. (An example where
stretch is provided by the action of gravity
is given in Fig. 8.5.) Objective quantitative
measurements are now becoming ever
more common, with controlled rates and
ranges of imposed limb displacements.

In deeply relaxed normal subjects, resistance to joint rotation is moderate and uniform at all speeds, and is probably produced mainly, if not solely, by passive
(viscoelastic) properties of the muscles and
joints. It is unlikely that stretch reflexes
contribute even minimally to tone of a
deeply relaxed subject. Yet, some uncertainty remains, because it has been impossible to evaluate the contributions of *all*
synergistic muscles acting on a joint. Tone
becomes stronger when stretch reflexes are
reinforced through mental concentration
or by muscular exertions such as making a
fist. When we become alert from deep re-

laxation, stretch reflexes are suddenly
turned on. In contrast, tense, nervous subjects cannot switch them off. Muscle tone
is clearly under the influence of diverse supraspinal descending systems. Since the
level of arousal is so important a governor
of tone, it is not surprising that it is heavily
influenced by the balance of cholinergic
and noradrenergic projections from the
forebrain and brain stem.

Joint rotation produces sustained muscle stretch, in contrast to the brief effect of
a tendon tap. The muscular response to
sustained stretch consists of an initial,
brief, intense "phasic" reflex, which declines to a longer lasting, less powerful,
"tonic" level. Both components contribute
to muscle tone. The phasic reflex is predominantly the output of the segmental
motor servo, which includes the actions of
spindles and tendon organs (groups Ia, II
and Ib afferent fibers; Figs. 4.8 and 5.1).
The longer duration of the tonic reflex
gives more opportunity for its supraspinal
modulation. Tonic stretch reflexes of red
muscles, such as the soleus, have lower
thresholds and generate greater force than
those of relatively pale muscles, such as
gastrocnemius. This is in accord with the
properties of tonic and phasic actions of
motor units innervated by small and large
MNs and with Henneman's size principle
(Figs. 4.1–4.3 and 4.5).

The contributions to tension development by the passive (viscoelastic) muscle properties has been assessed for voluntary, active contractions; it amounts to 15%. During maximal voluntary, active contractions, molecular ("crossbridge") bonding of muscles innervated by tonically firing MNs generates about 85% of the tension in the flexors of the human arm when contracting against stretches in their physiological control range (Fig. 8.1). The zone of reflex control is limited by the normal span of joint movement and by the way the muscles are inserted on the bones forming the joint. (In Fig. 3.5, for instance, the cat's leg was rotated through a range of 120 deg, that is, from 150 to 30 deg. By comparison, the physiological range of the human forearm is 150 deg.)

Figure 8.1 shows the functional, physiological limits of reflex control. The figure is based on measurements of active resistance of non-inserted muscles of amputees, and thus can compare "overstretched" values with those limited by normal insertions. All muscles exert maximal active force when they contract at their resting lengths (marked 0 in Fig. 3.6C), which is about 80 deg for the human elbow. It is therefore understandable that the patients declared the resting lengths of their muscles as the most comfortable ones for operating the prosthetic devices to which they could be attached.

Fig. 8.1. The physiological range of control *(shaded region)* set by the limits of joint movement covers about half the length to which muscle can be stretched. Length–tension characteristics of flexor muscles of the human forearm plot maximal voluntary muscle force (active + passive) produced in relation to muscle length. *Passive* curve shows force at corresponding lengths when muscles are entirely relaxed, as in Figs. 3.6A and 4.6A. Compare the physiological range of muscle lengths to those of proprioceptive sensitivities shown in Fig. 4.10. (Modified from Ralston et al., 1948; and from Houk and Rymer, 1981)

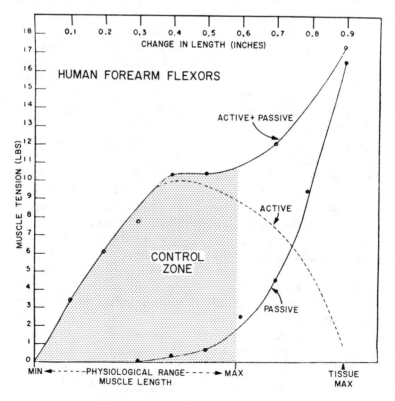

Returning to the stretch reflexes, we ask at what level of contractile effort do they start generating tone? There is no clear answer to this simple question for lack of direct measurements of any participating reflex. We learned in Chap. 4.1 that low-level tone is actively maintained by non-synchronous tonic discharge of small motor units, which respond to stretch at low thresholds and with slow, nonfatiguing contractions. Large, quicker motor units are recruited successively during bigger stretches. Figures 4.3–4.5 imply that slow, tonically active MNs suffice for the production of tone, and that they begin to contribute even with weak activation. This depends, however, on the strength of their supraspinal support: tone is created by alertness and motor set, discussed in Chap. 6.2, for which we lack direct measurements. At low tonic rates, individual twitches do not fuse into tetanic contractions (e.g., below 4 Hz for the slow, red soleus muscle of the cat and below 15 Hz for the fast, pale human dorsal interosseus muscle; Figs. 4.4 and 4.5). Even these low rates of tonic stretch reflex maintenance require support by descending facilitation, according to the model of cat reflexes. In the cat, tonic stretch reflexes are not maintained in relaxed, intact animals (or in spinal ones); but only during the extremely strong supraspinal support provided by decerebrate rigidity. This recalls the tensing of limbs by supraspinal long loops (Fig. 6.7), suggesting that normal muscle tone may be the consequence of the tonic control of joint stiffness by impulses in the long-loop paths, which are important devices for matching move and hold programs. They dampen oscillations, which can be caused by loading a limb (Figs. 6.8 and 6.9), and do so even before they can begin ("phase-advance"). Damping is caused by the proprioceptive velocity and acceleration sensitivities in the reflex pathway as well as the predictive timing of supraspinal influences.

The role of the fusimotor system in tone is unclear because of the paucity of relevant data. Tone can be mimicked experimentally in humans and in animals by evoking slow contractions of muscles by means of vibrating muscle tissue or tendons. In humans, this *tonic vibration reflex* resembles the tonic stretch reflex in many ways, including its responsiveness to cortical descending facilitation. Vibration mimics the output of the whole motor servo because it usually excites Ib and group II afferents besides group Ia (unless its amplitude is kept small with the most rigorous controls; See Figs. 4.8 and 5.1). At present, this method is the most useful tool for the study of tone.

The frustration with our ignorance of the extent of fusimotor participation in maintaining tone has led to various experimental approaches, all futile so far. One of the most widely used methods for studying spinal excitability has been the H-reflex (introduced in Chap. 5.1), which is evoked by electrical stimulation of a nerve through the skin. The resulting phasic reflex contains monosynaptic and polysynaptic components, operating under supraspinal control as discussed in Chap. 6.2. Thus, the H-reflex is not just a model of the tendon jerk, with a mere substitution of electrical for physiologically adequate stimulation. Since the two processes generate different afferent input patterns to the spinal cord, comparison of the two reflexes cannot tell us how much the fusimotor drive is engaged, as was formerly believed. Supposedly differential nerve block by procaine infiltration of the motor point has also turned out to be invalid because of difficulties in maintaining stable, local tissue concentrations. The H-reflex can, however, be used to test the excitability of alpha-MN pools, using classical conditioning-type testing techniques. Recurrent inhibition (Fig. 5.4) can be tested by double stimulation of a nerve at various intervals to plot the time course of the inhibition; "autogenic" Ib inhibition (Fig. 5.5) can be tested by stimulation of two synergistic nerves, and reciprocal Ia inhibition (Fig. 5.2) by stimulation of the nerves of a pair of antagonistic muscles. Similarly, reflex modulation by previous excitation of skin nerves can be tested. This may yet become useful for the study of some aspects of tone, since descending supraspinal systems modulate the cord through spinal INs (Chap. 5.2).

2. Abnormal Tone

Hypertonia: Abnormally High Tone

Tone may appear normal when a limb is tested with slow rotations, but at higher speeds active resistance, felt as a "catch," may suddenly become apparent. (A modern quantitative assessment of responses at different speeds consists of controlled mechanical oscillations of the limb at different frequencies.) This phasic component of the stretch reflex is usually found when there are disorders of descending tracts. We now need to define spasticity and rigidity, and to examine how far the fusimotor system is involved.

Spasticity is accompanied by an elevated state of tone in patients that present with "hyper-reflexia" of both tonic and phasic stretch reflexes. Spasticity becomes apparent only with tests at several speeds of imposed limb movements, because spastic resistance to applied stretch is proportional to the velocity of the applied stretch.

In *spinal spasticity,* after chronic section of the spinal cord, tendon jerks are exaggerated and can become oscillatory by re-excitation *(clonus).* In partial spinal sections, clonus, which can usually be obtained at the ankle, may be under bulbospinal facilitatory drive. (Mechanisms that normally help prevent clonus were discussed in Chap. 6.2; Figs. 6.7 and 6.8). In addition to clonus, flexor spasms are common in spinal spasticity. Responses to input from flexor reflex afferents (FRA) lead to exaggerated flexor facilitation and extensor inhibition when the descending moderation by the reticular and vestibular systems is cut off by spinal lesions. The re-

sulting reductions of spinal inhibitions and facilitations trigger the *clasp-knife phenomenon,* in which the ability of stretched extensors (e.g., at the elbow or knee) fails at a certain point of resistance. Typically, the resistive contraction of the extensor quadriceps tends to melt away when the knee is bent to 90 deg. Figure 8.2 indicates (for the decerebrate animal model) how spinal section removes the inhibition that normally descends to FRA INs through the dorsolateral reticulospinal tract, and the facilitation of alpha MNs by the lateral vestibulospinal tract. These two descending paths are spontaneously active in the decerebrate state, leading to decerebrate rigidity, discussed below. Spinal section removes the descending inhibition and excitation, but the spinal spastic state is not, as was once thought, caused by hyperactive fusimotor drive. Directly recorded

Fig. 8.2. Extensor rigidity is generated in the decerebrate cat by spontaneous activity of descending systems, now released from cerebral inhibition. Subsequent spinal section of the dorsal reticulospinal and lateral vestibulospinal tracts enhances FRA inhibition (and vestibulospinal facilitation) of extensor MNs. Sufficient stretch of the knee flexors brings on the pathological clasp-knife reflex inhibition of knee extensors, by afferent excitation of flexor stretch afferents (high threshold, groups II, III and IV), which facilitate FRA INs. Compare to Figs. 5.6 and 8.3. (From Houk and Rymer, 1981)

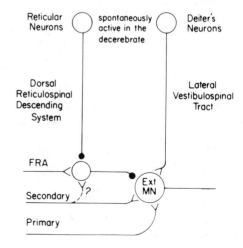

spindle responses to stretch, and their fusimotor support, are normal in patients with spinal spasticity.

Cerebral spasticity is the name for a variety of conditions caused by lesions rostral to (i.e., above) the brain stem. This condition exhibits fewer flexor spasms and less of the clasp-knife reflex (which may be absent entirely in the upper limbs), presumably because the uninterrupted dorsal lateral reticulospinal tract is functioning relatively normally, not being under direct cortical control. In contrast, the lateral vestibulospinal tract is disinhibited, which favors extension (particularly in "decerebrate rigidity" of cats, see below). In human hemiplegic spasticity, the effects are most severe in leg extensors and arm flexors. The tonic vibration reflex is depressed or absent. Tendon jerks are often exaggerated. As in the case of spinal section, the main effects in chronically affected patients and animal preparations are on alpha MNs. The primary impairment can be due to limited and prolonged recruitment during onset of agonist contraction and its delayed cessation at movement termination. Fusimotor drive is normal in human cerebral spasticity, as shown by recordings from single muscle afferent fibers (microneurography).

The most plausible current view is that human spasticity of supraspinal origin results from varying imbalanced facilitation and inhibition descending to the spinal cord from damaged or disconnected cerebral cortex. The cord is disinhibited by the interruption of the normal cortical excitatory input to the medullary reticular formation, whose output (through the lateral reticulospinal tract; Figs. 5.7 and 5.8) ordinarily *inhibits* antigravity (i.e., extensor) spinal reflexes and promotes voluntary (flexor) functions (Chap. 5.2). Thus there is spinal disinhibition of extensors. [This is equivalent to Magoun's original description of the action of the "inhibitory (medullary) reticular formation" in the cat.] In the human there is, in addition, facilitated promotion of extensor reflexes by the *fa-*

cilitatory pontine reticulospinal and vestibulospinal tracts, which are less affected by cortical lesions because they lack direct cortical controls (see Chap. 5.2). Magoun had described excitatory drive from the caudate nucleus of the basal ganglia to the cat's "facilitatory" reticular formation, whose identification as a single structure is now being splintered by more searching, new techniques. The multiple functions of these descending systems, discussed in Chap. 5.2, warn us to think of spasticity as the net result of supraspinal and spinal causes. A promising animal model, with normal spindle responses to stretch, has been developed by Tasker through bilateral lesions of monkeys' areas 4 and 6 (that disconnect their descending projections to the brainstem; Fig. 5.9).

The situation resembles, but is not the same as, that in the *decerebrate cat* prepared by acute midbrain section, because fusimotor drive is elevated in that animal model. Figure 8.3 shows how cortical disconnection releases bilateral reticular facilitation of spinal extensors that outweighs unilateral reticular inhibition. In addition, extensor MNs are driven by the vestibulospinal system [originating in the lateral vestibular (Deiter's) nucleus: Figs. 5.8 and 8.2] which is under direct cerebellar and indirect cortical control. The importance of extensor facilitation by the vestibulospinal system is borne out by the collapse of reflex-standing and the lowered tone after interruption of the vestibulospinal tracts. After decerebration, peripheral input to the lateral extensor facilitatory area (rostral and lateral to the pontine facilitatory area; see Fig. 5.8) remains and adds extensor facilitation to the disinhibition. Both tracts act on alpha as well and as on gamma MNs, but the relative effect is greater on the (smaller) gamma MNs that are recruited first. Thus, in contrast to the chronic human condition, the acutely decerebrate cat has abnormally high gamma activity that in turn affects the input from muscle receptors, as proved by the loss of extensor tone after section of the dorsal roots. This reasonably coherent view of the acute animal model does not, however, implicate tonic fusimotor drive in the maintenance of normal muscle tone in normal animals and humans. The role of the fusimotor system in tone is still elusive.

Rigidity in patients with Parkinson's disease is characterized by hypertonia (mostly in the flexors of arms and legs) that is not closely related to velocity of muscle stretch. Tonic reflexes are elevated, the tonic vibration reflex may be increased, and phasic stretch reflexes are normal. Fusimotor drive is no higher than that in healthy subjects who are as nonrelaxed as a patient with parkinsonism.

Rigidity (as well as chronic human spasticity) has often been compared to acute decerebrate rigidity of the cat, discussed above. We now see that the fusimotor aspect of this animal model does not correspond to either of these two clinical entities. Spasticity was characterized above by imbalanced descending supraspinal controls. The main abnormality of patients with Parkinson's rigidity is the saturated, high gain of medium-latency (M2) responses to muscle stretch. Long-loop responses are set at the upper limit of their physiological range and thus cannot be modulated voluntarily. This is apparent in the EMG records of Fig. 8.4B when compared to those in Fig. 8.4A of normal M1, M2 and M3 responses followed by voluntary activity (cf. Fig. 6.1). In Fig. 8.4B, M2 and M3 are fused and very large. When resistance to stretch is unwanted, they do not abate as in normal subjects, but instead remain as large during passive stretch as during active resistance. Quantitative comparison of normal and parkinsonian M2–M3 long-loop responses requires that they are set into perspective (calibrated) in terms of initial velocities of the test movements and of the background EMG levels.

Fig. 8.3. Diagram of the major pathways involved in decerebrate and decerebellate rigidity. Midbrain (mesencephalic) transection (along *broken line* **A**) produces decerebrate rigidity. Additional disruption (*line* **B**: by occlusion of carotid arteries to produce "anemic decerebration") of inhibition from the cerebellum onto Deiter's nucleus and fastigial nuclei produces decerebellate rigidity. Facilitation and inhibition indicated by (+) and (−). (From Carew, 1981)

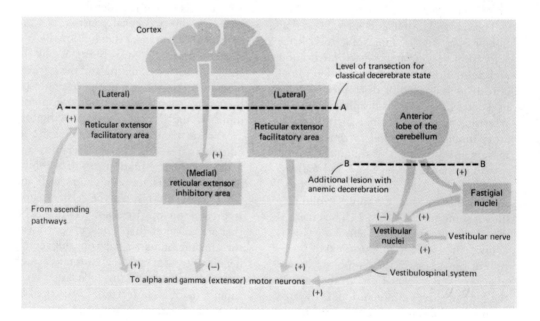

Values obtained from patients with Parkinson's disease rise well above the normal range (Fig. 8.4C).

The clinical picture is matched by findings with a useful animal model for Parkinson's disease: monkeys intoxicated with phenothiazine. The results suggest that the basal ganglia normally regulate the gain of long-loop, transcortical responses. The result is in line with the suggestion, made in Chap. 6.2, that long-loop responses may function in the normal maintenance of muscle tone. Their involvement is most likely mediated through spinal interneurons (INs). These neurons form circuits that perform integrative functions at the spinal level, such as adjusting the action of descending controls

and the relative strengths of opposing muscles (Chap. 5.1). These circuits become inoperative when spinal INs are put out of action, for example by ischemia of the spinal cord. This is, in fact, a very effective method for producing experimental rigidity.

Hypotonia: Abnormally Low Tone

This condition may develop with cerebellar disease, but is not always observed because it may regress after some weeks. Figure 8.5 illustrates how muscle tone on the affected side can be assessed from the angle that the hands make with the forearm in the relaxed position. Depressed discharges of spinal gamma MNs and elevated stretch

Fig. 8.4. Patients with Parkinson's disease have excessively large long-loop (M2 + M3) responses to muscle stretch. Responses of the wrist to abrupt load changes (at 0 time on abscissas) in normal (A) and rigid parkinsonian (B) subjects. Long-loop responses remain large in patients even when they are passive. (C) Normalized display of large M2–M3 (= M2 + M3) components for four parkinsonian patients (see symbols), made comparable by corrections for background EMG and initial velocities, plotted on the abscissas. The normal range is displayed three dimensionally by the tilted slab. [(A,B) From Lee and Tatton, 1978; (C) from Lee, Murphy and Tatton, 1983; as presented at the International Conference on Neurophysiological Basis of Motor Disorders, Chicago, 1982]

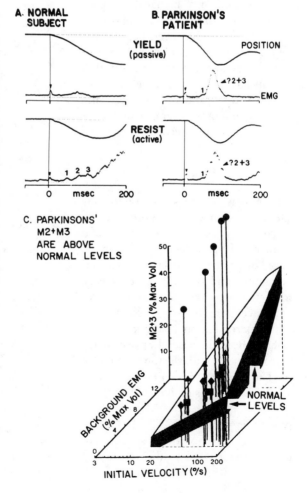

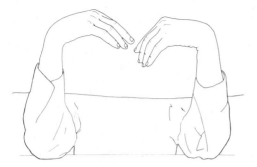

Fig. 8.5. The pull of gravity on relaxed hand postures reveals hypotonia of a patient with cerebellar disease on the left side. (Traced from Lance and McLeod, 1981)

thresholds of muscle spindles in acutely decerebellate monkeys have led Gilman to suggest that decreased gamma bias is a major cause of experimentally produced cerebellar hypotonia. Whether this applies to the hypotonia of the chronic patient is still open to doubt, however, because the level of gamma drive is higher than normal in the acute preparations. Another suggestion has been that cerebellar hypotonia may be a by-product of the dysfunction, or loss, of motor programs, with consequent deficient premovement tensing of muscles.

3. Summary

Muscle tone is the resistance offered by muscles to continuous stretch produced by (imposed) passive flexion or extension of a joint. In deeply relaxed subjects, tone is produced by passive viscoelastic properties of the muscles and joints. In alert subjects, stretch reflexes contribute to tone, under the influence of motor set. The extent of fusimotor participation in the generation of tone is uncertain. Useful answers may come from studies with the tonic vibration reflex. The H-reflex, which evokes phasic responses, is a less suitable tool for this study.

Hypertonia occurs clinically as spasticity and rigidity. Spastic resistance to stretch is proportional to the velocity of applied stretch. Chronic spinal spasticity is characterized by clonic tendon jerks and by flexor spasms, of which the clasp-knife reflex is a variant. Flexor release is caused by descending disinhibition of the FRA. Cerebral spasticity has less flexor release, and is probably due to disinhibition of spinal MNs from normally descending reticulospinal inhibition. Fusimotor drive is normal in both types of chronic human spasticity. Rigidity is characterized by hypertonia (mostly in flexors) that is not closely related to the velocity of joint displacement. Fusimotor drive is no higher in patients with parkinsonism than it is in normal humans who are equally unrelaxed. Parkinsonian rigidity is marked by abnormally strong long-loop (M2–M3) responses to passive limb displacements, even when no resistance is offered. The raised fusimotor levels in acutely decerebrate cats make them unsuitable as animal models for spasticity or rigidity.

Hypotonia may develop after cerebellar disease, but it may regress after some weeks. It is uncertain whether cerebellar hypotonia is caused by depressed fusimotor drive. Alternately, hypotonia may be a by-product of the dysfunction of motor programs.

References

Brodal, A. 1981. *Neurological anatomy. 3rd ed.* New York: Oxford Univerity Press.

Brooks, V. B. 1979. Control of intended limb movements by the lateral and intermediate cerebellum. In *Integration in the nervous system*, eds. V. J. Wilson and H. Asanuma, pp. 321–358. Tokyo: Igaku-Shoin.

Burke, D. 1983. Critical examination of the case for and against fusimotor involvement in disorders of muscle tone. In *Motor control mechanisms in health and disease*, ed. J. E. Desmedt. *Adv. Neurol.* 39:133–150.

Burke, D., Hagbarth, K. E., Wallin, B. G., and Loefstedt, L. 1980. Muscle spindle activity induced by vibration in man: implications for the tonic stretch reflex. In *Spinal and supraspinal mechanisms of voluntary motor control and locomotion*, ed. J. E. Desmedt. *Prog. Clin. Neurophysiol.* 8:243–253.

Carew, T. J. 1981. Descending control of

spinal circuits. In *Principles of neural science,* eds. E. R. Kandel and J. H. Schwartz. New York: Elsevier/North-Holland. [Fig. 8.3]

Desmedt, J. E. 1983. Mechanismsm of vibration-induced inhibition or potentiation: tonic vibration reflex and vibration paradox in man. In *Motor control mechanisms in health and disease,* ed. J. E. Desmedt. *Adv. Neurol.* 39: 671–683.

Dimitrijevic, M. R., Fanagel, J., Lehmkuhl, D., and Sherwood, A. 1983. Motor control in man after partial or complete spinal cord injury. In *Motor control mechanisms in health and disease,* ed. J. E. Desmedt. *Adv. Neurol.* 39:915–926.

Gauthier, G. M., Roll, J. P., Hugon, M., and Martin, B. 1983. Motor dyscontrol as a hazard in massive body vibration in man. In *Motor control mechanisms in health and disease,* ed. J. E. Desmedt. *Adv. Neurol.* 39:685–697.

Gilman, S. 1969. The mechanism of cerebellar hypotonia: an experimental study in the monkey. *Brain* 92:621–638.

Gottlieb, G. L., and Agarwal, G. C. 1978. Sinusoidal oscillation of the ankle as a means of evaluating the "spastic" patient. *J. Neurol. Neurosurg. Psychiatry* 41:32–39.

Herman, R. 1970. The myotatic reflex: clinico-physiological aspects of spasticity and contracture. *Brain* 93:273–312.

Houk, J. C., and Rymer, J. C. 1981. Neural control of muscle length and tension. In *Motor control.* Sect. 1, vol. 2. *Handbook of physiology,* ed. V. B. Brooks, pp. 257–323. Bethesda, Md.: American Physiological Society. [Figs. 8.1 and 8.2]

Katz, R., and Pierrot-Deseilligny, E. 1982. Recurrent inhibition of alpha-motoneurons in patients with upper motor neuron lesions. *Brain* 105:103–124.

Lance, J. W., and McLeod, J. B. 1981. *A physiological approach to clinical neurology.* London: Butterworths. [Fig. 8.5]

Lance, J. W., de Gail, P. and Neilson, P. D. 1966. Tonic and phasic spinal cord mechanisms in man. *J. Neurol. Neurosurg. Psychiatry* 29:539–544.

Landau, W. M. 1974. Spasticity: the fable of a neurological demon and the emperor's new therapy. *Arch. Neurol.* 31:217–219.

Lee, R. G., and Tatton, W. G. 1978. Long-loop reflexes in man: clinical applications. In *Cerebral motor control in man: long-loop mechanisms,* ed. J. E. Desmedt. *Prog. Clin. Neurophysiol.* 4:320–330. [Fig. 8.4A,B]

Lee, R. G., Murphy, J. T., and Tatton, W. G. 1983. Long-latency myotatic reflexes in man: mechanisms, functional significance, and changes in patients with Parkinson's disease or hemiplegia. In *Motor control mechanisms in health and disease,* ed. J. Desmedt. *Adv. Neurol.* 39:489–508. [Fig. 8.4C]

Nashner, L. M. 1979. Organization and programming of motor activity during posture control. In *Reflex control of posture and movement,* eds. R. Granit and O. Pompeiano, *Prog. Brain Res.* 50:177–184.

Neilson, P. D., and Lance, J. W. 1978. Reflex transmission characteristics during voluntary activity in normal man and patients with movement disorders. In *Cerebral motor control in man: long-loop mechanisms,* ed. J. E. Desmedt. *Prog. Clin. Neurophysiol.* 4:263–299.

Ralston, H. J., Inman, V. T. Strait, A. and Shaffarth, M. D. 1948. Mechanics of human isolated muscle. *Am. J. Physiol.* 151:612–620. [Fig. 8.1]

Sahrmann, S. A., and Norton, B. J. 1977. The relationship of voluntary movement to spasticity in the upper motor neuron syndrome. *Ann. Neurol.* 2:460–465.

Tasker, R. R., Gentili, F., Hwang, P. and Sogabe, K. 1980. Animal models of spasticity and treatment with dentatectomy. In *Spasticity: disordered motor control,* ed. R. G. Feldman, R.R. Young and W. P. Koella, pp. 155–177. Chicago: Year Book Med. Publishers.

Veale, J. L., Rees, S., and Mark, R. F. 1973. Renshaw cell activity in normal and spastic man. In *Human reflexes, pathophysiology of motor systems, methodology of human reflexes,* ed. J. E. Desmedt. *New Devel. Electromyogr. Clin. Neurophysiol.* 3:523–538.

Wiesendanger, M. 1985. Is there an animal model of spasticity? In *Clinical neurophysiology in spasticity,* eds. P. J. Delwaide and R. R. Young, pp. 1–12, Amsterdam: Elsevier Science Publishers BV (Biomedical Division)

Wiesendanger, M. 1972. *Pathophysiology of muscle tone.* Berlin: Springer Verlag.

9
Postural Control

The control of posture provides good examples of how the brain coordinates reflexes into behavioral patterns. We begin this topic by refreshing our memory about the classical "postural reactions" discovered by Magnus, his co-workers, and those who followed them. We conclude the topic by integrating their findings into the recent, rational approach by Nashner and his associates. One important aspect of postural control is emphasized throughout: the use of multiple backup controls. Posture is safeguarded by multiple inputs and outputs. It reflects the care that evolution has bestowed on the capability to adjust the body to the direction of gravity, and parts of the body in relation to each other. Since we depend heavily on visual orientation, particular care is given to how we keep our gaze directed to where it is needed—how we "keep our eyes on the ball," so to speak.

The most telling indication that postural adjustments are programmed is the timing: we coordinate muscle tensions before beginning a postural task such as righting ourselves, or bending to lift an object. A whole array of postural subprograms will be presented, many of which can generate acceptable postures without assistance of the others. The object of postural control is the functional end result; there is no single preferred "controlled

variable." The CNS uses any strategy and tactic that works to achieve the intent of the individual under the circumstances of the moment. As the chapters that follow will show, these comments apply to voluntary movements as much as to postural adjustments.

Many practical implications derive from the study of posture. The recognition that the positions of the head and the eyes, as well as of the body and the limbs, are all interdependent is widely used. This knowledge has led to improved industrial designs of the environment for work and to more rational plans for the execution of many sports. The aims in both areas are to optimize muscular peak efforts and to reduce fatigue. They are equally important in daily activities such as preserving a good posture when walking, sitting or lying down, or, for example, when driving a car. The clinical importance was stressed at the beginning of this part: it affects orthopedics, the clinical neurological sciences, and rehabilitation, and it offers great opportunities to occupational and physical therapy.

1. Righting Reactions

The head is ordinarily righted by the neck muscles under visual guidancy by *optical* and *labyrinthine* righting "reflexes." The latter are activated by the vestibular apparatus, which provides "dynamic" sensors for rotations (i.e., angular acceleration) in the semicircular ducts and for linear acceleration (such as gravity) in the otoliths, as well as "static" position sensors in the utricle and saccule. These sensory structures for interstitial receptors and the cochlea, sketched in Fig. 9.1, are filled with endolymph whose movement bends the hair cells in the sensory epithelium (called macula). The sensors of each duct are located in enlargements near the utricle, from which the ducts begin and to which they return. The macula in the utricle is oriented roughly in parallel with the ground, while that in the saccule is more or less vertical. Both structures (called otoliths) serve to detect changes in head position, which is accomplished by changes of pressure exerted by calcium carbonate crystals embedded in the tissue above the sensory cells. Their signals initiate the *static vestibular* "reflexes." In the absence of vision, normal head posture is preserved by the neck muscles under the influence of the

otoliths, which can reflect static head orientation accurately within a range of 30 deg of "static tilt" from the direction of gravity. These labyrinthine reflexes not only thus help vision define the vertical, but they also help to damp movement oscillations. The semicircular canals signal the angular velocity of the head, and stabilize it by evoking postural reflexes that also activate appropriate antigravity limb muscles (see Fig. 9.7). The vestibulospinal tract has already been introduced (in Chap. 5.2) as the path through which extensor, antigravity muscles are adjusted in relation to the position of the head. The postural role of the vestibulospinal system was stressed, since it promotes segmental standing reflexes. Vestibulospinal facilitation of static gamma MNs was suggested as a mode of activating postural, isometric adjustments of muscle tension and slow, small self-initiated movements. In other words, the postural actions of the vestibulospinal system may be brought about in part by servo-assistance of muscle spindles.

Postural "reflexes" are really a series of

Fig. 9.1. Vestibular and auditory structures. The utricle and saccule contain receptors that measure "static" position as well as linear acceleration (e.g., gravity). The three semicircular ducts contain "dynamic" receptors that measure rotation, that is, angular acceleration. The auditory cochlear duct is connected with these structures, which all contain endolymph. (From Barr and Kiernan, 1983)

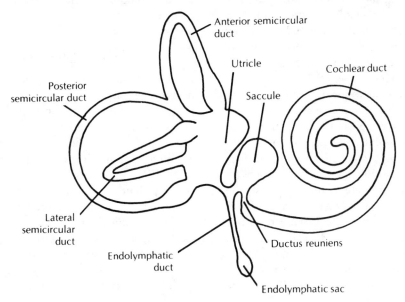

reactions that are coordinated by central connections that include the vestibular nuclei. The reflexes continue after interruption of sensory inflow to neck muscles and joints. Vestibular reflexes for adjustment of the neck *(vestibulocollic)* form a closed loop, because the labyrinths receive feedback about the resulting head movement. Labyrinthine and neck reflexes stabilize the head by acting in opposite directions, thus canceling for head movements as long as the trunk is fixed. During head tilt, eye position (gaze) is maintained by similar reflexes of the extraocular muscles. The central pathways for the expression of vestibular integration have been detailed in Chap. 5.2 (see Fig. 5.7). The vestibulospinal tracts (Fig. 9.2) relay two important aspects of head orientation: static information from the utricle and saccule is carried by the lateral one (LVST), and phasic information from the semicircular canals is carried by the medial tract (MVST). Integrative vestibular signals reach the spinal cord also through the reticulospinal tract, because there are many interactions between the vestibular nuclei and the reticular formation. The reticulospinal output is integrated by the cerebellum by virtue of its input from the lateral reticular nucleus (LRN, Fig 5.5B and Chap. 13), which coordinates macular and neck afferents. The anatomical contiguity and the similar actions of the vestibulospinal and the medial reticulospinal tracts were noted in Chap. 5.2, and the apposition of their nuclei is stressed in Figs. 5.8 and 9.2.

Another system for righting the head depends on nonsymmetrical contacts with the body surface. This can continue to function without visual or labyrinthine inputs. The body contacts trigger peripherally and centrally interlocked stretch reflexes that terminate in adjustments of the neck. The are called *body-righting reflexes acting on the head.* All of these reactions can be demonstrated in decorticate animals, with the exception of optical righting that depends on intact visual cortex. The reactions, however, normally also use

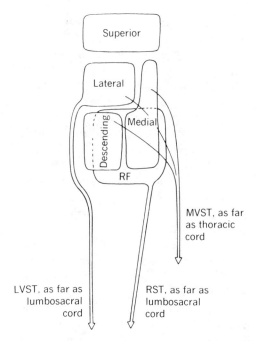

Fig. 9.2. Diagram of the origin of lateral and medial vestibulospinal tracts (LVST and MVST) in the vestibular nuclei and of the extent of their spinal descent. Also shown are the pontine and medullary reticulospinal tracts (drawn together as RST), which originate from the pontine and medullary reticular formation (RF). Compare to Figs. 5.7 and 5.8. (From Wilson, 1975; in Wilson and Peterson, 1980)

cerebral support, without which they become deficient.

2. Eye–Head Coordination

Reflexes elicited from the semicircular canals compensate for changes in eye or head position to maintain a constant direction of gaze. This is another instance where overall programs guide the object of greatest attention, in this case the eyes (see Chap. 7.1). If a person is rotated in a revolving chair, the resulting reflexes turn the eyes and head in the direction opposite to the rotation through the angle of rotated displacement. If rotation continues so as to drive the eyes to the limits of their movement range, the eyes snap back quickly (in a saccade-like movement) to a fixation point, from which the slow counter-rotation begins again (nystagmus). The slow component is driven from input arising in the labyrinths, and the quick reset is brought about by the same brain stem nuclei that generate voluntary saccades. Since the labyrinths do not receive feedback about eye movements, the *vestibulo-ocular reflexes* (VOR) operate in the "open loop" (or "feedforward") mode.

When we take a look at a stationary object, the eyes and head cooperate to keep the gaze fixated on the target. The cooperation is organized through vestibulo-ocular reflexes that monitor head movements and adjust saccadic eye movements to cancel any deviation of central (foveal) vision from the target. This reflex action ensures that we always have the greatest freedom for adjustment of vision. The reflex clears the stage for independent programming of head and eye movements, because any mismatch is automatically corrected, particularly at high frequencies. At low frequencies, gaze control is aided in addition by visual receptors that sense slippage of the retinal image (*optokinetic reflex*, OKR). This measure of visual accuracy activates the same brain stem nuclei as the vestibular speedometer. The gaze is kept on target, no matter whether the head turns first (VOR) or the eyes turn first

(OKR). In either case, gaze is achieved by the summed eye saccades plus head movements.

Conscious vision is suppressed during eye saccades, so our perception of the visual environment remains stationary. Foveation is followed by smooth pursuit, operated for small adjustments by head adjustments. Figure 9.3 demonstrates the remarkable similarity between the eye saccade (A), which has to do all the work when the head is prevented from turning, and the same result achieved by the sum of saccade and head movement (B) when both are free to move. The inverse situation applies to some patients with Parkinson's disease, who cannot make large saccades and therefore turn the head instead. The same cooperation between head and eye movements occurs in sequential examinations of stationary and moving targets. Figure 9.3 is a good example of how multiple sensory inputs can serve the same purpose in postural control, providing backup means of achieving an essential result. When repetitive action is called for, the vestibulo-ocular reflex adapts for optimal performance. This adaptation will be related to movement adaptation and to cerebellar function in Chap. 13.6. Cooperation between two systems, such as head and eyes, is the rule rather than the excep-

Fig. 9.3. Eye and head movements cooperate to maintain the direction of gaze. (A) Eye saccade to a suddenly appearing target, made by a monkey whose head is prevented from moving. (B) When head is free to move, gaze (G) equals the saccade from (A), but it now consists of the sum of the eye saccade (E) and head movement (H). (From Morasso, Bizzi and Dichgans, 1973; in Bizzi, 1981)

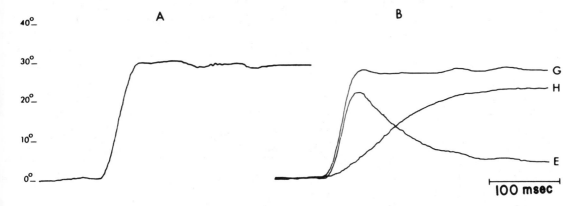

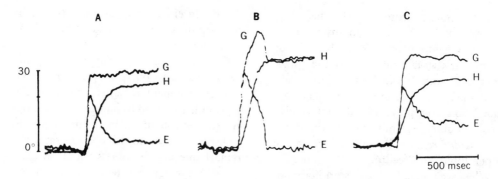

Fig. 9.4. Eye and head movements can compensate for loss of labyrinthine reflexes. (A) Normal eye–head coordination of a monkey (conditions and labels as in Fig. 9.3). (B) Coordination 40 days after bilateral labyrinthectomy, when gaze overshoots but is corrected by saccade. (C) Coordination 120 days after labyrinthectomy, when performance has returned close to normal. (From Dichgans, Bizzi, Morasso and Tagliasco, 1973; in Wilson and Peterson, 1980)

tion: the jaws and the lower lip, for instance, work together to keep the sum of their displacements constant in the production of speech.

The programming of head and eye movements presupposes that the brain has "reference" information about the positions of the head and of the eyes in their orbits. Head position is signaled by the labyrinths and neck proprioceptors, and eye position is computed from comparison of visual input and knowledge of head position. (Eye position may also be signaled by spindle-like receptors in the extraocular muscles to the superior colliculus, but it is uncertain if this initates reflex head adjustments.) Commands for eye positions are encoded by neurons in the cortical frontal eye fields and in the midbrain and brain stem. Visual and vestibular inputs are coordinated by the cerebellum after confluence in the nucleus reticularis tegmenti pontis (NRTP; Chap. 13). Eye movements thus involve complex calculations. For moving targets, the perceived target velocity is signaled to those parts of the CNS that govern movements of the head and eyes. This lets the extraocular muscles take over if the head cannot follow, as in Fig. 9.3A, without a (visually appreciated) break in gaze accuracy.

The neck plays a very important part in postural control. Afferent information from neck proprioceptors, particularly the numerous spindles in the perivertebral neck muscles, is used for adjusting the positions of the eyes as well as of the limbs. *Cervico-ocular reflexes* move the eyes in the direction of body displacement if it occurs while the head cannot move, as in Fig. 9.4A. The plasticity with which the brain can achieve a goal is well illustrated by the ability of these reflexes to direct and steady the gaze in the absence of labyrinthine function. Pathological gaze overshoot, but corrected by a saccade, after a month in that condition is illustrated in Fig. 9.4B. Essentially normal function has returned 3 months later (Fig. 9.4C).

Head movements toward a previously learned target are corrected after perturbations. These corrections can be made entirely with feedforward guidance. Figure 9.5 illustrates how a chronically vestibulectomized monkey makes visually triggered head movements (Fig. 9.5C) toward a position where a familiar target had been shown briefly before movement onset (Fig. 9.5A). When an impeding load caused the head to stop short of the target ("undershoot"), the correct final position was reached after the load was removed. Figure 9.5B demonstrates that the same result was achieved even after that monkey's neck re-

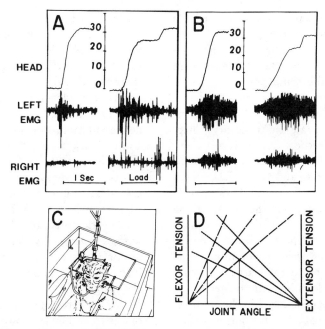

Fig. 9.5. Corrections of head position to a learned target can be made accurately without postural reflexes or visual guidance. (A) Visually triggered head movements made by a chronically vestibulectomized monkey to an (unseen) learned target position. Records on the right in each panel show corrections after adding and removing a load. (B) Same final end position is obtained after deafferentation of the neck. (C) Monkey in task chair, with head attached to torque motor through which loads can be applied. (D) Schematic representation of how muscle length–tension curves can determine angular positions of a (hinge) joint. Compare to Figs. 3.4 and 7.7. [(A,B) From Bizzi, Dev, Morasso and Polit, 1978; in Bizzi, 1981; (C) from Bizzi, Polit and Morasso, 1976; in Bizzi, 1980; (D) from Bizzi, Accornero, Chapple and Hogan, 1982; in Bizzi and Abend, 1983)

flexes were abolished by section of the cervical and thoracic dorsal roots, in addition to the previous removal of vestibular reflexes. Figure 9.5D diagrams a plausible explanation of this remarkable approximation to Fel'dman's mass-spring system in operation (see Figs. 3.4 and 4.6). The brain seems to remember the equilibrium lengths of muscles participating in learned movements, as we have already seen in Figs. 7.7 and 7.8. In this case they are the neck muscles that previously had brought the head to the correct position. The brain can program alpha MNs (to make muscles assume previously successful length–tension relations) with feedforward commands in the absence of proprioceptive and vestibular inputs.

The accuracy of this feedforward guidance system is good enough for reaching relatively wide (i.e., easily learned) target positions. This explanation would account for the undershooting of movements in the right records of Fig. 9.5A,B, when the head was made to turn against unexpected loads that could not be sensed because of deafferentation and vestibulectomy. Load compensation, discussed in Chap. 6.2, must in this experiment be the result of feedforward commands and of the visco-elastic properties of the contracting muscles.

This experiment illustrates a common rule, introduced in Chap. 6: usually tonic muscle actions are commanded by tonic spinal discharges, and phasic actions by phasic bursts. An example of the rule, and an exception to it, are illustrated in Fig. 7.5B,C. Movement end points are determined by tonic muscle actions, while the trajectory (i.e., the path to be followed at a certain velocity) is determined by phasic muscle actions. Such phasic and tonic actions combine as one rides on the other. In this instance, the tonic position ("hold") commands cannot specify velocity: that is accomplished by the phasic "move" commands that integrate the trajectory (Chap. 6.2 and 6.4). We know that trajectory compensation is implemented by phasic stretch responses (Fig. 6.6, and Chap. 7.1), which are inoperative in these monkeys because the afferent path from the neck to the spinal cord had been cut. In this condition, they cannot combine the learned movement with a new velocity, or movements to new end points at the learned velocity, because motor learning requires feedback. The slow movement speed in the right record of Fig. 9.5B, against an impeding load, may be due partly to postoperative weakness and perhaps also in part to the dependence of all feedforward programs on updates by peripheral feedback, which here are cut off by denervation. In this "open-loop" experiment, long-loop responses, discussed in Chap. 6.2 and visibly active in the EMG records of Fig. 9.5, cannot be servo-generated and therefore are programmed (triggered, reaction-time) responses instead. In the normal situation they probably are a mixture of both types.

Overall guidance of a goal to be attained has also been demonstrated for speech movements, which depend primarily on the jaws and lips (as well as the tongue, chest wall, vocal cords, and glottis). Speech is a planned activity, which depends on successive individual, "continuous" lip movements. We manage to generate normal speech gestures despite unexpected mechanical interference with the jaw or lips. Measurements have been made of the action of the jaw muscles, lower-lip depressors and upper-lip depressors and elevators, for instance when the lower lip has to overcome unexpected loads. Compensatory responses of lip movements with a variety of facial muscles have been de-

scribed by Abbs, analogous to the head and eye movement compensations described above. Kinematic and EMG data suggest that the corrections that preserve intended speech gestures are made with feedforward as well as feedback controls.

A rare example of human peripheral deafferentation, documented by Marsden and co-workers, confirms the operation of the rules established by animal experiments (Figs. 7.6, 7.7, and above). Figure 9.6 provides a comparison of the performance of a normal person and of a patient who was deafferented by a severe peripheral sensory neuropathy that, however, spared motor functions. The patient could perform many familiar motor acts, even change gears while driving his car. Yet, he could not carry out subtle, daily activities that involve somatosensory updating, such as feeding himself and drinking, writing, and fastening buttons to get dressed. Vision cannot compensate for loss of tactile sensations when small objects are manipulated between the fingers. The most striking defect was an inability to maintain a constant muscular contraction. The patient could not hold a *constant* contraction of his thumb, for instance, against a constant force or at a given position, for more than a second or so without visual information. This is caused by loss of proprioception, because normal subjects with anesthetized skin and joints, but functioning muscle sense, can maintain such constant muscular force (not illustrated). (The deafferented monkey in Fig. 9.5 could point toward the learned target, but only if it was fairly wide, certainly much wider than that managed before deafferentation. Furthermore, it preferred to use co-contractive steadying of the arm, a sign of incomplete, nonupdated programming.)

The deafferented patient reveals the functional importance of sensory updating for the correction of subtle, programmed motor activity. This is as true for small movements as it is for accurate postures of the digits. Such small movements are more

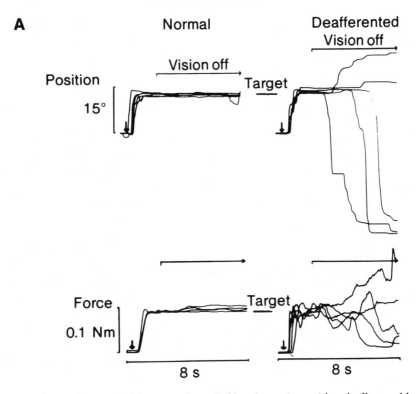

Fig. 9.6. Comparison of a normal human subject *(left)* and a patient with a deafferented hand and forearm *(right)* in the maintenance of a constant thumb position *(upper traces)* and exertion of a constant force *(lower traces)*. After some practice with two alternating levels displayed on an oscilloscope, normal subject can perform both tasks without seeing the position or force "target" display, while the deafferented patient must substitute vision for lost somatosensory input. Without either input, the patient's thumb starts moving randomly shortly after visual feedback is removed. Compare to Figs. 9.3–9.5. (From Marsden, Rothwell and Day, 1984; based on Rothwell, Traub, Day, Obeso, Thomas and Marsden 1982)

likely to stray from the intended end point if their afferent input is cut off or if their reference point is moved by disturbing the limb. It seems probable that loss of updating is responsible in either case (cf. Fig. 7.8). (Chapter 12 will show that motor cortex neurons that are task-related to small movements are more dependent on peripheral feedback than neurons related to large movements.)

3. Static Postural Reactions

Effects arising from neck proprioceptors and descending to the body are known as *tonic neck reflexes*. They coordinate body attitudes for movement readiness according to the position of the head. Tonic neck and other postural reactions are genetically inherited subprograms of the sort discussed in Chap. 1.1. The term reflexes, as mentioned before, is inappropriate, because they are a series of coordinated, triggered reactions whose adequate stimuli are normally *internal* to the CNS, namely the preceding "reflex." Evidence for that view comes from the observation that during limb adjustments after a perturbation, joints are stabilized successively at intervals of only 20 msec—too short a time for round trips involving peripheral conduction and muscular contraction. Only the first of the series needs to begin with its adequate peripheral stimulus: stretch of neck muscles. This analysis also applies to the "supporting reactions" starting with ankle movements (see below and Figs. 9.10 and 9.11). Postural adjustments can also be brought about by the therapist through manipulation of the head, which elicits tonic neck reflexes—an example of the clinical importance of these reactions cited in the introduction to this part of the text.

If the head is rotated, extensor tone is exaggerated on the side to which the head is pointing and diminished on the other side. Such *asymmetrical tonic neck reflexes* (ATNRs) occur in daily life, probably accounting for assumed postures such as those illustrated in Fig. 9.7. The same sort of steadying changes follow tilting of the head: bending it forward causes flexion as well as relaxation of the forelimbs and simultaneous extension and increased tone of the hindlimbs. Opposite changes apply if the head is bent backwards (Fig. 9.8). The proprioceptive origin of the reactions was proved by Magnus through their persistence in labyrinthectomized, decerebrate animals, although ordinarily labyrinths play their part as well. Figure 9.8 presents a graphic summary of the task-oriented nature of tonic neck reflexes for animals and humans. The middle column shows only proprioceptive reactions because the head is kept level, and hence there is constant, nonchanging input from the otoliths. Conversely, *otolith-evoked "static" reflexes* appear in the left and right pictures of the second row. Both inputs are activated together in the situations cartooned in the four corners.

4. Support and Attitude Reactions

Stance is an integral part of maintaining an upright posture. It includes the stiffening of the legs by co-contraction of antagonistic muscles and the presence of attitudinal and righting reflexes. None of these integrative properties are present in "reflex standing" of acutely decerebrate or bul-

bospinal animal preparations, discussed in Chap. 5.2. Yet, in the natural state, the reactions to be described may be heavily dependent on subcortical programs operating with support of the middle level of the motor hierarchy. This includes input–output specifications by the sensorimotor cortex, coordination by the basal ganglia and fine adjustments by the cerebellum.

Stance is achieved by a group of interactive stretch reflexes called the *supporting reactions*. They are "subprograms" comprising the successive triggering of the "reflex" components, like the postural neck reflexes. A pillar-like state, suited to the circumstances of the moment, is brought about by the "positive supporting reaction," which is triggered by contact of the feet with the ground ("magnet reaction"), and by the consequent stretch of the flexors of the distal joints, including the ankle. This, in turn, fixes the limb for standing by triggering coordinated co-contractions of opposing muscles around the involved joints, which includes the back. Limbs become movable again when the original stimulus ceases (e.g., when the foot is lifted off the ground) and when a "negative supporting reaction" is triggered

Fig. 9.7. Positional responses are often used in ordinary voluntary activities. Note how the orientation of the head influences that of the limbs, presumably through tonic neck "reflexes." Compare to Fig. 1.1. (Traced from Fukuda, 1961; in Brookhart, 1979)

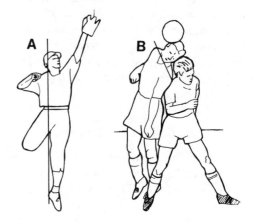

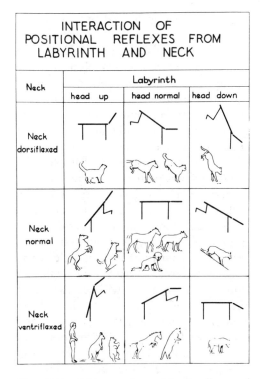

Neck	Labyrinth		
	head up	head normal	head down
Neck dorsiflexed			
Neck normal			
Neck ventriflexed			

INTERACTION OF POSITIONAL REFLEXES FROM LABYRINTH AND NECK

Fig. 9.8. Scheme of combined effects of ("static") positional responses from the neck and the otoliths on the stance of a stylized quadruped (stick figures), of some animals, and of the human in two positions. (From Roberts, 1967, 1975; in Wilson and Melvill Jones, 1979)

by stretch of the distal joint extensors. ("Physiological extensors" are muscles that normally oppose gravity, although their anatomical action may be flexion. We can oppose gravity, for instance, by exerting torque against the ground when flexing our toes. See Chaps. 5.2 and 6.6.)

5. Placing and Hopping Reactions

We now contrast the reactions discussed above with highly integrative, programmed sequences that specifically depend on the motor cortex and its adjustments by the cerebellar circuit (see Fig. 2.2). The *placing reactions* become obvious in the absence of the usual, visual modes of adjustment. An animal normally places the forefeet on any firm surface that it encounters with the feet and adjusts the

leg muscles so as to support the body; it does not do so with nonsupporting soft surfaces. (A similar aspect of postural reactions in humans is described in relation to Fig. 9.11.) A number of touch stimuli elicit placing reactions: touch of the chin brings the paw up to the chin, followed by leg extension into stance. Touch of the vibrissae causes the feet to be placed on the touching object. If the feet of a cat, in any position, are pushed over the edge of the supporting surface, they are replaced on that surface immediately. If a leg of a standing cat is pulled away without being supported, stable stance is regained at once by leg adduction. Although placing is abolished by lesions disconnecting the motor cortex, chronic spinal cats can regain the ability for tactile placing.

Quadruped stance is organized by central programs that support the animal's center of mass by coordinating diagonally opposite limbs. Unexpected loss of support by one limb does not displace the center of mass from the line between diagonally opposite limbs. The overall program involves the motor cortex, because stance is no longer adjusted by leg placing after precentral lesions, and also because precentral stimulation can trigger appropriate adjustments. A different strategy is used by cats when they lift one paw voluntarily, without involving the diagonal limb. In this case, weight changes are restricted to the forelimbs, and the vertebral column bends toward the side of the supporting, weight-bearing limb.

Hopping reactions are corrective leg movements, triggered by horizontal displacement of the body. The leg hops in the direction of the displacement, so that the foot is kept under the shoulder or hip; that is, the center of mass is kept between the supporting legs. These complex sequences are assisted by lower level subprograms that we encounter in other motor situations. Supporting tone in the leg, for instance, disappears before hopping (we described premovement relaxation in relation to Fig. 1.3). Placing and hopping re-

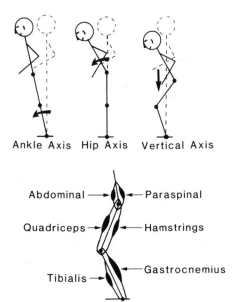

Ankle Axis   Hip Axis   Vertical Axis

Abdominal ——→ ◆ ←—— Paraspinal

Quadriceps ——→ ◆ ←—— Hamstrings

                         ←—— Gastrocnemius

Tibialis ——→ ◆

Fig. 9.9. Mechanics of human stance. The upper stick diagrams illustrate the coordinate axes of an abstract three-dimensional space for body positions in the sagittal plane (illustrated in Fig. 9.13). The lower diagram illustrates the approximate geometry of action of six representative ankle, thigh, and trunk muscles. (From Nashner and McCollum, 1986)

actions depend on the contralateral cortex from which movements of the involved muscles can be elicited. They disappear when such cortex is inactivated, and they survive removal of all other cortex. Although contact placing is not observed in the human, patterned responses of muscles and limbs are emitted as automatic postural reactions that depend on functioning sensorimotor cortex (e.g., Fig. 9.10). Those involving support by antigravity muscles can resemble partial placing reactions by depending on contact with a firm surface (Fig. 9.11).

6. Human Postural Control Programs

The task of staying upright usually begins with muscular actions at the support base. First the ankle joints are adjusted, after which the body moves like an inverted

pendulum that is hinged at the ankles. This concept, originally developed by the Russian group of Gurfinkel, Fel'dman and others, has led to fruitful analysis by combining biomechanical and other techniques. The current paradigm is to examine kinematic and muscular responses to perturbations of individuals who are standing on a platform with built-in force sensors. Nashner has shown that when the human body is perturbed in the anterior–posterior plane, it flexes at the ankles as well as at the knees and the hip, for which three pairs of opposing muscles suffice as a minimum (Fig. 9.9). An important property of the control of these muscle synergies, or patterns, is that their overall amplitudes are governed without change of their relations one to another, through action of the basal ganglia (cf. Figs. 7.1 and 7.2). Cerebellar control also contributes to the preservation of the patterns (Fig. 6.4A). The postural reactions described above (except placing and hopping) contribute to overall postural programs that actively preserve balance. Those overall programs can use all available sensory inputs, and activate automatic sequences of muscular action patterns, beginning normally at the distal joint (or joints).

Postural coordination depends on how the body is supported. For instance, when a subject is made to sway on a flat surface, the ankle joints are stabilized first. Figure 9.10 shows that muscle activation progresses proximally from the support base up. The figurines and the EMG traces on their right show that action begins at the ankle after an initial latency of 100 to 120 msec. Those latencies mark these responses of synergistic muscle groups to postural imbalance as being most probably "long-loop" (or "functional stretch") responses, which we know require a functioning sensorimotor cortex in human subjects (cf. Chap. 6.2). That the muscular patterns are programmed is suggested also by the fact that they always appear in the same combinations of graded intensities and timing for the same perturbations, for instance as in Fig. 9.10, top left. The amplitudes of functional stretch responses adapt within a few trials in a task-related manner according to whether they serve a useful purpose or not. More proximal joints are activated successively at intervals of only 10–20 msec. These short intervals indicate programmed linkage within the CNS, because of inadequate round-trip time to the periphery and back after muscular contraction. The upper row shows that the combinations of all the muscles acting on a joint (called "synergies") depend on the direction of the displacement, starting with gastrocnemius for forward sway and tibialis anterior for backward sway. Similar synergies are used for similar imbalances, no matter whether they are unexpected, involuntary occurrences or expected ones produced by voluntary effort. Comparison of the upper and lower rows in Fig. 9.10 demonstrates the similarity of the muscle patterns responding to similar perturbations, no matter whether we are balanced solely by firm stance or whether we assist by holding onto a support with our hands. In this connection we recall the parallels drawn in Chap. 6.4 between the production of long-loop responses and voluntary movements.

Postural adjustments always involve both sides of the body, and can be brought into action by programs using a number of postural devices either in concert or separately, as described in this chapter so far. Figure 9.11 illustrates the coordinated, task-related manner in which even very slight perturbations of one arm can trigger functional stretch responses in the *opposite* arm. Two conditions are contrasted in the left and right figurines in the top row. In both cases the subject pulls with his left wrist against a load that may change slightly and thus perturb the position of that hand by a few millimeters. On the left, this subject is trying to balance a cup of tea with his right hand, while on the right he grips the tabletop for support. The instructions for the subject are to move against all perturbations, while trying to balance on

his knees. The subject is preoccupied with steadying himself against the pull on his left wrist. The load on the left wrist could increase to reverse the movement toward the left, stretching the left biceps slightly in the process, or it could increase just enough to bring his pull to a halt. It could stay steady as a control, or it could release sufficiently to let his ongoing pull move his left wrist a few millimeters to the right.

The long-loop responses of triceps in the right arm present a striking illustration of task-related adaptation: in the left column they tend to steady the position of the teacup in space, while in the right column they firm up the supporting posture of the arm against the table. The cumulative, integrated EMGs of the right triceps are shown in the upper row (A), where upward and downward slopes of the traces mean increases and decreases of triceps EMG. (Stretch responses of the pulling left biceps

Fig. 9.10. Human postural motor programs to combat sway with "functional stretch responses" are similar for body displacements by movement of the supporting platform (*upper row,* in the direction of the *arrows* beneath the feet), and for voluntary displacements by arm pull and push against a firm bar (*lower row,* at first 100-msec timer). *Left and right columns* compare reactions in each case for forward and backward sway. Figurines at the left of EMG traces show geometry of participating muscles. Medial gastrocnemius, **G**; hamstrings, **H**; paraspinals, **P**; anterior tibialis, **T**; rectus femoris belly of quadriceps, **Q**; abdominals, **A**; arm biceps, **Bi**; triceps, **Tr**. See Fig. 9.9. (From Nashner, 1977; Cordo and Nashner, 1982)

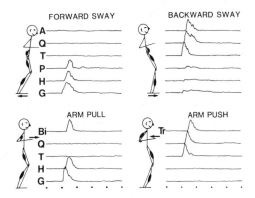

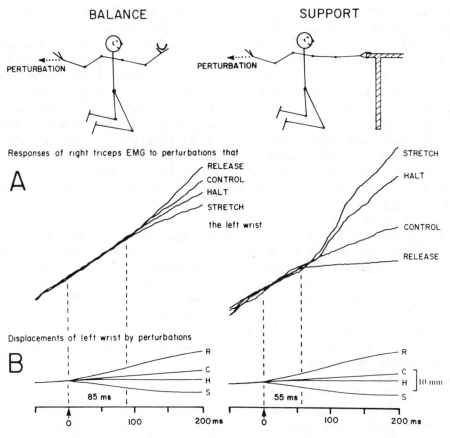

Fig. 9.11. Postural functional stretch responses are task oriented. Perturbations of the left wrist, while the right arm balances a teacup *(left column)* evoke gentler and later long-loop responses in the right triceps brachii muscle, compared to the oppositely directed ones evoked when the right arm supports the body *(right)*. The figurines illustrate the postural reactions that generate the cumulative, integrated, rectified EMG of right triceps brachii, row (A), during displacements of the left wrist, row (B); perturbation labels correspond to those in row (A). (Modified from Marsden, Merton and Morton, 1981. Figurines added.)

are not illustrated.) When the left wrist is released, letting it move toward the right, the right triceps contracts to steady the right arm holding the teacup. When the left wrist is pulled toward the left, the right triceps relaxes. In contrast, when the right arm is used for support of the hand gripping the table, *oppositely* directed and more vigorous reactions are evoked by the same perturbations. Now the usual postural reactions are seen: release of the left wrist relaxes triceps of the right arm, and pull on the left wrist evokes contraction of the right triceps. The laten-

cies of the supportive responses are briefer by 30 msec than those of the balancing ones, suggesting that these more practiced ones are emitted in predictive, phase-advanced fashion.

The teacup experiment (which was actually also carried out with a surrogate cup, by having the right hand supported against gravity in a sling and touching a dangling 100-g weight) shows that the crossed arm can make at least two different types of automatic, postural responses. The subjects reported that the choice was not conscious. Responses appropriate for

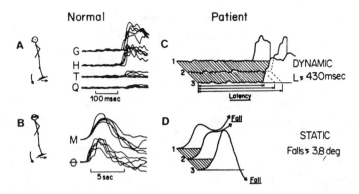

Fig. 9.12. Vestibular function tests, consisting of induced sway with stabilized ankles, of normal subjects (A,B) and of patients with loss of function of the semicircular canals, shown as three successive trials [(C) *dynamic* loss, resulting in delayed balance, with gastrocnemius latency beyond 430 msec] or of the utricular otoliths, tested with subjects (B,D) blindfolded [(D) *static* loss, resulting in drift followed by fall at 3.8-deg tilt]. EMGs in (A–D) are from gastrocnemius (**G**); in (A,B) also from hamstrings (**H**); tibialis anterior (**T**); and quadriceps (**Q**). **M,** Moment exerted by ankle muscles upon platform; **θ,** body sway angle. (From Nashner and Grimm, 1978; in Brooks and Thach, 1981)

supporting the body were made only when the support surface was felt to be firm, and that they found it difficult, after having experienced a yielding surface as an alternative, to consciously reestablish supportive reactions in triceps. This description matches the observed behavior of cats during tactile placing on a yielding surface, described earlier.

Some subjects do not evince functional stretch responses to postural imbalance, but instead rely on vestibular input for voluntary corrections. This can be tested on a force platform by preventing ankle adjustments (through constraints) while subjects are made to sway by backward movement of the platform, as in Fig. 9.10, but with added upward rotation of the platform (Fig. 9.12A). Although this increases the amplitude of sway, normal subjects without functional stretch reflexes can remain stable, even with their eyes closed (Fig. 9.12B). In the absence of ankle use, the semicircular canals normally initiate dynamic stabilizing adjustments, followed by maintenance of stance with the aid of input from the utricular otoliths. Patients

with loss of semicircular canal function (Fig. 9.12C) fall rapidly, making either no response or a very late dynamic response. In contrast, patients with dysfunction restricted to the otoliths (Fig. 9.12D) respond with normal latency to the fall, but then show a static instability, consisting of a slow drift over the next 5–10 seconds, ending in a fall.

A promising hypothesis for understanding postural adjustments has been proposed by Nashner and McCollum. Figure 9.13A shows how a perturbation, in their scheme, makes the upright-standing body fall when it is perturbed after tilting about the ankle and hip joints (ankle and hip axes in Fig. 9.13A). The joints bend progressively along the lines radiating out from the equilibrium center of the hip-ankle plane (as indicated in the figurines, and also in Fig. 9.9). When we are perturbed into anterior–posterior sway, we regain our equilibrium by activating stereotyped muscle synergies, mostly at the ankle and hip (e.g., Fig. 9.10). Upright stance can be maintained by certain combinations of ankle and hip angles that are

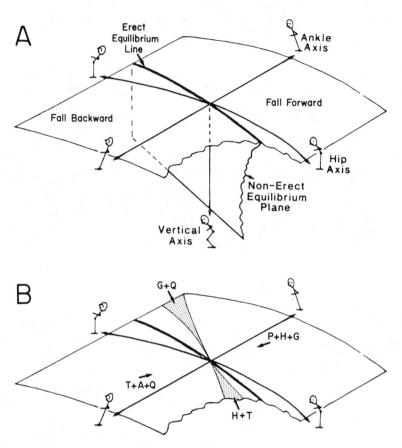

Fig. 9.13. Postural corrections are made by economical programs. (A) Body positions (see figurines) are defined in an abstract three-dimensional space. The horizontal plane defines ankle–hip relations with knees fully extended (erect). The vertical surface provides equilibrium with knees bent; its top *(thick line)* denotes where the body is in erect equilibrium. (B) The ankle–hip plane is divided into four regions characterized by different minimal combinations of muscles that, when contracting together, accelerate the body toward the origin, that is, completely erect postural equilibrium. Muscles are labeled by initial letters of names given in Fig. 9.9; also see Fig. 9.10. (Modified from Nashner and McCollum, 1986)

denoted by the heavy line in Fig. 9.13A,B. Stooping reactions of the knees to regain equilibrium are plotted downward in the vertical nonerect plane of Fig. 9.13A.

The stereotyped muscle synergies are simple and few in number, on the simplifying assumption that only the six muscles shown in Fig. 9.9 are used. In that case, merely two or three muscles suffice to restore body balance from any region of dis-

equilibrium. Figure 9.13B displays the calculated regions in which different muscle synergies can restore our upright stance. (The calculations combining the gravitational field, which increases radially along the arrows of the hip–ankle plane, with the fields of muscle action are not illustrated here.) The muscles are labeled by their initial letters as in Fig. 9.9. The scheme is an abstract representation of events we have already encountered. The top row in Fig. 9.10 illustrates opposition to forward sway by means of **P + H + G**, and to backward sway with **A + Q + T**. The method has predictive power, because it allows calculations of what could happen in untried situations, giving it investigative and therapeutic potential. It is based on tests with normal human subjects whose use of discrete synergy programs for particular imbalances were learned from previous experience.

Use of learned programs relieves the brain from having to calculate the consequence of many combinations of muscles, which exemplifies Bernstein's concept of the economy of hierarchical function. The economy extends also to the sensory side of postural adjustments, because we balance ourselves without unnecessary switching between different synergies, which once more economizes use of calculations in having to detect, and react to, more than a minimal number of regions of imbalance. Bernstein was the first to recognize that CNS organization of postures and movements is constrained by their physical forces. This led him to view the CNS as a hierarchy that coordinates mechanically sound reflexes at the behest of higher centers. The coordinating structures were thought to govern motor actions in the context of task requirements by running simple, self-adapting programs. The most widely considered system, the *mass-spring model*, which was proposed by his scientific descendents in 1966 (see Figs. 3.4, 4.6A,B, and 9.5D), is currently undergoing rigorous testing and revision. It has now become clear that changes of limb position involve going through a series of length–tension curves, rather than just snapping, springlike, from one to another (cf. Fig. 7.8). The importance of feedback assistance for these transitions is now well recognized, particularly for changes of small amplitude where spindle servo-assistance might transmit feedforward commands. We concluded in Chap. 4.2, also, that servo-assistance may

be useful in the installation of motor programs.

Humans use different strategies for standing on different surfaces, such as the ground compared to a narrow beam. The feet cannot exert sufficient torque on the beam surface, and balance is therefore preserved by body rotation about the hips (hip axis in Fig. 9.13A). The proportionate contributions from various muscles in the synergy are always the same for a particular strategy, which, moreover, may be used in postural adjustments as well as in locomotion. For instance, the strategies of starting with ankle or hip adjustments are used equally for standing *as well as* walking on a particular surface. Postural contractions in leg muscles are superimposed on normal step-related activities. These mechanisms, not illustrated here, are discussed further in Chap. 10.

How do we deal with different sensory messages, such as visual and vestibular inputs, when they give conflicting information about the orientation of the body? Conflict of visual and proprioceptvie inputs produced by muscle vibration may result in panic and autonomic reactions, although there is rational disbelief about the perceived limb position and an absence of pain (Chap. 3.1). It is common knowledge that motion sickness can result from conflict of visual and vestibular inputs on board ship, and from conflict of gravitational and angular vestibular inputs on board a spacecraft. Similarly, normal subjects experience illusions about the position of the ground while performing kneebends in excessive gravity (Chap. 1.3), and conversely, limbs seem excessively heavy in normal gravity for stroke patients with impaired commands from motor cortex (Chap. 7.4).

How do we deal with sensory conflict about balance? Rational views and previous experience may not resolve conflicts, as has been related with regard to feline or human placing of a limb on unstable surfaces that may evoke doubts about their ability to support the limb and/or the body (cf. Fig. 9.11). Normal adults assign different degrees of importance ("weight") to various sensory inputs ahead of time, and *suppress sensory conflict* within about five trials. For patients with vestibular dysfunction, however, this suppression frequently fails, causing them to respond to inappropriate motion cues. This general line of testing has led Nashner to the hypothesis that the brain senses the location of the body's center of mass in relation to various regions of imbalance, and reacts by activating appropriate postural strategies. (Selections of strategies and tactics were introduced as functions of the highest and middle levels in Fig. 2.4.) These strategies are composed of sequential automatic postural movements, some of which we encountered, for instance, in units 3 and 4 of this chapter.

This line of research has great therapeutic potential. Movement strategies can be devised, for instance, for patients with postural problems, using the posture model to define the limits within which particular movements can orient the patient's body. It has been possible to identify appropriate help for some children with cerebral palsy. Ataxic children are destabilized by sensory conflict, although they exhibit normal muscular coordination. In contrast, those with spastic hemiplegia deal normally with sensory conflict but have abnormal patterns of muscular coordination.

Comparison of normal and spastic sway correction provides a good example for success and failure of a motor program. Figure 9.14 shows two stages of the normal program that is initiated by contraction of gastrocnemius, shown in the first figurine in the left diagram. The filled arrows symbolize the thrust generated by the muscle action, an the open arrows indicate the mechanical reactions to those forces. Thus, gastrocnemius generates a backward thrust of the leg with respect to the ground, which in turn creates a forward thrust by mechanical (intertial) coupling at the knee and hips. The second figurine in that diagram shows that this allows the body to move back to a vertical position approximately as a rigid mass. The right-hand diagram in Fig. 9.14 illustrates that spastic hemiplegics do not follow the usual distal-to-proximal progression of automatic postural movements. Instead, the reverse ensues: a proximal-to-distal sequence, which is marked by abnormally variable amplitudes of synergic muscle pairs. The thigh muscles (hamstrings) contract first, which tends to extend the hip and flex the knee, as indicated by the filled arrows in the left-hand diagram. This is followed by a delayed and slow gastrocnemius contraction that cannot support the buckling knee, shown in the right-hand diagram. Too little torque is exerted on the ankle too late, and the knee collapses when the abnormal sequence fails to support the center of mass. The heightened phasic-stretch reflexes at the ankle of spastics (Chap. 7.2) are of no avail when they are not employed in a properly timed sequence. Normal posture can only be maintained by normal motor programs.

The postural task system includes, among other items, the cerebral cortex, basal ganglia and the cerebellum. Patients with Parkinson's disease are imbalanced because they have no consistent strategy of using either the ankle or the hip as the initial fulcrum about which to right the body: the caudate "complex" circuit seems to be not functioning (Fig. 2.7). Patients with cerebellar disease have different problems: their vestibular reactions are not integrated, their muscle patterns are not composed consistently. The two diseases recall the two levels of sensorimotor "packaging" with which we introduced task systems in Chap. 2.3. Furthermore, cerebellar patients do not adapt to changing circumstances because of deficient use of a special cerebellar input nucleus, the inferior olive (Chap. 13.7).

We stated above that postural and locomotor programs use the same muscle patterns. This means that these programs converge after having been organized by different parts of the brain. Movements are

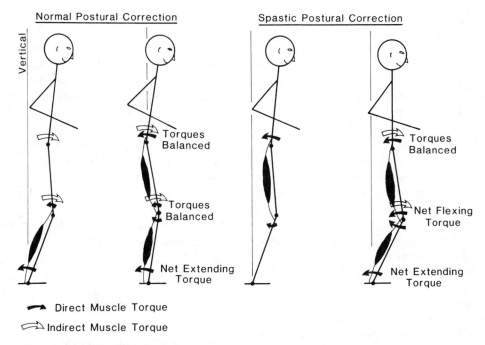

Fig. 9.14. Correct operation and failure of a postural motor program. *(Left)* Normal correction of forward sway begins with contraction of gastrocnemius (the support base) and stabilizes the knee, which restores the vertical position of the body. *Filled* and *open arrows* characterize muscular and mechanical, reactive forces, respectively. *(Right)* Abnormal attempt at correction of forward sway by a spastic hemiplegic patient begins with hamstrings (well above the support base), which causes the knee to buckle. (From Nashner, Shumway-Cook and Marin, 1983)

preceded by postural adjustments—of joint stiffness before joint movement, and of the position of the head, body and limbs before they are moved. Postural adjustments are carried out by the middle level of the motor hierarchy (Fig. 2.3), after preparations by the highest level to blend postures and movements into one smooth sequence by matching move and hold programs (Chap. 6.2). Muscles pull on joints to produce actions (filled arrows in Fig. 9.14), which lead to opposite reactions (open arrows). This interaction prescribes the range of postures from which movements can spring and to which they can return while still maintaining body equilibrium.

7. Summary

Postural reactions are programmed sequences that are triggered by muscular, vestibular or visual cues about body imbalance. Some function as closed loops, such as the vestibular (vestibulocollic) reflexes that adjust the neck because the labyrinths receive feedback about the resulting head movement. In contrast, vestibulo-ocular reflexes function as open loops, since the labyrinths do not receive feedback about eye movements, which instead is computed by the brain from comparison of visual input and knowledge of head position. Movements of the eyes and head can be coordinated by reactions that are triggered by various senses, but they can succeed for previously learned movements in entirely open-loop fashion. In the absence of proprioceptive as well as vestibular input, the brain remembers the equilibrium lengths of the neck nuscles that previously had brought the head to the correct position, and programs alpha MNs accordingly.

Attitudes of the body and limb are coordinated by static postural reactions. Tonic neck reflexes arise from neck proprioceptors and adjust the body and limbs through a series of internally triggered reactions. Only the first of the series begins with a peripheral adequate stimulus: stretch of neck muscles or otolith discharge due to static tilt. Stance is achieved also by a series of interactive stretch reflexes, which cause co-contraction of opposing muscles to stiffen the limb. This "positive supporting reaction" is triggered by contact of the foot with the ground, and ceases at the end of such contact. All the reactions mentioned above are operated by subcortical mechanisms, although they normally use support by the cerebral cortex. In contrast, placing and hopping reactions depend on normal function of motor cortex and its adjustments by the cerebellar circuit. The aim of quadruped stance reactions is to stabilize the body's center of mass between the legs.

Human postural control programs aim to keep the body's center of mass in line with the support base. They incorporate the postural reactions described above (except placing and hopping), and they depend on normal cortical and cerebellar function. Human postural adjustments can be modified by instructions, they are predictive unless instructions change, and they are adaptive to the circumstances of the moment. They begin either as long-loop (functional stretch) responses triggered by muscle stretch, or as responses to visual or vestibular input. Normally, adjustments begin with the joints closest to the support surface (e.g., the ankles). The body is then balanced like an inverted pendulum by a series of interactive, internally triggered stretch reflexes, which coordinate a minimal number of muscle groups (synergies) in repeatable patterns according to the stance of the body and the surface on which it stands. If the feet cannot exert sufficient torque on the ground, balance is achieved by replacing the ankle strategy with one based on hip move-

ments. The sequences, which can involve many successive joints on both sides of the body, including bending of the knees, are task oriented and adapt within a few trials. A current theory posits that the brain senses how the body is disequilibrated and, in response, emits learned simple synergies to regain body balance. The "mass-spring" model is still the most useful for consideration of central feedforward ("hold") programs for limb end positions. Combinations of force platform tests and EMG recording are beginning to make it possible to calculate what type of movements can assist patients with their postural problems.

References

Abbs, J. H., Gracco, V. L., and Cole, K. J. 1984. Control of multimovement coordination: sensorimotor mechanisms in speech motor programming. *J. Motor Behav.* 16:195–231.

Abrahams, V. C. 1979. Proprioceptive influences from eye muscle receptors on cells of the superior colliculus. In *Reflex control of posture and movement,* eds. R. Granit and O. Pompeiano. *Prog. Brain Res.* 50:325–344.

Anderson, J. H., Soechting, J. F., and Terzuolo, C. A. 1979. Role of vestibular inputs in the organization of motor output to forelimb extensors. In *Reflex control of posture and movement,* eds. R. Granit and O. Pompeiano. *Prog. Brain Res.* 50:413–421.

Barr, M. L., and Kiernan, J. A. 1983. *The human nervous system.* 4th ed. Philadelphia: Harper & Row. [Fig. 9.1]

Bizzi, E. 1980. Central and peripheral mechanisms in motor control. In *Tutorials in motor behavior,* eds. G. E. Stelmach and J. Requin. *Adv. Psychol.* 1:131–143. [Fig. 9.5C]

Bizzi, E. 1981. Eye–head coordination. In Sect. 1, vol. 2. *Motor control. Handbook of physiology,* ed. V. B. Brooks, pp. 1321–1336. Bethesda, Md.: American Physiology Society. [Figs. 9.3 and 9.5A,B]

Bizzi, E., and Abend, W. 1983. Posture control and trajectory formation in single- and multi-joint arm movements. In *Motor control mechanisms in health and disease,* ed. J. E. Desmedt. *Adv. Neurol.* 39:31–45. [Fig. 9.5D]

Bizzi, E., Accornero, N., Chapple, W., and Hogan, N. 1982. Arm trajectory formation in monkeys. *Exp. Brain Res.* 46:139–143. [Fig. 9.5D]

Bizzi, E., Dev, P., Morasso, P., and Polit, P. 1978. Effects of load disturbances during centrally initiated movements. *J. Neurophysiol.* 41:542–556. [Fig. 9.5A,B]

Bizzi, E., Polit, P., and Morasso, P. 1976. Mechanisms underlying achievement of final head position. *J. Neurophysiol.* 39:435–444. [Fig. 9.5C]

Brookhart, J. M. 1979. Convergence on an understanding of motor control. In *Posture and movement*, eds. R. E. Talbott and D. R. Humphrey, pp. 295–303. New York: Raven Press. [Fig. 9.7]

Brooks, V. B., and Thach, W. T. 1981. Cerebellar control of posture and movement. In Sect. 1, vol. 2. *Motor control*. V. B. Brooks, *Handbook of physiology*, ed. pp. 877–946. Bethesda, Md.: American Physiological Society. [Fig. 9.12]

Chaikin, A. 1984. Sick in space. *Science 84* 5(5): 50–55.

Chan, C. W. Y. 1983. Tonic labyrinthine reflex control of limb posture: reexamination of the classical concept. In *Motor control mechanisms in health and disease*, ed. J. E. Desmedt. *Adv. Neurol.* 39:621–632.

Cordo, P. J., and Nashner, L. M. 1982. Properties of postural adjustments associated with rapid arm movements. *J. Neurophysiol.* 47:287–302. [Fig. 9.10]

Dichgans, J., Bizzi, E., Morasso, P.,and Tagliasco, V. 1973. Mechanisms underlying recovery of head–eye coordination following bilateral labyrinthectomy in monkeys. *Exp. Brain Res.* 18:548–562. [Fig. 9.4]

Evarts, E. V., and Granit, R. 1976. Relations of reflexes and intended movements. In *Understanding the stretch reflex*, ed. S. Homma. *Prog. Brain Res.* 14:1–14

Fuchs, A. F. 1981. Eye–head coordination. In *Motor coordination*, eds. A. L. Towe and E. S. Luschei, Vol. 5. *Handbook of behavioral neurobiology*, pp. 303–366. New York: Plenum Press.

Fukuda, T. 1961. Studies on human dynamic postures from the viewpoint of postural reflexes. *Acta Otolaryngol. [Suppl.] (Stockh.* 161:1–52. [Fig. 9.7]

Gahery, Y., and Massion, J. 1981. Co-ordination between posture and movement. *Trends Neurosci.* 4:199–202.

Granit, R., and Pompeiano, O., eds. 1979 *Reflex control of posture and movement*. Vol. 50. *Progress in Brain Research*. Amsterdam: Elsevier/North-Holland Biomedical Press.

Gurfinkel, V. S., and Shik, M. L. 1973. The control of posture and locomotion. In *Motor control,* eds. A. A. Gydikov, N. T. Tankov, and D. S. Kosarov. pp. 217–234. New York: Plenum Press.

Hayes, K. C. 1982. Biomechanics of postural control. *Excerise Sports Sci. Rev.* 10:363–391.

Magnus, R. 1926. Some results of studies in the physiology of posture. *Lancet* 211:531–585.

Marsden, C. D., Merton, P. A., and Morton, H. B. 1981. Human postural responses. *Brain* 104:513–534. [Fig. 9.11]

Marsden, C. D., Rothwell, J. C., and Day, B. L. 1984. The use of peripheral feedback in the control of movement. *Trends Neurosci.* 7:253–257. [Fig. 9.6]

Massion, J. 1984. Postural changes accompanying voluntary movements: normal and pathological aspects. *Hum. Neurobiol.* 2:261–267.

Miles, F. A. 1984. Sensing self-motion: visual and vestibular mechanisms share the same frame of reference. *Trends Neurosci.* 7:303–305.

Morasso, P., Bizzi, E., and Dichgans, J. 1973. Adjustment of saccade characteristics during head movements. *Exp. Brain Res.* 16:492–500. [Fig. 9.3]

Nashner, L. M. 1982. Adaptation of human movement to altered environments. *Trends Neurosci.* 5:358–361.

Nashner, L. M. 1977. Fixed patterns of rapid postural responses among leg muscles during stance. *Exp. Brain Res.* 30:13–24. [Fig. 9.10]

Nashner, L. M., and Grimm, R. J. 1978. Analysis of multiloop dyscontrols in standing cerebellar patients. In *Cerebral motor control in man.* ed. J. E. Desmedt. *Prog. Brain Res.* 4:300–319. [Fig. 9.12]

Nashner, L. M., and McCollum, G. 1985. Organization of postural human movements: a formal basis and experiments synthesis. *Behav. Brain Sci.* 8:135–172. [Figs. 9.9 and 9.13]

Nashner, L. M., Shumway-Cook, A., and Marin, O. 1983. Stance posture control in select groups of children with cerebral palsy: deficits in sensory organization and muscular coordination. *Exp. Brain Res.* 49:393–409. [Fig. 9.14]

Richmond, F. J. R., and Abrahams, V. C. 1979. What are the proprioceptors of the neck? In *Reflex control of posture and movement,* eds. R. Granit and O. Pompeiano. *Prog. Brain Res.* 50:245–254.

Roberts, T. D. M. 1975. The behavioral vertical. *Fortschr. Zool.* 23:192–198. [Fig. 9.8]

Roberts, T. D. M. 1967. *Neurophysiology of postural mechanisms.* London: Butterworths. [Fig. 9.8]

Rothwell, J. C., Traub, M. M., Day, B. L., Obeso, J. A., Thomas, P. K., and Marsden, C. D. 1982. Manual motor performance in a deafferented man. *Brain* 105:515–542. [Fig. 9.6]

Sanes, J. N., and Evarts, E. V. 1983. Effects of perturbations on accuracy of arm movements. *J. Neurosci.* 3:977–986.

Wilson, V. J. 1975. The labyrinth, the brain and posture. *Am. Sci.* 63:325–332. [Fig. 9.2]

Wilson, V. J., and Melvill Jones, G. 1979. *Mammalian vestibular physiology.* New York: Plenum Press. [Fig. 9.8]

Wilson, V. J., and Peterson, B. W. 1980. The role of the vestibular system in posture and movement. In *Medical physiology,* ed. V. B. Mountcastle, pp. 813–836, 14th ed. St. Louis: The C. V. Mosby Co. [Figs. 9.2 and 9.4]

Zee, D. S., and Leigh, R. J. 1983. The neural control of eye movements. In *The clinical neurosciences.* Vol. 5. *Neurobiology,* eds. W. D. Willis, Jr., and R. N. Rosenberg, pp.519–546. New York: Churchill Livingstone.

10

Locomotion

In this chapter we step from posture to locomotion, an activity that is *programmed as patterns* by the brain. Humans learn to manage at different speeds of locomotion, to push the legs against the ground at the correct angles and with the correct forces, in coordination with appropriate body postures as well as arm swings. Below, we examine the process of locomotion and its management by the central nervous system.

1. Running and Walking

The purpose of locomotion is to transport the body across the ground. It entails repeated patterns of using, abandoning, and regaining a balanced stance on the ground successively with the alternate legs. (We follow here the expositions by Grillner and by Winter.) The development of running styles from the toddler through juvenile stages to the adult are illustrated in Fig. 10.1, and the adult walking cycle is explained in Fig. 10.2A. During walking and running, the objects of greatest attention for the CNS are the movements of the feet. We can follow them, in Fig. 10.2A for instance, in walking, from the moment the toes of one leg push off the ground behind the trunk to that when the heel of that leg strikes the ground in front of the trunk. This step is called the swing phase, and it is followed by the stance (support) phase, consisting of the adjustments to support the body weight on the plantar surface of the forward foot. The stance phase includes a flexion–extension–flexion sequence of the standing knee, while the other leg goes through its swing, ending with the heel of the swinging leg striking the ground. At the end of stance, the supporting leg is once more behind the trunk with the toes poising for pushoff. Now the walking cycle can begin anew. The two steps, from a heel contact (or strike) of one leg to its next one, together constitute the adult *walking cycle*, which begins and ends with both legs in the same relative positions to each other. The step cycle is a basic unit of locomotion, but the walking cycle completes the pattern, assuring smooth transportation as well as posture. The sequence recalls the unity of movements and postures of arm movements (Fig. 1.3).

The programs for "plantigrade" gait, with heelstrike followed by plantar sole placing (which we do, like very heavy quadrupeds, such as elephants), are acquired gradually during the first year of life, at which time humans still place the feet with the toes first when supported under the arms ("digitigrade gait" like the lighter quadrupeds, such as cats and dogs). As the nervous system matures and muscles become stronger, the infant pattern is abandoned in favor of "toddling" (illustrated in the top line of Fig. 10.1). This evolves into a steadier form of walk during the first 4 years, followed by learning to use the legs with digitigrade gait for running, which gains speed but sacrifices stability. Adult patterns for walking and running are acquired during the teens and mature in late adolescence. We note here that the power patterns in jogging (not illustrated) are very similar to those in walking. Nearly three-quarters of all joggers land with heelstrike (plantigrade gait), and only one-quarter land on the ball of the foot (digitigrade gait).

The adult walking cycle is illustrated in

Fig. 10.1 Development of locomotor movements in humans. Programmed walking and running develop gradually from the unstable gait of a child that has just started to walk. (From Bernstein, 1967; in Grillner, 1981)

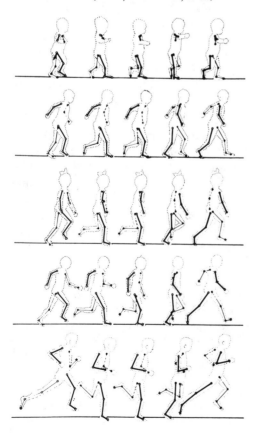

Fig. 10.2A. Successive swing and stance phases overlap slightly with those of the opposite leg, at which time the body is supported by both limbs instead of just one. The duration of one walking cycle is the time taken for one stride (e.g., one step from the left to the right leg and the succeeding one from the right to the left one). In Fig. 10.2A the right leg goes through a complete walking cycle that begins and ends with the right heel striking the ground in front of the body. At the end of the first (right–left) step of the cycle, the right leg touches the ground with the toes behind the body. After pushoff (when the toes have left the ground, slightly after midcycle, that is, 50–60% of the stride), the right leg swings forward to let the right heel strike the ground once more, but it is now one stride length ahead of the original start position. Stride length is the linear distance in the plane of progression between successive points of foot-to-floor contact of the same foot, composed of the step lengths for the left and right feet.

The rapidity with which steps are taken is called the "cadence" of walking, which is related inversely to the duration of the walking cycle. When we walk at different speeds (cadences), we reproduce the pattern of the walking cycle described in Fig. 10.1A faster or slower than normal. Cadence is controlled by the vigor of the pushoff, which can increase leg acceleration and thus decrease swing time. This way of looking at speeds of locomotion, stressed by Herman, is analogous to slow and fast arm movements, illustrated in Fig. 7.5A,B. Faster acceleration is matched by faster deceleration and more vigorous energy absorption when the leg accepts the weight of the body. The leg makes a "harder" landing during faster locomotion (cf. Chap. 1 for the analogy to flight). Walking programs are normally updated by peripheral feedback about joint angles and velocities, just like those for arm movements (Figs. 7.7 and 7.8).

Walking movements are programmed as *patterns* that involve at least three principal joints: the ankle, knee, and hip. These patterns are preserved at different speeds for leg movements just as they are for arm movements (cf. Figs. 7.1–7.4). This is easy to understand because the object of greatest attention for the CNS is always the action of the legs. The natural measure of movements therefore is the walking cycle (composed of two steps), and all activities should be scaled to its completion, as is indicated by the "% stride" values in Fig. 10.2AB. The patterns are in fact preserved so well that the leg joints always assume the same characteristic angles at any particular phase of the walking cycle, whether we progress at slow, natural, or fast cadences. The preservation of order between the patterns using ankle, hip, and knee at various cadences is best explained by the mechanical coordinating actions of those muscles that cross two joints ("biarticulate" muscles; see Fig. 9.9). When the cadence is the controlled variable, the pattern and the successive angles of the participating joints are regulated, just as for arm movements (i.e., kept constant; see

Fig. 10.2. Patterns of leg action in human gait are the same at all speeds when scaled in relation to stride length. (A) Definition of alternate stance and swing phases, with slight overlaps for each leg, in relation to steps and to stride length (expressed as percentage of stride). (B) Identical actions of one leg at slow, natural, and fast stride cadences (expressed as percentage of stride length, averages of 15 subjects). The three resultant speeds of joint rotations are given in degrees per second. *Arrows* indicate torques about joints, as in Fig. 9.14. Preservation of stride pattern is similar to that of handwriting shown in Fig. 7.2. [(A) From Murray, 1967; (B) from Winter, 1983]

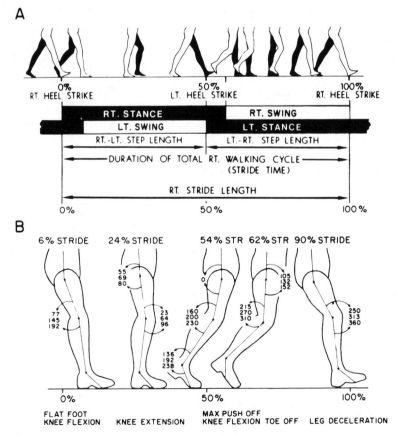

Chaps. 4.2, 6.3, and 7.1). Also, just as for arm movements, the actual joint velocities are by-products (Chap. 7.1). Typical values for slow, natural, and fast walking cadences are noted for each joint in Fig. 10.2B (plotted in units of the action sequence).

The speed of walking is governed by the intensity of leg muscle action. We would expect this from our study of arm muscle actions that govern the speed of arm movements (Figs. 1.3 and 7.5). And in further analogy, agonist and antagonist actions must be scaled in appropriate relations to each other if the leg is to land the body smoothly to reach equilibrium. Motor patterns for the walking cycle are adjusted so that vigorous pushoffs are followed by appropriate absorption of energy. Winter has pointed out that cadence cannot be altered by just speeding up the sequence generators in the CNS without adjustments of power because swing and stance phases would remain unadjusted, causing the body to collapse as the legs fail to stabilize the harder landings (see above). Instead, walking patterns for increased cadences are preserved by increasing the power bursts whereby the muscles generate and absorb energy.

Typical patterns of power bursts for pushoff and weight acceptance at fast and slow cadences are shown in Fig. 10.3, obtained by cinematographic analysis and measurements of walking on force-recording platforms. These methods permit calculations of energy use for the ankle, hip, and knee joints in terms of torque (moments of force) as well as their energy use (power). Power equals work/time = force × velocity, since work = average force × distance. Power is calculated here as net angular force (torque, or moment) × angular velocity (cf. Chap. 7.2). Each line depicts the main events in three walking cycles, from one heel contact (HC, at about 90% of the stride; see Fig. 10.2A,B) to the next one of that leg. Both lines are plotted on the same scales for time (abscissa) and power (ordinate). The sequences begin with the adjustments described above from heelstrike to weight acceptance by the knee, that is, energy absorption by the knee extensors, which is expressed as a negative power burst (**K1,** at about 10% of the stride). The stance phase concludes with the major positive burst of mechanical energy for pushoff into the swing phase as the ankle plantarflexes (**A2,** near 50% of the stride), which propels the toes off the

Fig. 10.3. Patterns of power bursts are preserved when walking at different speeds. Lines depict three strides, each terminated by a heel contact (**HC**); other letter symbols are explained in the text. Positive (+ve) and negative (−ve) power bursts are plotted up and down, respectively, on ordinate, against real time (seconds) on abscissa. Graphs are calculated from the same data as Fig. 10.2B. Note similarity to Fig. 7.2, which shows preservation of velocity patterns when writing at different speeds. (Adapted from Winter, 1983)

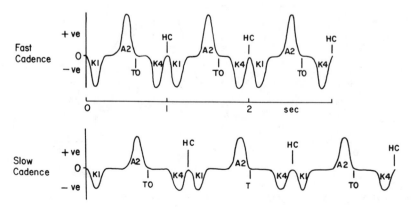

ground (**TO,** near 60%). Another negative burst occurs at the end of the swing phase as the swinging knee and foot are decelerated by the knee flexors (**K4,** near 90% of the stride) prior to heel contact.

There is a striking similarity between the preservation of patterns for walking (Fig. 10.3) and for writing (Fig. 7.2). Both show semiautomatic movements made at various cadences, one for the legs and the other for the arm. In both cases *the controlled variable is a transient rate of change of a parameter in relation to its steady state.* In Fig. 10.3 the controlled variable is power and in Fig. 7.2 it is writing speed (both are plotted against real time scaled in seconds). In both cases changes of cadence require changes of intensity of the transient alterations (which are angular velocities $\times$ torque in Fig. 10.3 and angular velocities in Fig. 7.2). Power bursts and velocities both reflect accelerations produced by the activation of muscle motor units; that is, they are both indicators of the motor program being carried out by the spinal cord. Recall that the same point was made in comparing isotonic and isometric arm movements (Fig. 7.5). The EMG patterns, indicating use of the underlying motor programs, are identical in Fig. 7.5B and D for the quick achievement of controlled force, whether the limb is moved by the force (Fig. 7.5B) or is prevented from moving (Fig. 7.5D).

Patterns can be preserved because phasic uses of muscles are fitted automatically to the background level of muscle tension. Thus the use of the same programs, and hence the unity of isotonic and isometric movements, follows from Henneman's size principle of spinal recruitment, because it expresses the transformation of properties of the spinal cord to those of the muscles served by the motoneurons. The genetically inherited recruitment order adjusts the intensity of spinal corrections to their background levels, smoothing changes from one level to another. The recruitment order dictates the input/output relations of the stretch reflex and with it

those of the motor servo (Chaps. 3.2, 4.1, and 5.1). At this point we are ready to consider the neural control of locomotion.

2. Central Pattern Generators

Locomotion, like many postural reactions described in Chaps. 9.1–9.4, does not require control by the cerebral cortex; it is managed by subcortical and spinal centers, which of course are subject to cortical intervention. (In this unit we largely follow the expositions by Grillner.) Our point of departure is the fact that "spinal" animals (whose spinal cords have been disconnected from their brains) can emit patterns of gait as long as their weight is supported and the ground is moving under their feet (which is also true for infants).

Patterns for locomotion are generated in the spinal cord by "central pattern generators" (CPGs) that operate in a flexible manner under supraspinal control. The most complex controls, emanating from the cerebral cortex, the cerebellum, and the brain stem, initiate and maintain patterns of optimal activity by making predictive adjustments based on the circumstances of the moment. One example is the predictively programmed deceleration of the legs during stepping, which leads to a smooth landing for stance in preparation for the next step. Melvill Jones and his associates have shown that the long-loop functional stretch response appears in the EMG of the human gastrocnemius muscle about 140 msec *before* contact with the ground (Chap. 6.2). Long-loop responses are an output of the cerebrocerebellar circuit (cf. Chap. 6.2). The cerebellum, for instance, is involved in normal locomotion as witnessed by the walk-related, bursting rhythms of many neurons in the dorsal and ventral spinocerebellar paths (DSCT, VSCT) and some of its cortical output neurons, the Purkinje cells, as well as some neurons in its medial and intermediate output nuclei, the fastigial and interposed nuclei (see Chap. 13.3–13.5). However, the cerebellum is not essential for the generation of movement synergies, because decerebellate animals can walk, albeit clumsily. Related efferent paths also contain neurons that fire in rhythm with locomotion, for instance in the vestibulospinal, large reticulospinal, and rubrospinal paths (see Chap. 5.2). The afferent spinoreticular paths also contain such neurons. The coordinated rhythmic movements of the legs as two separate units was stressed in Figs. 10.2 and 10.3, but the detailed control during locomotion makes it most likely that the CPGs govern their component parts rather than the entire leg.

Although theoretical models abound, the nature of pattern generation is still uncertain because the exact connections of only a few spinal INs are known with certainty: Ia INs, R cells, VSCT cells, and spinobulbar cells connecting to LRN (Figs. 5.2, 5.4, and 5.5). The aforementioned neurons are driven by the CPGs or indeed could be parts of them (except those in DSCT). All these neurons help shape the motor output without dominating the production of rhythms, however. The ease with which locomotion is adjusted to changing circumstances makes it likely that CPGs are arranged as flexible networks of local control centers (or "unit CPGs"), each of which governs individual muscle synergies (e.g., knee flexors or ankle extensors). The control centers are coordinated by signals of central and/or peripheral origin. These rules apply not only to locomotion but also to other rhythmical movements that can be engaged voluntarily. Breathing is a prime example and, to a lesser extent, mastication is another.

We know that locomotor patterns are programmed, because *neural control signals for locomotion are emitted even in paralyzed animals* (e.g., with curare, the neuromuscular blocking drug). During normal locomotion, spinal MNs are modulated by reflexes of the sort discussed in Chap. 4, and the central drives of CPGs are adjusted by other reflexes that are sensitive to the speed of the treadmill (even in spinal animals). Motor performance is measured and improved by sensory feedback, which can be adjusted by the CPGs and their central controls during movements. (Control of ascending information was discussed in Chap. 5.2). Loads are monitored probably by Golgi tendon organs and group III (FRA) afferents; hip position as well as the direction of joint movements are monitored by afferents in muscles and joints. Most of our insights into neural control of locomotion have been obtained from studies with cats, building on the large fund of known connections accumulated over the years. Remarkably detailed information about feedback control has been garnered from records of single afferent fibers in chronically wired animals that can walk freely or on a treadmill.

The basic ingredient for alternate discharge of two CPGs is their tendency to fire in bursts and to inhibit each other so that only one is active at a time. Firing of bursts can be a consequence of the membrane properties of the discharging neurons. Cellular pacemaker activity ("autorhythmicity") can result from slow afterpotentials that lead to reexcitation during recovery from burst. A reciprocal arrangement of two CPGs that controls extensors (E) and flexors (F) is represented in Fig. 10.4, which also indicates their tendency to fire in bursts by arrows on the perimeter of the CPG circles. Figure 10.4 is a simplified, abstract version of the segmental spinal circuit shown in Fig. 5.2B that illustrates alpha–gamma coactivation and the interactions of R cells and Ia INs. Recall that R cells not only inhibit the synergists of their parent alpha MNs but also disinhibit antagonist MNs by inhibiting the Ia INs projecting to those antagonists.

Alpha–gamma coactivation may depend on CPGs, because it occurs in spinal animals in which descending monoaminergic paths have been activated by administration of dopa, although it may be absent in freely moving animals (cf. Chap. 5.2). Such preparations reveal how central locomotor rhythmicity can be evoked. This is called

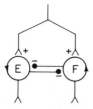

Fig. 10.4. A simple scheme to generate alternate extensions and flexions of a limb. Diagram of two central pattern generators (CPGs), which are both driven by tonic excitatory input (+) and are linked in reciprocal inhibition (−). CPGs fire spontaneous bursts, indicated by *arrowheads* on circumferences of their circular symbols. (Adapted from Grillner, 1981)

"fictive" locomotion when movement is prevented by paralysis. For instance, Fig. 10.5 shows diagrammatic examples of step-linked responses of spinal INs to stimulation of FRA afferent nerves (cf. Chap. 5.1). The horizontal lines indicate the durations of IN discharges, which are promptly followed by responses in flexor and extensor nerves. This is not the only possible pattern, however, because differ-

Fig. 10.5. Coordinated stepping signals can be generated in the spinal cord. Schematic representation of activity periods of a spinal interneuron (IN) related to ipsilateral flexor activity (i. fl.) during fictive locomotion of spinal cat treated with dopa. Ipsilateral extensors (i. ext.) and contralateral flexors (c. fl.) discharge after IN burst whose peak time (in seconds) is indicated in separate line. (Adapted from Edgerton, Grillner, Sjöström and Zangger, 1976; in Grillner, 1981)

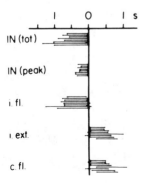

ent INs (not illustrated) are active in different phases of the step cycle.

It is of advantage to the individual to be able to uncouple particular muscles from the CPGs under certain circumstances. For instance, extensors can maintain tonic tension while flexors contract rhythmically, or there may be changes in the timing (phase) relationship between muscle groups. Figure 10.6 presents a hypothetical scheme by Grillner for coupling unit CPGs that control extensors and flexors of the hip, knee, ankle, and foot, as well as a short toe flexor. It is an enlarged version, drawn for the cat, of the basic scheme shown in Fig. 10.4. As before, the ability of each unit to fire in bursts is represented by arrows along their circumferences, and coordination between units is indicated to depend on their excitatory and inhibitory connections. How they might function is shown in the examples in Fig. 10.6B, where **Ex 1** depicts the uncoupled, independent operation of three unit CPGs. **Ex 2** illustrates how mutual inhibition between units 1 and 2, and mutual facilitation between units 2 and 3, synchronizes all three but puts 1 out of phase with 2 and 3. **Ex 3** shows how two alternating unit CPGs could both inhibit a third, causing it to fire a burst each time it is disinhibited, that is, between the bursts of each of the other two. The three examples in Fig. 10.6B for the connective scheme in Fig. 10.6A could explain the alternation between flexors and extensors at the hip and ankle, the coordination between different extensors, and the common double bursts in the knee flexors as well as the burst in the short toe flexor (of the cat).

Coordination between different limbs is of central origin, because it occurs even in spinal, paralyzed animals. It could be produced most simply for four limbs by the central interaction of four coupled generators, one for each leg. The coupling could be of the sort illustrated in Fig. 10.6A for the ankle and foot, and would be assisted by internal, corollary discharge along the VSCT. Such a scheme could provide the

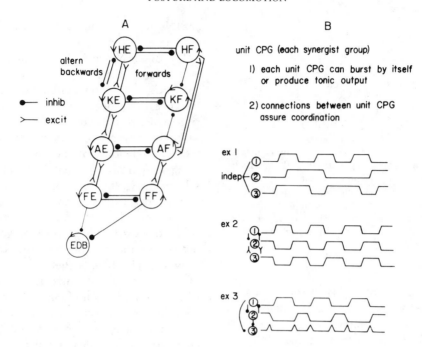

Fig. 10.6. Scheme of a limb CPG, composed of unit CPGs that each can fire bursts, based on simple arrangement shown in Fig. 10.4. Connections between unit generators decide the relative phase of different muscle groups and how they are used in locomotion. (A) Connections that could produce locomotor output of a quadruped like the cat. (B) Possible correlations (see text). Abbreviations: E, extensor; F, flexor; H, hip; K, knee; A, ankle; F, foot; EDB, short toe flexor, extensor digitorum brevis. (From Grillner, 1981)

integration needed for walking along a curved path, where the stance phase has to be shortened for the leg walking along the outer, fast side and lengthened for that on the inner, slow side of the curvature. Forward and backward motion could be produced by this network by reversing hip–knee coordination through switching from excitatory to inhibitory connections. Thus, a forward walk would be switched to a backward direction by descending commands that preferentially excite paths for reciprocal inhibition (see Chap. 5.1 and 5.2). Most importantly, Grillner points out that the concept of unit CPGs opens up simple ways for parts of the generator network to be used in motor acts that are not related to locomotion. We are now ready to consider the supraspinal centers that send descending commands to the CPGs.

3. Supraspinal Control

Which parts of the brain are needed for locomotion? The answer to this questions is the same as that for movements in general: it depends on the extent to which the action is purposeful (Chap. 2.3). Locomotion, and its adjustments by vision and proprioception, can continue without use of the high-level cortex and limbic system, but judgements about its purpose are diminished or lost. Removal of prefrontal cortex, for instance, leads to restless locomotion without apparent purpose. If the refinement of cortical processing in all areas of association cortex is abolished by bilateral removal of the basal ganglia, cats lose all discrimination of interest and follow any moving object (cf. Fig. 2.7, Chap. 2.2). If the limbic projections toward the brain stem and spinal cord are damaged (by lesions of the interpeduncular nucleus in the midbrain; cf. Chap. 2.1), the animals lose their expression of purpose as well as the ability to adapt to obstacles in their path: they continue to walk in "obstinate progression" even when pushing up against a wall.

Removal of control by the sensorimotor cortex over the putamen loop of the basal ganglia by section through the caudal part of the hypothalamus (along line I in Fig. 10.7; also see Fig. 2.7) leaves cats able to initiate locomotor activity but unable to avoid obstacles. This lesion disconnects the subthalamic nucleus, whose stimulation induces locomotion together with other motor activity. This nucleus (STN, discussed in relation to Fig. 14.2) lies within an area named the subthalamic motor region (SLR) by Orlovsky because its connection to the spinal cord is needed for modulated locomotion. More caudal disconnections, along line III in Fig. 10.7, leave only episodic periods of locomotion after recovery from the postoperative disfacilitation. All spontaneous locomotion ceases after disconnections of the limbic mammillary bodies from their spinal targets (along the intermediate line II in Fig. 10.7; cf. Chaps. 2.1 and 11.2). The mesencephalic motor region (MLR, Fig. 10.7) receives a projection from the basal ganglia, specifically from the nucleus accumbens in the ventral striatum, via the pallidum (Chaps. 11.2 and 14.1). The nucleus accumbens thus links the limbic and the locomotor systems, making the MLR a critical gate for locomotion under limbic drives. Electrical stimulation of the MLR evokes locomotion, as does stimulation of the more caudal pontine region (PLR). These areas, which might function like "command neurons" do in invertebrates, transmit their control signals to the spinal cord through reticulospinal fibers in the dorsolateral funiculus (cf. Chap. 5.2). The locations of these structures in the cat's diencephalon—that is, the part of the brain

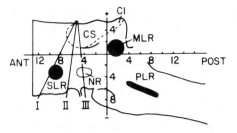

Fig. 10.7. Spinal CPGs can be driven by stimulation of some centers in the midbrain and brain stem. Locations of subthalamic (SLR), mesencephalic (MLR), and pontine (PLR) locomotor regions in cat brain, drawn against stereotaxic coordinates (in millimeters) in rostrocaudal plane. Compare to Fig. 2.1C. Abbreviations: ANT, anterior; POST, posterior; CS and CI, colliculi superior and inferior; NR, nucleus ruber (red nucleus); lines I, II, and III refer to brain transections explained in the text. (From Grillner, 1981)

that contains the thalamus and hypothalamus—are shown in sagittal section in Fig. 10.7 (compare to Fig. 2.1C).

The MLR lies in the caudal pole of the cuniform nucleus, whose location is shown in coronal section in Fig. 5.8. That nucleus is well connected to affect locomotion because it projects to the raphe nuclei and the gigantocellular and magnocellular nuclei of the brain stem (which give rise to reticulospinal fibers in the ventrolateral funiculus; Fig. 5.8), to the reticular nucleus of the thalamus (Fig. 11.14), to the pontine precerebellar nuclei and the inferior olive (Fig. 13.2), and to the striatum, the input of the basal ganglia (Fig. 14.2).

The location of the cuneiform nucleus also coincides with the dorsorostral pole of the locus ceruleus, which is an important modulator of the effectiveness of synapses elsewhere by virtue of its release of noradrenaline (NA). NA modulates by synaptic transmission of nearby cells, increasing the membrane potentials which raises the effectiveness of their other inputs by one-quarter to one-half for 0.5 to 1 second. Recall that spinal MNs tend to fire twice within 2 to 3 msec ("doublets") at the onset of stepping movements. Such high "instantaneous" frequencies speed the rise of muscular force (cf. Fig. 3.5A). NA synthesis and liberation is increased by provision of its metabolic precursor, dopa, whose effects on locomotion were discussed in the preceding unit. The locus ceruleus is thus as active a modulator for locomotion as it is for muscle tone (Chap. 8.1). The importance of the "locomotor strip" down to PLR (Fig. 10.7) has been documented above, but the strip is not indispensable. Stimulation of MLR can elicit fictive locomotion in paralyzed animals, and real locomotion in braintransected animals if their feet receive the adequate stimulation of a moving treadmill. The brain stem is a very important relay in supraspinal control, as already mentioned. Activity of the corticobulbar component of the pyramidal tract, for instance (cf. Fig. 5.12), probably adjusts natural, ongoing locomotor activity.

The cerebellum is an important guide for locomotion, although it is not essential for its initiation, as noted at the beginning of Chap. 10.2. Cerebellar activation may also be involved in the action of the MLR, because its most effective point of stimulation is in, or near to, the brachium conjunctivum that carries connections to the cerebellum. Yet, MLR stimulation can evoke locomotion even after cerebellectomy by exciting the vestibulospinal, rubrospinal, and reticulospinal paths (Figs. 5.7–5.9). Hindlimb flexion during stepping, by the cat, is controlled through cerebellar projections via reticulospinal and rubral paths, and leg extension through vestibulospinal fibers originating in Deiter's nucleus (cf. Chap. 5.2). Figure 10.8 outlines how feedback about peripheral events reaches the cerebellum through the DSCT. Internal feedback (efference, or corollary, discharges) about flexor muscle activity ascends in the VSCT, and about extensor activity in the spinoreticulocerebellar tract (SRCT). Their phasic signals arise even during fictive locomotion, which proves their central, corollary nature. External and internal feedback trig-gers rhythmic discharges of the output cells in the medial and intermediate cerebellar cortex, the Purkinje cells, which in turn is reflected in phasic firing of the cerebellar output nuclei and their projection paths (cf. Chaps. 2.3 and 5.2). Climbing fiber inputs to the cerebellum, to be described in Chap. 13.5 and 13.6, are not involved in generating locomotor rhythms but instead are crucial for their adaptations to environmental changes.

4. Reflex Actions

Reflexes of the sort outlined in Chap. 5.1 act on spinal MNs and INs. Their participation in locomotion was already referred to at the beginning of Chap. 10.2. These reflexes can be distinguished from those acting on CPGs, because the latter kind persists in spinal, paralyzed animals. Reflexes affect CPGs according to the position of the limbs and the direction of their movements. This is a spinal equivalent to the state-dependent, long-loop control of direction as well as speed in relation to the path traversed (Fig. 6.6). For spinal locomotor control, motor set and trajectory formation by the cerebrocerebellar circuit are replaced by simple polysynaptic reflexes. The spinal task system is a simpler entity that, most importantly, lacks the ability to adapt and learn (cf. Figs. 6.4B and 9.12).

Fictive locomotion responds to peripheral information about leg position and its direction of movement. Thus, fictive bursts vary according to the hip position when the leg is moved passively. Flexor activity is favored during passive, imposed flexion up to the position where extension would normally begin in the step cycle, when flexor activity is replaced by extensor activity. Conversely, during passive extension, extensor activity is evoked up to a certain point and then replaced by flexor activity. Thus, reflexes providing positive feedback are replaced by negative feedback appropriate for the programmed, upcoming support phase inherent in the

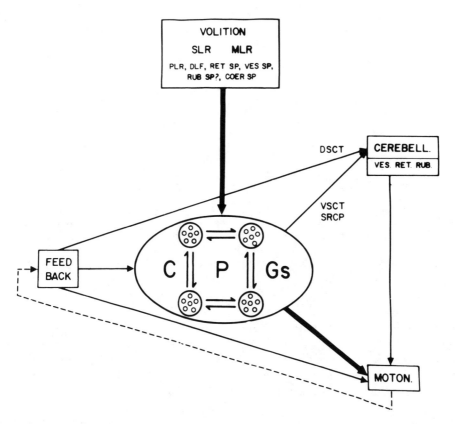

Fig. 10.8. Central pattern generator (CPG) networks are at the core of locomotor control system. A significant part of these networks is in the spinal cord, but they are normally controlled from higher centers (volition). CPGs drive spinal motoneurons (MOTON, MN). Peripheral feedback acts on CPGs, MNs, and cerebellum (via dorsal spinocerebellar tract: DSCT). Cerebellum also receives internal efference copy from CPGs (via ventral spinocerebellar and spinoreticulocerebellar path: VSCT, SRCP). Cerebellum influences spinal MNs via vestibulospinal (VES SP), reticulospinal (RET SP), and rubrospinal (RUB SP) systems. COER SP, ceruleospinal; DLF, dorsolateral funiculus; other locomotor regions as in Fig. 10.7. (From Grillner, 1981)

arrangement of the CPGs. These arrangements (schematized in Fig. 10.6) also coordinate the joints of a moving limb, even if those joints are denervated except, for instance, the hip joint, which can then still provide reference bearings for the CPGs. Similarly, increasing the load on a moving leg prolongs its swing in the ongoing direction, which assists *recovery from stumbling*. When an obstacle is encountered during extension, flexion is prolonged in order to reach a smooth, safe landing. If extension is obstructed close to the ground, landing the foot is aborted and the

leg is pulled upwards once more by flexion to try for a better landing. We must remember that the actual duration of touchdown support on a foot lasts less than one-tenth of the time of a step (i.e., about 50 msec; Figs. 10.2A and 10.2B). Reflex adjustments are therefore only useful if they occur early enough to allow for the phase lag inherent in electromechanical coupling (that is in excess of 0.1 second; Chap. 3.2). The *reflex reversals* described above provide a primitive form of motor set that also coordinates the contralateral limbs (cf. Fig. 9.11 for an example of reversal op-

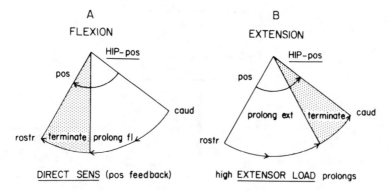

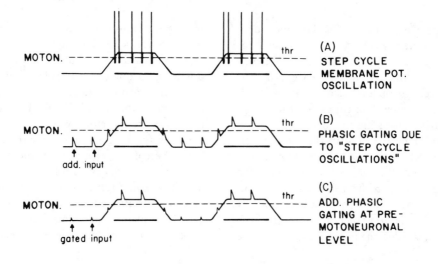

Fig. 10.9. Reflexes drive CPGs within the anatomical framework of normal locomotion patterns. (A) and (B) Diagrams showing effects that may be important during hip flexion (fl) and extension (ext). Obstructions to movements prolong those phases (positive feedback) until hip reaches position at which alternate step would ordinarily be initiated. At this position, reflex reverses and terminates ongoing movement (negative feedback). (From Grillner, 1979, 1981)

erated by higher motor set). The effects of reflexes on CPGs are shown schematically in Fig. 10.9.

If the moving leg is stopped in the support phase (during dopa-induced fictive locomotion), persistent extensor activity ensues, although the other leg continues to walk. These reflexes rely on afferents in muscles as well as in joints, but they can operate with only one input or the other.

Multiple modes of feedback are universal in the central nervous system (cf. Figs. 9.3 and 9.4). Directional sensitivity exerts effects during dopa-induced fictive locomotion that are analogous to the effects during imposed, passive movements. During fictive flexion, added loads facilitate flexor activity, and vice versa for extensors. The positive-feedback effects terminate when movement directions are reversed. These

Fig. 10.10. CPGs gate spinal MNs and their inputs. (A) Membrane potential oscillations during step cycle. In most depolarized part (i.e., above threshold: thr), cell is spiking. In (B) and (C), spikes have been omitted; only their durations are indicated by *horizontal bar*. (B) shows that additional input (add. input) is gated out by step-cycle oscillations. (C) shows that additional input may be gated out also through diminution at a pre-MN site. (From Grillner, 1981)

considerations of limb reflexes triggered by sensors of limb position and direction recall the proposal that postural adjustments depend on sensing when particular motor synergies can or cannot support the body in the erect plane (Fig. 9.13). Presumably the same wide range of inputs are used to control locomotion as well as posture in the intact individual.

Finally, we may ask how the CPGs influence spinal MNs, how they "gate" reflex actions. In this context CPGs can be regarded as spinal devices under the influence of the brain stem centers discussed above. Two probable mechanisms are known: a postsynaptic one influences the responsiveness of MNs to its inputs, and a premotoneuronal one depresses the amplitude of those inputs. The postsynaptic effect consists of rhythmic raising and lowering of the membrane potential of MNs, making them respond better by depolarization and respond less well by hyperpolarization. This is illustrated in Fig. 10.10 as potential steps, drawn as solid lines. In Fig. 10.10A the cell is firing bursts as its membrane potential threshold has fallen below threshold (indicated by the horizontal broken line). The membrane oscillations and threshold are the same in Fig. 10.10B,C, but the bursts are not shown. Instead, Fig. 10.10B presents an additional, subthreshold input that is ineffective in discharging the MN. Figure 10.10C indicates the depression of this input before it reaches the MN, making it even less effective. An example of such possible premotoneuronal mechanism is the suppression of low-threshold cutaneous inputs by activation of the dorsolateral reticulospinal tract (Fig. 5.6B).

5. Summary

Walking and running consist of patterned leg actions that balance the body while transporting it across the ground. The legs assume the same relative position throughout the walking cycle at different speeds by adjustment of the bursts of power emission during pushoff and of power absorption during weight acceptance. The preservation of patterned leg use at different speeds implies that the same programs are used by the central nervous system at all speeds to control transient changes of power in relation to its steady state. This closely resembles the preservation of writing patterns at different speeds and of patterned muscle use in isotonic or isometric arm movements. Patterns can be preserved because Henneman's size principle of spinal recruitment fits phasic muscle use automatically to its steady base level.

Locomotor programs are produced by central pattern generators (CPGs) that are located in the spinal cord. Programs can be emitted even from spinal, paralyzed animals (fictive locomotion). Normally, however, they are used flexibly under the direction of higher center. CPGs for control of a whole limb are probably made up of networks of small unit generators that control simple muscle synergies. CPGs drive spinal motoneurons (MNs) by raising and lowering their membrane potentials rhythmically, which causes the MNs to fire in bursts. Alternating activity of two opposing muscles can be produced by the mutual reciprocal inhibition of two such burst-firing CPGs. The excitability of CPGs is governed strongly by locomotor centers in the midbrain and brain stem that are under limbic as well as higher control. For instance, intact connections between the limbic system and the association cortex are essential for judgements about purposeful locomotion.

Peripheral and internal feedback regulate the CPGs as well as the motor servos under their control. Peripheral feedback arises from afferents in muscles and joints that are sensitive to the positions of the limbs and the directions of their movements. These messages can generate spinal reflexes that prevent stumbling by prolonging or terminating leg movements according to where that leg ordinarily switches from flexion to extension or vice versa (reflex reversal). Internal feedback consists of efference copies carried by the ventral spinocerebellar tract to the cerebellum, which exerts important supraspinal control over the CPGs.

References

Beninger, R. J. 1983. The role of dopamine in locomotor activity and learning. *Brain Res. Rev.* 6:173–196.

Bernstein, N. 1967. *The coordination and regulation of movements.* Oxford:Pergamon Press. [Fig. 10.1]

Conrad, B., Benecke, R., Carnehl, J., Höne, J., and Meinck, H. M. 1983. Pathophysiological aspects of human locomotion. In *Motor control mechanisms in health and disease,* ed. J. E. Desmedt. *Adv. Neurol.* 39:717–726.

Edgerton, V. R., Grillner, A., Sjöström, A., and Zangger, P. 1976. Central generation of locomotion in vertebrates. In *Neural control of locomotion,* eds. R. M. Herman, S. Grillner, P. Stein, and D. G. Stuart. *Adv. Behav. Biol.* 19:439–464. [Fig. 10.5]

Fel'dman, J. L. , and Grillner, S. 1983. Control of vertebrate respiration and locomotion: a brief account. *Physiologist* 26:310.-316.

Forssberg, H. 1982. Spinal locomotor functions and descending control. In *Brainstem control of spinal mechanisms,* eds. B. Sjolund, and A. Bjorklund. Fenstrom Foundation Ser. 1, pp. 253–271. Amsterdam: Elsevier Biomedical Press.

Forssberg, H., Grillner, S., and Rossignol, S. 1977. Phasic gain control of reflexes from the dorsum of the paw during spinal locomotion, *Brain Res.* 132:121–139.

Grillner, S. 1981. Control of locomotion in bipeds, tetrapods and fish. In *Motor control.* Sect. 1, vol. 2. *Handbook of physiology,* ed. V. B. Brooks, pp. 1179–1236. Bethesda, Md.: American Physiological Society. [Figs. 10.4–10.10]

Grillner, S. 1979. Interaction between central and peripheral mechanisms in the control of locomotion. In *Reflex control of posture and movements,* eds. R. Granit and O. Pompeiano. *Prog. Brain Res.* 50:227–235. [Fig. 10.9]

Herman, R. M., Wirta, R., Bampton, S., and Finley, F. R. 1976. Human solutions for locomotion. I. Single limb analysis. In *Neural control of locomotion,* eds. R. S. Herman, S. Grillner, P. G. Stein, and D. G. Stuart. *Adv. Behav. Biol.* 18:13–49.

McMahon, T. A. 1984. *Muscles, reflexes, and locomotion.* Princeton, N.J.: Princeton University Press.

Mogenson, G. J. 1984. Limbic-motor integration—with emphasis on initiation of exploratory and goal-directed locomotion. In *Modulation of Sensorimotor activity during alterations in behavioral states.* ed. R. Bandler, pp. 121–137, New York: Alan R. Liss.

Murray, M. P. 1967. Gait as a total pattern of movement. In *An exploratory and analytical survey of therapeutic exercise,* eds. E. C. Wood, D. E. Voss, and H. D. Bouman. *Am. J. Phys. Med.* 46:(1) 290–333. [Fig. 10.2A]

Pierrot-Deseilligny, E., Bergego, C., and Maieres, L. 1983. Reflex control of bipedal gain in man. In *Motor control mechanisms in health and disease,* ed. J. E. Desmedt. *Adv. Neurol.* 39:699–716.

Shik, M. L., and Orlovsky, G. N. 1976. Neurophysiology of locomotor automatism. *Physiol. Rev.* 56:465–501.

Smith, J. L. 1980. Programming of stereotyped limb movements by spinal generators. In *Tutorials in motor behavior,* eds. G. E. Stelmach and J. Requin. *Adv. Psychol.* 1:95–115.

Stein, P. S. G. 1978. Motor systems, with specific reference to the control of locomotion. *Ann. Rev. Neurosci.* 1:61–81.

Wetzel, M. C., and Howell, L. G. 1981. Properties and mechanisms of locomotion. In *Motor coordination,* eds. A. L. Towe and E. S. Luschei, Vol. 5. *Handbook of behavioral neurobiology,* pp. 567–625. New York: Plenum Press.

Wetzel, M. C., and Stuart, D. G. 1976. Ensemble characteristics of cat locomotion and its neural control. *Prog. Neurobiol.* 7:1–98.

Winter, D. A. 1983. Biomechanical motor patterns in normal walking. *J. Motor Behav.* 15:302-330. [Figs. 10.2B and 10.3]

Winter, D. A. 1979. *Biomechanics of human movement.* New York: John Wiley & Sons.

Winter, D. A. 1984a. Kinematic and kinetic patterns in human gait: variability and compensating effects. *Hum. Movement Sci.* 3:51-76.

Winter, D. A. 1984b. Moments of force and mechanical power in jogging. *J. Biomechanics* 16:91-97.

IV

The Middle Level of the Motor Hierarchy

In this part we consider the hierarchical middle level, its connections and components, how they are guided by "higher" levels, and how they interact with the "lower" spinal cord (Chap. 2.2). We deal with neural connections and the meaning of their messages, beginning with an introduction designed to orient us. Chapter 11 is an overview of the main components of the middle level and their connections, extending the outlines begun in Chaps. 2 and 5. Building on that foundation, we then consider how motor commands are fashioned and implemented by the motor cortex, the cerebellum, and the basal ganglia, in Chaps. 12–14.

INTRODUCTION

The middle level consists primarily of the sensorimotor cortex, the cerebellum, and the putamen circuit of the basal ganglia (Fig. 2.7), including the thalamic connections of these structures as well as some parts of the brain stem. This level receives instructions about *what* to do (by making strategic decisions, motor plans; Chap. 2.2) and dispenses commands about *how* to carry them out. It does the motor control "staff work" for the higher level "headquarters" that determine the relevance of the incoming messages and the optimal responses to them (Fig. 2.4). The middle level implements behavioral decisions by making tactical adjustments to suit the circumstances of the moment; that is, the middle level chooses and updates motor programs. These programs (Chap. 2.2) are timed and scaled to fulfill the behavioral intent. Toward this end the brain needs translations of "intent" and of the coordinates of the sensory reflections of the world around us into those of the world within us. How intent is encoded in abstract form still remains a mystery. We have seen examples of translation into coordinates of muscular function, for instance, in the scaling of hold programs—that is, how to maintain the positions of our limbs at particular angles and with particular stiffness (Figs. 7.7 and

9.5)—and of the scaling of move programs as reference trajectories (Figs. 6.6 and 6.10, and 7.8). Such examples also document how the timing of the brain is adjusted to accommodate the delays caused by the conduction of messages within it, and especially by their (electromechanical) coupling to mechanical action.

Behavioral relevance for intended motor acts is established by interaction of the limbic system (cf. Fig. 2.3) and the high-level cerebral association cortex (e.g., prefrontal, temporal, and parietal areas). The prefrontal cortex is necessary for formulating integrated behavior that is relevant to contextual, goal-oriented action, particularly in novel situations. One of its functions is to reject irrelevant inputs. The association areas project to the premotor cortex (lateral area 6) and the supplementary motor area (SMA; medial area 6), which organize the principal output stage of the middle level, the sensorimotor cortex. From area 6 onwards, "premotor" instructions are converted into specifications of how motor acts are to be carried out. The cortical areas are identified by name in Fig. 2.1A,C and by their numbers in Fig. 11.1. Parietal association cortex includes area 7 (and the secondary projection area 5 in some classifications). The temporaral areas include 40, 39, 22, and 23, and the prefrontal areas are those rostral to area 8.

Just how are behavioral commands transformed into sensorimotor actions? The pyramidal, corticospinal system receives and processes three major kinds of information: feedforward instructions for motor acts, internal feedback (efference copies), and external sensory feedback for guidance of the resultant movements (Chap. 2.2, Fig. 2.5, and Chap. 5.2). "Higher," feedforward instructions from the prefrontal, as well as posterior parietal and temporal, association areas reach the premotor cortex (area 6) through transcortical projections. The motivational and emotional components are provided by the limbic system, which consists of the hypothalamus and its extended connections in the CNS (Fig. 2.7). Limbic influences are examined in Chap. 11.2; here we just take a quick glimpse. The crucial fact about limbic steering of sensorimotor activities is its multiple method of control. It is exerted through association cortex, nonprimary motor areas, and subcortical motor centers, because the sensorimotor cortex has few direct limbic inputs. The limbic system projects to association cortex through the caudal part of the cingulate gyrus, and through its rostral part to circuits concerned more closely with motor activities. This multiple limbic steering of sensorimotor activities presumably provides more versatile control than might be achieved by exclusive direct projection to pericruciate cortex, because motivation is brought to bear on the parts of the brain that decide *what* to do as well as on parts that carry out those orders. In addition to their corticocortical connections, both parts of the cingulate cortex connect with at least two subcortical structures of vital importance for motor control, the basal ganglia and some pontine nuclei that project to the cerebellum, which also receive ascending subcortical limbic connections

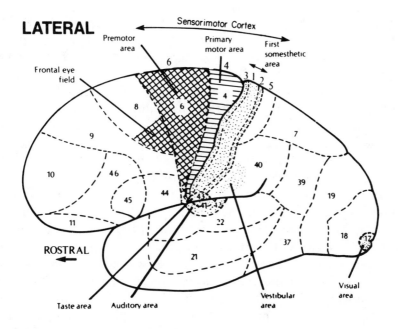

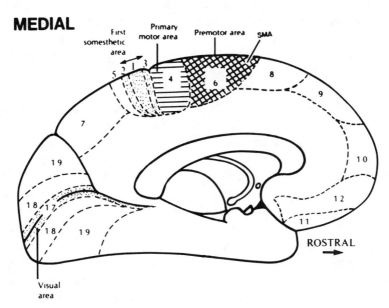

Fig. 11.1. Locations of the major areas of the cerebral cortex, which can be distinguished by distribution criteria of cellular types (cytoarchitectonic classification of Brodman). Compare to Fig. 2.1. SMA, Supplementary motor area. (Slightly modified from Barr and Kiernan, 1983)

(Fig. 2.2, 2.5, and 2.7). These double connections may be parts of corollary loops to control the effectiveness of limbic orders.

The major routes for information flow to premotor cortex are sketched in Fig. 11.2, which stresses the central position of the premotor and the supplementary cortices as gateways in programming of the pri-

mary motor area. Once the caudate loop of the basal ganglia has enabled
the higher level cortex to form overall motor plans, movements are initiated through the influence of the lateral cerebellum on the premotor
and primary motor cortices. In addition, movements are managed by the
putamen loop of the basal ganglia, the intermediate cerebellum, the red
nucleus, and the medullary reticular formation (RF). Figure 11.2 is a
modification of the seminal scheme proposed by Allen and Tsukahara
over a decade ago. Cerebellar connections are drawn to the sensorimotor
cortex (as in Fig. 2.7), which includes area 5, not shown here. The cerebellum is not connected by direct tracts to the (higher order) association
cortex, which occupies most of the white areas in Fig. 11.1. Figure 2.7
features the contribution of the limbic system, together with the two
recently recognized separate circuits through the dorsal basal ganglia.
Figure 11.2 indicates connections of the superior colliculus, a nucleus for
integration of somatosensory input with behaviorally relevant visual information. Collicular integration yields coordinated visual and body orientation toward a visual target. The reticular part of the substantia nigra
is one of its important inputs. The integrated collicular output is projected to the premotor cortex and the adjacent frontal eye field (Fig. 11.1).
The colliculus receives specially processed visual information from parietal area 7, which deals with task-related, directed visual attention.
These examples of translation from one local brain "language" to another indicate how the premotor cortex is instructed by the "hidden
masters" in limbic and association cortex.

The middle level receives instructions of various complexities through
transcortical projections, a theme that was introduced in Chap. 2. Overall plans (or "complex programs") for related motor acts are prepared
with the aid of the caudate circuit of the basal ganglia. Such a motor
plan could be exemplified by the sequence of getting up to greet a friend
and then offering the hand in greeting. Orders for such sequential or
simultaneous actions (as part of a repertoire) are apparently routed
through the prefrontal cortex, since this type of performance suffers
equally where there are lesions of either the caudate nucleus or the prefrontal cortex. The caudate circuit is thus part of the "higher" hierarchical level, in as much as it enables their plans to be translated into
motor action. The connections of the caudate loop (paralleling transcortical projections to the prefrontal cortex) suggest that it controls the effectiveness of corticocortical processing. Instructions for simpler acts
within the overall performance, such as the extension of the arm when
offering the hand, reach area 6 through the putamen circuit of the basal
ganglia that probably scales the amplitudes of the patterns of motor action. The two circuits, through the putamen and through the lateral cerebellum (Fig. 11.2), convey motor "intent" at the simpler level of its
implementation.

Both circuits of the basal ganglia are thought to participate in modulating the overall intensity of cerebral action, one with respect to overall

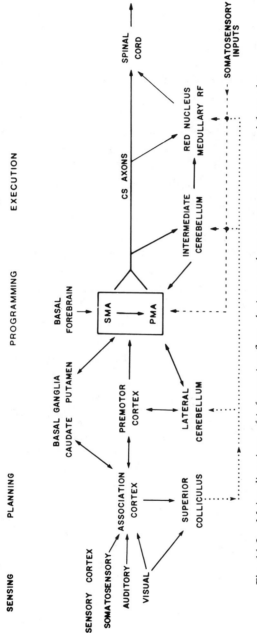

Fig. 11.2. Major directions of information flow, during a voluntary movement, to and from the primary (PMA) and supplementary motor areas (SMA). Only some of the connections of the superior colliculus are shown. CS, Corticospinal; RF, reticular formation. For details see text. Compare to Figs. 2.7, 5.9, and 5.10. (Modified from Humphrey, 1983; after Allen and Tsukahara, 1974; DeLong, Georgopoulos, and Crutcher, 1983)

plans and the other with respect to their constituent postures and movements. The putamen circuit scales muscular responses without altering their relative strengths; that is, they scale the amplitudes of complex and simple output patterns as a whole in relation to the task context (e.g., Figs. 7.1 and 7.2). The cerebellum particularly determines the correctly timed execution of programmed responses, their updating, and also their skillful adaptation (Chap. 13). Instructions for complex and simpler acts cooperate to prepare the sensorimotor cortex before movements begin. The resulting modulation of muscular excitabilities is further modified by feedback about the circumstances that affect the required effort at any given time (see Figs. 5.9–5.12 for pathways). The sensorimotor cortex receives such feedback from the periphery through the sensory systems, as well as from within the CNS through corollary efference signals about movement commands at different levels (Fig. 2.5).

Diagrams of brain circuits usually are a mixture of anatomical charts and information flow sheets. They are useful because they direct our attention to some special aspect, but of course none can show even all major connections because of their complexity. Figure 11.2, discussed above, is no exception. Figure 11.3 is a compromise between the two aims. Many paths are left out and laterality is ignored as in previous diagrams, but it is useful for reorientation about the overall connections. The terms "tract" and "path" have been used interchangeably. The

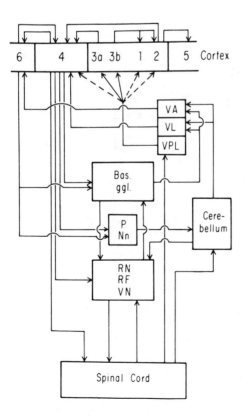

Fig. 11.3. A condensed flowchart of signals in some of the main pathways connecting components of the motor system. Cerebral cortical areas numbered as in Fig. 11.1, and thalamic nuclei named as in Fig. 11.14. Other abbreviations: Bas. ggl., basal ganglia; P Nn, pontine nuclei; RN, red nucleus, RF, reticular formation; VN, vestibular nuclei. (From Somjen, 1983)

stricter distinction between them is that tracts make direct connections between two structures, while paths are less direct because they relay through synaptic connections. The two loops through the dorsal basal ganglia are combined into one, and the separate projections from that and the cerebellum to the supplementary and premotor cortices are shown just as "area 6" without much distinction of the thalamic nuclei involved. (Those points are illustrated in greater detail in Figs. 11.9 and 11.11.)

11

Overview of the
Middle Level

The purpose of this chapter is to gain an understanding of the *anatomical basis of sensorimotor integration*. The chapter is a selective summary by necessity, dealing with the flow of information in the circuits of Figs. 11.2 and 11.3. Beginning with "high-level" input from the association cortex, we continue with input from the limbic system, and then go on to integration within the "middle level," considering inputs from the cerebellum, basal ganglia, and sensory afferents.

This order of presentation reflects the fact that task orientation is imposed on the motor cortex by grouping its output neurons into appropriate input–output units. Inputs, which are of many kinds from the periphery and from within the CNS, are grouped functionally by transcortical and thalamocortical mechanisms. The middle level activates appropriate muscle synergies by forming task-oriented cell assemblies in the cerebral cortex and in its related structures. This crucial function in motor control involves the use of association cortex (Fig. 11.2) and of subcortical sensorimotor circuits looping through the dorsal basal ganglia as well as the cerebellum. These loops course back to sensorimotor cortex (i.e., areas 6, 4, 3, 1, 2, and 5) through separate thalamic nuclei (see Figs. 11.1 and 11.9, later). Functional organization of the middle level is brought about by four devices, of which three are under-

stood reasonably well: the cerebellum, the basal ganglia, and cortico(trans)-cortical connections, including input from high-order association cortex. The fourth device, the limbic system, is still a bit mysterious; it is the best hidden of the "masters" referred to in the introduction to this part.

1. "High-Level" Inputs

How is sensory information integrated to be most useful for motor action? How is its relevance for motivated action recognized and translated into appropriate motor activity? Sensorimotor integration is made possible by cortical summing of information, but integration does not consist of simple summation. Integration is brought about by selective, "conditional" summations. Such summations occur in many parts of the CNS. The higher the species, with humans at the top, the greater is the number of alternate pathways in the CNS to the distributed foci for such summations. The frontal lobes are the most important structures for abstract thought and the organization of independent behavior with regard to future goals. The prefrontal cortex is linked reciprocally with the parietal cortex which, in turn, is linked to the premotor cortex. This will be considered below.

Let us consider the example of how "*di-*

rected attention" is brought to bear on the even-shifting visual scene. The desire to attend to a particular, selected visual object requires orienting the body and eyes toward the object of attention. Desire begins with projections from the limbic system (Figs. 2.2, 2.3 and 11.7). Two transcortical projections from the cingulate gyrus are relevant: to the cortical frontal eye field (which is needed for "voluntary" quick eye movements, Fig. 11.1) and indirectly to the sensorimotor cortex through transcortical connections via area 7, of the posterior parietal cortex, which is needed for visually directed attention. Further, there are cingulate connections to the motor cortex, and subcortical limbic connections to the superior colliculus as well as to the basal ganglia (Chap. 5.2 and Figs. 11.2 and 11.4).

Area 7 (part of which is named area PG in Fig. 11.4) is of central importance for directed visual attention. Electrical stimulation of this area evokes eye movements and head turning in the same direction. If this area in the inferior parietal lobule is injured or diseased, human subjects or monkeys suffer from "contralateral neglect," a diminished ability to integrate visual and tactile sensory information. As a consequence there is deficient orientation of the body in space and a disability to execute purposeful movements in space. This is an example of impaired purposeful movements (apraxia). The effects of the lesions are explained by the properties of the lost neural organization. Mountcastle has shown in experiments with monkeys that many neurons in area 7 are light sensitive and discharge only when the eye sees a relevant target. These cells reflect the attention of the animal. Other, similar cells also discharge under these conditions but only before voluntary quick eye movements (saccades, Figs. 9.3 and 9.4). Their responses depend, however, on the *state* of the animal rather than on the details of the viewed object. The most important of these states is whether the subjects direct their visual attention to an object with interest in a task-related manner. Another is

the general attentiveness of the subject (which requires arousal by the ascending reticular activating system and the nucleus basalis in the forebrain; Figs. 5.8, 11.2, and 11.4). Task-related interest and motivation depend mostly on limbic signals that a desired reward has been identified as available. Arrival of such signals in association cortex leads to task execution. In our example, these signals govern whether or not to foveate the target and to proceed with vision-related motor tasks. The conditional consent involves the special light-sensitive and task-dependent neurons in area 7, described above. (They operate as "gates" between interest and saccadic eye movements. Examples of other gating functions were described in Chap. 5.1 for spinal INs.) Visual attention can progress to manual reaching with the assistance of a group of light-insensitive neurons in area 7 that discharge before and during task-related arm activity as long as the animal is in a task-related state of attention. Like the visuomotor neurons, these neurons are related to limb functions but not with respect to the details of motor action.

State-dependent "manipulatory" neurons in the secondary sensorimotor area (area 5, located in the superior parietal lobule) also seem to open links to motor action. Projections from area 5 to area 6 and further direct connection to the primary motor cortex (area 4) presumably trigger detailed precentral enactment of the intended action (Figs. 11.5 and 11.6). Furthermore, area 4 accesses the motor-oriented subcortical loop of the basal ganglia through the putamen, and that of the cerebellum through the pons.

The parietal cortex apparently provides three kinds of information for motor programming to the premotor and supplementary motor cortex: (1) the demanded direction of motion in "extrapersonal" space, which is related to the body's proprioceptive reference systems, (2) the body's position in space, and (3) the starting position of the limbs to be moved. Area 5 receives its main inputs from the primary sensory area (but is also reciprocally connected with the premotor cortex and the SMA) and projects to area 7 (Fig. 11.5). The actions of association cortex are never of just one kind. For instance, one-third of the neurons in area 5 issue central commands for neurons in area 4 before movement onset, while two-thirds follow up on the correct direction of the ongoing movement. They encode direction much like precentral neurons, but those neurons in area 5 fire after movement onset instead of before. The later firing group is highly sensitive to peripheral input, while the command group responds only to central signals. Electrical stimulation of this area produces components of complex orienting movements involving the head, shoulders, and limbs. Lesions of this area in monkeys lead to tactile avoidance; that is, the animal presents only the healthy side for contact and automatically withdraws a limb from tactile contact.

A theory by Denny-Brown proposes that the parietal cortex controls exploration of the environment through its influence on subcortically mediated, extensor-oriented "grasping" responses. The "instinctive tactile grasping reaction" is an orientation of the hand or foot in space such as to bring a light contact stimulus into the palm (or sole) when very facile grasping occurs. The reaction is essentially an exploratory palpation directed vertically into space from the point of contact. The parietal influence is thought to be balanced by the frontal control of subcortical (flexor-oriented) "avoidance" responses. Parietal lesions therefore "release" the frontally supported avoiding reaction, and conversely, frontal lesions (of areas 8, 6, or 24) release the parietally supported grasping responses. Grasping is reinforced by precentral-related thalamic lesions, for instance in the ventrolateral nucleus (VL). Patients (or monkeys) with parietal lesions exhibit "tactile avoiding," which includes withdrawal of the limb in response to contact with any part of the fingers or hand, even just a few hairs. It appears as if the unpleasant attributes of every stimulus are emphasized at the expense of pleasant or interesting features.

The limbic influence on this reaction is confirmed by its reinforcement through lesions of the anterior thalamic nuclei, which relay to the medial surface of the frontal lobe and to the cingulate and hippocampal cortices (Figs. 2.4 and 11.12). Movements and postures thus acquire an exaggerated emotional component, which can lead to abnormally persistent attitudes, such that attempts by the examiner to displace the limb meet increasing resistance (dystonia). Denny-Brown concluded that the balance between grasping and avoiding actions depends on correct function of area 4 (which is also essential for exploratory reactions with the hands or fingers, foot, or lips to contact stimuli), because this balance is not recovered after precentral lesions. He deemed the precentral gyrus as essential for movements directed into extrapersonal space that accurately orient the hand or foot to a target, but not essential for retraction from a touch contact or a painful or visual stimulus. Support for this view comes from properties of neurons in area 4, which will be considered in the next chapter.

The dysfunctions described in this chapter show what we can learn from the study of lesions. Lesions reveal what the brain can still do without an excised part. They reveal residual functions after loss of specific information or commands, or of a functional balance. For instance, destruction of the cerebellum reveals what the cortex and the basal ganglia can still do, and destruction of the basal ganglia show the residual capabilities of the cerebrocerebellar circuit. "Release" of abnormal functions can teach us (as in the apparent paradox caused by loss of frontal and parietal cortices) about the controls exerted by the removed tissue. The results of lesions, considered in isolation, do not necessarily reveal much about the essential functions that are normally performed by the excised tissue.

Visually guided movements depend heavily on the superior colliculus (Fig. 11.2) which participates in directed visual attention. It keeps the visual field intelligible despite altered views presented to the retina during movements of the head and body. It receives visual signals from the retina and, in addition, is reciprocally connected with the visual cortex, the frontal eye field, and area 7 (Fig. 11.4). When the eye foveates a target of interest with the intent for visuomotor action, the discharge intensity of collicular neurons is enhanced. The same is true for neurons firing before voluntary saccades in related areas such as the frontal eye field and the posterior parietal cortex. The basal ganglia are involved in this alerting function, as judged by the preceding neural discharge in the reticular part of the substantia nigra (SNpr). We will meet a form of enhancement again as a property of task-related neurons in the motor cortex (Chap. 12). It is the parietal connection that endows the colliculus with its ability to steer vision to objects of interest. "Steering" also invokes the need for participation of the cerebellum, which is apprised of visual events through the pontine connections of the visual as well as parietal cortex and of the collicular tectopontine tract (Chap. 5.2).

Figure 11.4 summarizes the connections of area 7 (PG) that make it a focus for selective action. It filters out uninteresting objects and events from the ever-shifting scene described in terms of shapes, motion, space, and color. This kind of exclusion is an important principle in the operation of the interpretative, "higher order" brain. The prefrontal cortex, which projects to premotor area 6, also inhibits the transmission of irrelevant material. Prefrontal lesions in monkeys lead to indiscriminate, hyperactive tactile motor explorations, and in humans and monkeys alike also diminish the appreciation of time and how to deal with it, causing an inability to plan ahead and to organize tasks in time. Even after much elaboration of the visual input

in the main visual pathway, it says nothing about the significance of the visual scene.

The recognition of the *significance* of an object (with regard to food, for instance) appears in a limbic structure, the amygdala, and is reflected in the activity in temporal and orbitofrontal cortex. Bilateral lesions of the temporal lobes in monkeys produce excessive visual exploration during which objects are picked up but not recognized for what they are. The lack of recognition (agnosia) is caused by dysfunction of the inferior lobe, which receives projections from the parietal, prefrontal, and limbic cortices. These descriptions of some of the consequences of lesions in association cortex display the loss of their normal *selective* actions. We might think of the normal accentuation of relevance by the association cortex as an editorial function (Chap. 3.1), perhaps as in a news magazine which directs our attention to selected items that are deemed to be of special interest. It stands in contrast to the broad-band reporting of the main line systems such as the somatosensory medial lemniscal system or the visual geniculostriate system. They publish "all the news that's fit to print." The diagram of the posterior (inferior) parietal connections in Fig. 11.4 is to the point.

Let us view Fig. 11.4 (half-seriously) as a conference of the senior editors of a magazine. The (sensory) news has already been sorted and sifted by various departments (the high-order association areas), and only the most relevant items come to the table, together with some background material provided by special (thalamic) correspondents. The implications of what is politically important and has readership appeal have been recognized by the (limbic) analysts, and their senior decides what should be stressed and how much. Copy composition is kept going by the (reticular) press chief, who has his eye on the clock and sees to it that coffee is served right at the conference table.

This whimsical description is perhaps

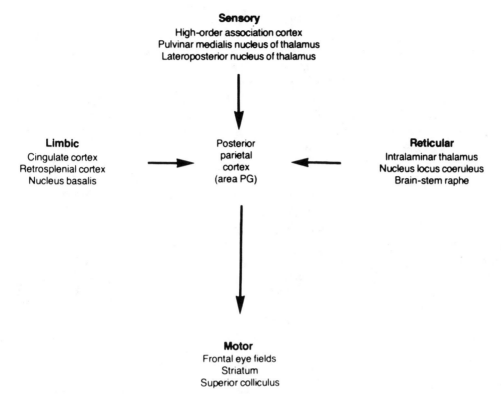

Sensory
High-order association cortex
Pulvinar medialis nucleus of thalamus
Lateroposterior nucleus of thalamus

Limbic
Cingulate cortex
Retrosplenial cortex
Nucleus basalis

Posterior
parietal
cortex
(area PG)

Reticular
Intralaminar thalamus
Nucleus locus coeruleus
Brain-stem raphe

Motor
Frontal eye fields
Striatum
Superior colliculus

Fig. 11.4. Summary of connections of the dorsal part of the inferior parietal lobule (area 7, part PG) that are relevant to directed attention. For details see text. (From Mesulam, 1983)

not too far off the mark, and it is not dis-respectful of the scholarship behind the diagram. How does the edited, general activity in area 7 lead to specific motor action? Scientific views evolve constantly as new methods reveal new aspects, including, of course, motor control. The diagram of "motor" output from PG correctly links it to the input of the basal ganglia (the striatum, which contains the putamen and the caudate nucleus), which was once thought of as a general reentrant path to motor cortex. We now recognize, however, that area 7 connects with the caudate loop, which returns to association cortex and not to motor cortex (which is connected with the movement-related putamen loop, Figs. 2.7 and 11.2). The main line of communication of this headquarters with its staff seems to be through

transcortical projections from prefrontal cortex to area 6.

How the association areas of the cerebral cortex acquire their "associative" properties becomes intelligible when we consider their anatomical connections. Figure 11.5 presents a scheme, based on the work of Jones and Powell that is thought to serve the buildup of sensory associations by synaptic convergence. The main points are the successive outward projections from somatosensory and visual cortex. (A few of the more recently discovered connections have been added. The corresponding links of the auditory system are not shown.) The projections from the three primary sensory areas converge in the quaternary links, which include the prefrontal cortex (shown as area 46) and the superior temporal sulcus (STS). Multiple convergences create associative levels of "higher" orders, but they lose their detailed somatotopy after leaving the secondary layer (e.g., areas 4, 6, and 5, which are still organized and connected somatotopically). What is lost are the detailed descriptions of the world around us and within us (somatotopy). What is gained is the ability to emit selective responses that can be triggered by a variety of meaningful stimuli.

The ability of neurons in the higher association cortex to respond to "abstractions" also means that stimuli can elicit different actions than they would have before processing in this cortex, which has already received some emotionally meaningful inputs from the limbic, cingulate gyrus and the amygdala. Somesthetic, visual and auditory association areas each project to the cingulate cortex and to the parahippocampal areas. This might help to channel biological drives into activities that depend more on the conditions of the society in which the individual lives, a distinction shared by the human species with the higher primates. Elaborations of emotionally meaningful inputs are projected back to the hypothalamus by way of the amygdala (cf. Figs. 2.3, 2.4, and 2.7) and hippocampus, which is involved in processing memories. Limbic and non-limbic information converges partly in the basal ganglia. Exactly how and where this occurs is still unknown. The limbic system *enables* the elaboration of task-related motor acts by channeling its commands to the association cortex and the sensorimotor system.

Fig. 11.5. Diagram of cascaded, stepwise, outward projections to the limbic system from somatosensory (A) and visual (B) areas of the cerebral cortex, numbered as in Fig. 11.1. Equivalent connections from auditory cortex are not shown. SMA, Supplementary motor area; PrCo, precentral cortex other than areas 4 and 6. Some recently discovered connections have been sketched in with broken lines. Also, it is now known that area 3 does not project to area 4. All sensory paths converge in the depths of the superior temporal sulcus (STS). TG, Temporal gyrus; OF, orbital surface of the frontal lobe. Most associative cortices project back to the amygdala and thus to the hypothalamus (limbic system). Compare to Figs. 2.8B and 11.14. (After Jones and Powell, 1970; modified from Popper and Eccles, 1977)

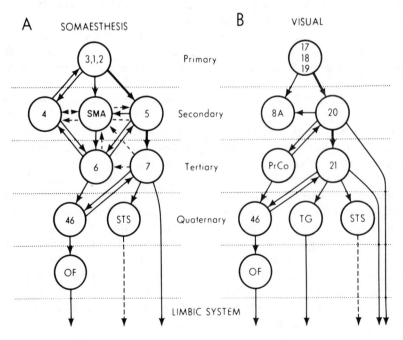

There is some direct indication that the SMA (medial area 6, the recipient of the output of the putamen loop of the basal ganglia) is involved in programming motor subroutines in relation to conscious intention. Its regional blood flow increases in the human brain while the subject *thinks* out, but does not carry out, a proposed motor sequence such as successive apposition of the fingers. In contrast, the premotor area (lateral area 6, which receives the output of the cerebellar loop) is activated when movements are made under guidance of sensory information. It is also activated during planning and executing well-learned finger movements. These tests of regional cerebral blood flow (rCBF), which are accurate to within 40 seconds, also show that the premotor cortex (lateral area 6) becomes active when voluntary movements are executed under the guidance of sensory information. Figure 11.6 presents Roland's summary charts of the selective activations of brain areas discussed in this chapter. It is possible to distinguish changes in rCBF caused by internal intention (Fig. 11.6A) as opposed to responding to external sensory input (Fig. 11.6B). Distinction is also made in Fig. 11.6 between actions involving intrapersonal space—that is, spaces of the body related to each other like the distances between our fingers, tested by their apposition (upper row)—as opposed to extrapersonal space, tested by pointing at objects located in front of the body (lower row).

Returning from the broad-spectrum view to a more detailed one, it should be pointed out that the specific correspondences between thalamus and sensorimotor areas are based on projections between small groups of cells in each, which are usually interspersed with other functional groups. The cortical cell groups are arranged in radial columns (at 90-deg angles to the cortical surface; Fig. 11.12). Functional outputs are served by many columns

Fig. 11.6. Conversion of intention into motor output. The medial and lateral aspects of the brain are shown on the left and right sides of both (A) and (B). The cortical areas shown (for which regional blood flow increased by more than 15% when subjects were executing voluntary movements) were not contingent on sensory information in (A), but were so in (B). All areas were activated bilaterally except MI and SI. MI, Primary motor area; SI, primary somatosensory area (1, 2, 3); SII, secondary somatosensory area; P, premotor area; F, frontal cortex; SMA, supplementary motor area; SS, supplementary sensory area; B, Broca area; other areas are identified by numbers; see Fig. 11.1. *, Not verified; **, only on the right side when subject responded from memory of extrapersonal space. Compare to Figs. 6.1 and 11.1. (From Roland, 1984b)

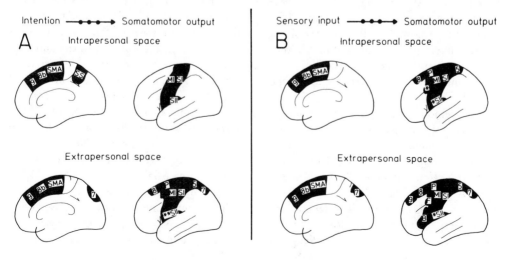

that are separated in small groups ("patches") located among others related to different outputs. The reason for the patchy distribution is the need to relate the outputs *(topography)* to the cross-filed, orderly layout of inputs *(somatotopy)*. Thus, each thalamic cell group projects to its own particular cortical area as well as divergently to several cortical areas. Each cortical column therefore receives convergent input from multiple thalamic inputs, including input from cells in rostrocaudally aligned columns that transcend thalamic nuclear borders. In addition, there are cortio-cortical connections, as shown in Figs. 11.3 and 11.5. The shared properties of functional cell groups, and also the specific organization of their work places (i.e., in thalamus and cortex), are preserved by their accurate interconnections. The work places of the brain appear to be uniform and tightly packed; when inspected with fairly coarse probes their dispositions resemble the benches and workers in an old-fashioned factory. Relatively coarse probes are the anatomical degeneration methods and electrophysiological recording of potentials from the surface or large volumes of the brain. Finer methods of inspection, however, reveal specialized groups that all relate to the same overall tasks but may be distributed in interspersed fashion, more like the teams in a modern production facility for large, complex products such as planes. Finer methods include cellular staining obtained by material transported by flow of axoplasm in nerve fibers and recording of unit potentials from identified cells. This cellular tissue arrangement is considered again in the next chapter.

The premotor and supplementary motor areas (lateral and medial area 6) are the recipients of much convergence and thus might be thought to "put it all together" in a *task-related* manner for area 4, the primary motor area (PMA in Fig. 11.2, area 4 in Fig. 11.3); but we still lack a simple scheme of information flow. The reason is not hard to find: our knowledge of

the connections is still sketchy. The SMA projects bilaterally to area 4 and to subcortical motor centers, which would fit it for preparation for complex movements, including postural and adjustments. This idea is supported by the slow, long-lasting movements evoked by its electrical stimulation. Many cortical areas, such as the premotor cortex that has been referred to as one entity so far, actually consist of several functional areas with distinct connections and properties. Furthermore, information flows not only in the directions indicated by the arrows in Figs. 2.7 and 11.2, but in many cases also in reverse through reciprocal connections that are omitted from the simplified diagrams. An example is shown in Fig. 11.7 for the relationships between the motor cortex (MI), the supplementary motor area (MII, medial area 6, labeled SMA in Fig. 11.1), and the premotor cortex (PM, the lateral part of area 6).

The lower part of Fig. 11.7 shows two important sets of connections that are analogous to some of the loops in Fig. 2.7. On the left we see the loop through the striatum (i.e., the input part of the basal ganglia), which projects to the SMA; and on the right the cerebellar loop, which, through its inputs in the pontine nuclei, projects to PM and MI. The simplified scheme refers to the putamen loop of the basal ganglia, which projects through the internal segment of the globus pallidus to the thalamic nucleus (VLo), and to the caudal and rostral parts of the cerebellar dentate nucleus, which project to thalamic nuclei (X and VPLo, VLc, respectively). Nucleus X is a part of the ventrolateral complex. [The thalamic nuclei are explained fully in Fig. 11.14. Details of the circuits of the cerebellum and of the basal ganglia are taken up in Chaps. 13.1 and 14.1. PM in Fig. 11.7 actually refers to a part of area 6 labeled APA in Fig. 11.8A; an acronym for arcuate premotor cortex, which is just caudal to the arcuate sulcus. The arcuate sulcus of the monkey has no direct human equivalent: it lies forward of the human precentral sulcus, as shown by comparison of Figs. 2.1A, 11.1, 11.8, and 11.14.]

Figure 11.7 makes three important points: (1) The three cortical areas (PM, MI, and MII) each have their own thalamic connections, that is, they each have special input–output modules. (2) The cortical areas are reciprocally connected. This arrangement creates multiple loops in which information can be routed in various ways to bring about a particular result. An intended motor act can thus, in theory, be brought about by orders that can reach their target neurons through more than just one compulsory path. Although neural messages create preferred paths by usage (Chap. 3.2), their common denominator is the address to be reached, that is, the topography. (Such "parallel processing" is used even more freely in the long-distance telephone system.) (3) The influences of the cerebellum and the basal ganglia not only converge in the motor cortex, but these two subcortical structures can influence each other through the interconnected cortical areas shown in Fig. 11.7. We already know from Fig. 5.9 that the primary (and supplementary) motor cortices send substantial projections directly to the spinal cord, while the premotor cortex sends most of its fibers to the medullary reticular formation, an origin of the reticulospinal tract. All three areas project to the small-celled part of the red nucleus, which connects to the precerebellar nuclei in the pons as well as in the inferior olive (although only fibers from area 4 relay to the large-celled part of the red nucleus that gives rise to the rubrospinal

Fig. 11.7. Summary of anatomical relationships between the cerebellum, basal ganglia, and motor cortical areas. Diagram illustrates (1) pathway from MI to the precerebellar nuclei in the pons and then to the *cerebellar* caudal and rostral dentate nucleus, respectively, to thalamic nuclei X, and VPLo as well as VLc, all connecting to the primary motor area (MI, area 4); (2) Pathways from MII to the striatum, and then to the internal segment of the globus pallidus of the *basal ganglia* to VLo and on to the SMA (MII, medial area 6); (3) Reciprocal connections between MI, premotor, and supplementary motor cortex; (4) reciprocal thalamocortical connections. Compare to Figs. 11.2 and 11.3. For abbreviations, see legend to Fig. 11.9. (Adapted from Wise and Strick, 1984)

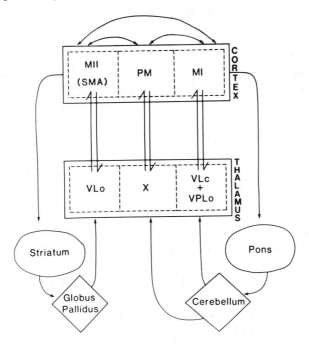

tract). *Links are thus provided by the supplemental motor area between the basal ganglia and the cerebellum, and by the premotor area between the cerebellum and the basal ganglia.* The distribution of interactive cortical components in Fig. 11.7 makes the "distributed" system more versatile than a simple hierarchy. This loosening up of schemes that were formerly thought of as rigid has important consequences. Multiple, alternate paths help to explain how patients might be able to partially overcome the damage left by some brain lesions in various ways, not just in one. Recognition of the distributed nature of the CNS will become of therapeutic value when we learn how to bypass and supplant nonfunctioning pathways by assisting alternate ones.

2. Limbic Inputs

The limbic system was introduced in Chap. 2 as a functional task system (rather than an anatomical entity) for relating sensory inputs to basic biological goals such as obtaining food and drink, reproducing the species, and attaching significance to past events. Limbic drives can be translated through subcortical connections into locomotion. More subtle activities, however, require correlations in areas of association cortex that are readily engaged by the limbic system through its widely distributed cortical projections. Figure 11.5 shows that all associative paths finally converge on the limbic system, in fact rather directly (through the amygdala) to the limbic mainspring, the hypothalamus. The two-way connections between the limbic and nonlimbic systems are presumably concerned with balancing the satisfaction of limbic demands (Figs. 2.4 and 2.7), but how this is controlled, monitored, and accomplished remains to be discovered. The general scheme suggests that the limbic system is organized, like the sensorimotor system (Chap. 2.3), to compare intended actions with their fulfillment. Limbic connections form an astounding set of circuits, whose functions we are just beginning to understand. The main ascending paths from the hypothalamus arise from one of its output nuclei, the mammillary body, and reach the limbic cortex (e.g., the cingulate gyrus) after relay in the anterior thalamic nuclei of which the largest in humans are the anterioventral nucleus (AV) and the medial dorsal nucleus (MD) (Figs. 11.8, 11.14B, and 11.15). Other paths link up through the amygdala (which is involved with the significance and emotional content of memories; Chap. 2.1), reaching the cingulate gyrus, the orbital surface and area 46 of the prefrontal cortex as well as the inferior parietal lobule (Figs. 2.2 and 2.7). The orbitofrontal cortex is linked to the brain stem system outlined in Fig. 2.3. Amygdaloid dysfunction leads to emotional over- or under reaction, and to loss of socialization.

The main intercortical distribution of limbic connections to the cerebral cortex originates from the central part of the limbic lobe, the cingulate gyrus (Figs. 11.8 and 11.15). The cingulate cortex also sends descending paths back to the medial dorsal thalamic nucleus (Fig. 11.15). Figure 11.8A gives a visual overview of the connections, which are summarized in Fig. 11.8B with emphasis on their reciprocities. The postcentral cingulate cortex (area 23) projects to the three higher associations areas (i.e. prefrontal, orbitofrontal, and temporal). The precentral part (area 24) reaches cortical areas that are more closely tied to motor integration. The two cingulate areas are reciprocally interconnected. The suggestion was made in Chap. 2.1 and also earlier in this chapter that the limbic system, like the sensorimotor system, gauges its achievements through comparison of the expected and the actual state of events. This probably involves comparator loops of the kind illustrated in Fig. 2.7. Perhaps the descending cingulate projections fulfill this comparator function when they synapse on cell groups or colonies that also receive ascending limbic connections in various parts of the brain. Furthermore, the

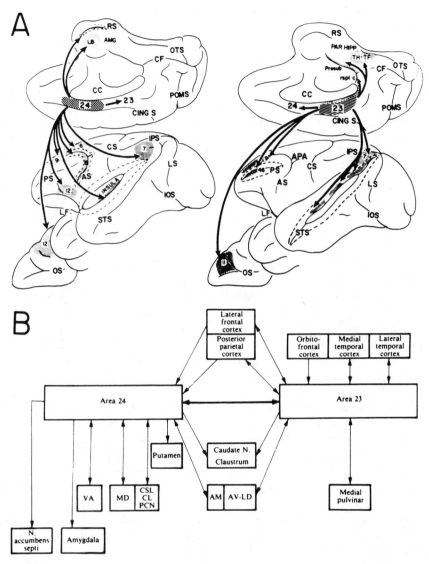

Fig. 11.8. Summary of the connections of areas 24 and 23 of the (limbic) cingulate gyrus. Projections from postcentral cingulate only go to high-order association cortex, and those from precentral cingulate reach other areas that are more closely linked to motor control, including motor cortex (not illustrated). (A) Projection patterns on the medial, lateral, and basal surfaces of the cerebral hemispheres. Compare to Fig. 11.14A(1). (B) Schematic representation of connections. Abbreviations: AM, Anteromedial nucleus; AMG, amygdala; AS, arcuate sulcus; APA, arcuate premotor area of premotor cortex; AV-LD, anteroventral–laterodorsal nucleus; CC, corpus callosum; CF, calcarine fissure; CING S, cingulate sulcus; CS, central sulcus; CL, central lateral nucleus; CSL, central superior lateral nucleus; INSULA, an area of cortex buried in the depths of the lateral sulcus; IOS, inferior occipital sulcus; IPS, intraparietal sulcus; LB, lateral basal nucleus of the amygdala; LF, lateral (sylvian) fissure; LS, lunate sulcus; MD, medialis dorsalis; OS, orbital sulcus; OTS, occipitotemporal sulcus; PCN, paracentral nucleus; POMS, parieto-occipital medialis sulcus; Presub, presubiculum; PS, principal sulcus; RS, rhinal sulcus; rspl c, retrosplenial cortex; STS, superior temporal sulcus; TH, TF, parahippocampal gyrus. [(A) From Pandya, Van Hoesen, and Mesulam, 1981; (B) from Baleydier and Mauguiere, 1980]

highest association areas of the cerebral cortex return their output to the amygdala and the hypothalamus, as mentioned above. The proposed limbic comparisons of demand and achievement may be carried out in loops between the cerebral cortex and subcortical structures, where ascending and descending limbic projections meet (Figs. 2.7–2.10 and 11.8B; and see in relation to Fig. 11.14). We take up further details of some limbic connections in relation to Fig. 11.15, after studying the thalamocortical system.

3. "Middle-Level" Integration

Normal sensorimotor integration requires correct operation of the basal ganglia as well as the cerebellum, neither of which can work effectively without the other. Their cooperation with the cerebral cortex was stressed in relation to Fig. 11.2, where the supplementary and premotor areas are highlighted as important portals for their influence on the motor cortex. What are the main cortical areas of the middle level concerned with movement?

The *sensorimotor cortex* is that part of the cerebral cortex through which movements can be elicited by its direct electrical excitation or by adequate peripheral sensory stimuli. It consists of three precentral and four postcentral areas identified in Fig. 11.9. The precentral parts are the primary motor cortex, area 4 (MI in Fig. 11.7; PMA in Fig. 11.2) and the supplementary motor area (SMA, medial area 6), whose corticospinal projections largely engage alpha and gamma MNs, as well as the premotor cortex, lateral area 6 (APA in Fig. 11.8). The postcentral parts are the primary somesthetic areas 3, 1, 2, and the secondary area 5, which all connect through transcortical fibers with the precentral cortex (Fig. 11.11) as well as subcortically to extrapyramidal structures or to INs in the spinal dorsal horn (Figs. 5.7–5.11).

There are two major *outputs of the motor cortex*: one descends as the pyram-idal tract, and the other projects to non-pyramidal targets such as the basal ganglia, thalamus, red nucleus, and reticular formation (Fig. 5.9). The functions of the pyramidal and extrapyramidal systems are interlinked because extrapyramidal information reenters the pyramidal system (Figs. 2.2 and 2.7). Locations of the sensorimotor cortex and its main connections along the neuraxis are identified in Figs. 11.1 and 11.2. Not shown in Fig. 11.2 are the symmetrical connections from the opposite hemisphere through the corpus callosum (which, however, exempt representation of the hands and feet; they are operated more independently). The corticospinal parts of the pyramidal system adjust the motor commands to be issued from the spinal cord. This, as shown in Chap. 5.2, is achieved in good part through direct action on spinal MNs by corticospinal neurons (CSNs) in the primary motor cortex. The cortical actions are highly coordinated, however.

Denny-Brown had already concluded that "damage to cortex of the pre- and postcentral gyrus caused a severe and permanent defect in all delicate spatial adjustments of movements of the hand and to a lesser extent on the foot and mouth. The small eversions, abductions, rotations that enable precise palpation and exploration or withdrawal, depend on the integrity of pre- and postcentral gyrus." In contrast to the inter-related losses after cortical lesions, spinal connections of CSNs can give the appearance of being "muscle-oriented" during artificial, minimal electrical stimulation of cortex. This appears to be so because such minimal stimulation can elicit contraction of individual muscles. Their normal physiological activation, however, occurs usually as part of muscle groups (synergies; see Figs. 9.7–9.13). Particular muscles are activated by the balance of cellular excitabilities in the cerebral cortex and in its connections, down to and including the spinal cord. How these balances are brought about is an important topic in this chapter, and it is a good example of the flexible use made by the brain of apparently fixed anatomical connections. Corticospinal activity integrates the excitability of spinal motor nuclei through the multiple axon branches of individual CSNs to several nuclei (Fig. 5.13A). Muscles acting on the same joint are activated in coordination with each other, not by exclusive, "private" corticospinal connections to particular spinal motor nuclei.

One of the main functions of the *cerebellum* and the *basal ganglia*, in concert with the cerebral cortex, has been characterized as "packaging" of different aspects of the motor "intent." The basal ganglia receive direct projections mostly from the cerebral cortex and none from the periphery (Figs. 11.2 and 11.3). They therefore coordinate central commands through feedforward and central feedback connections (efference copy, Fig. 2.5). The caudate circuit of the basal ganglia operates at the higher premotor level, presumably in the control of the formation of general motor plans that lead to middle-level coordination of complex motor tasks (Chap. 2.2). The putamen circuit, in contrast, operates at the middle level for premotor instructions, presumably involving the scaling of patterns of complex and simple motor acts, which includes the coordination of movements of the trunk with those of the eyes and limbs. The two basal ganglia loops pursue separate paths through the globus pallidus and substantia nigra, and they loop separately through the ventral anterior (VA) and lateral (VL) thalamus, respectively (Figs. 11.3 and 11.9).

The cerebellum, like the basal ganglia, operates with two distinct circuits, but both are linked to the middle level. The "higher" (prefrontal and temporal) cortical association areas project neither to the cerebellar input nuclei in the pons nor to those in the inferior olive. The lateral cerebellum issues premotor commands for movements details to motor cortex, not unlike the putamen circuit. The cerebellar circuit is essential for composing, timing, and grading the components of intended movements. This circuit was described in Chap. 7.1 as optimizing the trajectories of the objects of greatest attention for the central nervous system, such as the hand path for arm movements (Figs. 7.3 and 7.4). The lateral (neo-) cerebellar feedforward circuit is relatively unaffected by somatosensory input. The output of the lateral cerebellum reaches the motor cortex through two contiguous thalamic nuclei (VPLo and VLc, and the premotor cortex through nucleus X; Figs. 11.7 and 11.9). The second, more medial, cerebellar circuit does not issue premotor commands but instead guides motor execution in follow-up fashion. It feeds back reports about the progress of movements, particularly their velocity, for which it utilizes its strong somatosensory, proprioceptive input. This cerebellar follow-up circuit consists of two parts: an intermediate one whose output is directed partly to the motor cortex and partly to the red nucleus and the medullary reticular formation (Figs. 5.7–5.9), and a medial component that assists posture by sending processed spinal information for integration to the vestibular nuclei (Chap. 9).

The *motor cortex,* including the corticospinal system, has three major inputs: (1) in transcortical connections, (2) in the return loops from the cerebellum and the putamen loop of the basal ganglia, and (3) in somatosensory feedback paths. Somatosensory feedback to the motor cortex is used for sensorimotor integration, but it has no function in sensing. (Sensory perceptions are not impaired by lesions of the motor cortex, the basal ganglia, or the cerebellum.) The spinothalamic systems for pain, temperature, and some somatosensory appreciation reach all areas of the sensorimotor cortex. More specific and detailed somatosensory information is forwarded by the lemniscal system to the postcentral cortex through VPLc and to area 4 from the border of VPLo. (The two

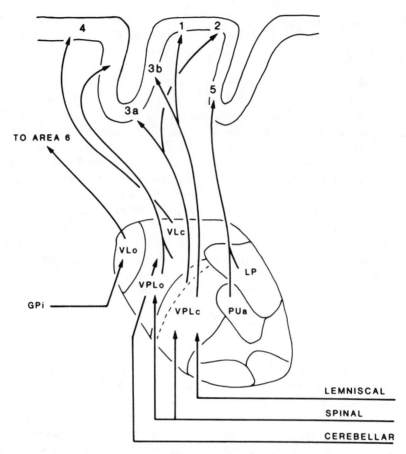

Fig. 11.9. Summary of thalamocortical projections to the sensorimotor cortex. The cytoarchitectonic regions of the cortex are indicated on a parasagittal view and the thalamic nuclei of interest below. Somatosensory inputs reach the VPLc nucleus over both lemniscal and spinothalamic pathways, and the VPLo nucleus by a spinothalamic route; inputs from cutaneous receptors terminate in the central core of the nucleus, those from deep receptors in a surrounding shell zone (drawn above the *broken line*). They have separate projections to areas 3b and 1 and areas 3a and 2. Cerebellar inputs terminate in the VLc and VPLo nuclei, to anterior and posterior parts of area 4. (Area X , between VPL and MD, is not included; compare to Figs. 11.7 and 11.14.) Abbreviations: GPi, internal segment of the globus pallidus; VLo, VLc, nucleus ventralis lateralis oralis or caudalis; VPLo, VPLc, nucleus ventralis posterolateralis oralis or caudalis; PUa, anterior pulvinar nucleus; LP, nucleus lateralis posterior. Compare to Fig. 11.3. (Modified from Jones and Porter, 1980; also see Jones, 1983; from Humphrey 1983)

spinal ascending systems, the lemniscal and the spinothalamic one, are shown separately in Fig. 11.9, but in Fig. 11.3 they are combined into one line leading to an undivided VPL nucleus.)

The postcentral afferent projections are very specific in their representation of the sites (somatotopy) and types of adequate peripheral stimuli (modalities) needed to evoke responses. The hallmark of sensory

cortex is its detailed somatotopy. The sizes of receptive fields reflect the density of peripheral innervation: the fields are small where there are many sensory nerve endings, for example on the fingers. Figure 11.10 provides an example for a human thalamic neuron on the path to the primary sensory cortex (Figs. 11.3 and 11.9). It shows the spatial (static) outline of the small peripheral receptive field on the fin-

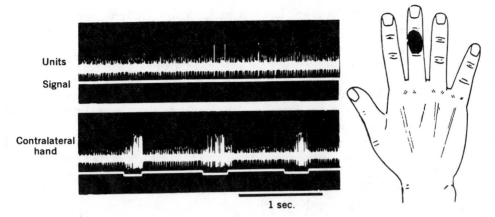

Fig. 11.10. Records, obtained during microelectrode exploration of thalamus of waking human subject during brain surgery, of discharges of a single neuron in the posterior portion of the ventral thalamic group. The neuron was activated by light tactile stimulation of area of skin on dorsum of contralateral middle finger, shown in black. (upper record) Spontaneous activity of thalamic units; (lower record) acceleration of discharge during three light strokes across receptive field, indicated by signal line. (From Jasper and Bertrand, 1966; in Mountcastle, 1980)

ger, a property of the medial lemniscal system, and the time-varying (dynamic) alterations of neural discharge when the field is brushed lightly. The neuron of Fig. 11.10 is located in the ventral thalamic group (which is the homolog of the ventrobasal complex in monkeys; see VPL in Figs. 11.3 and 11.14B, b).

The prevalence of particular peripheral inputs to various areas of the sensorimotor cortex is indicated in Fig. 11.11. It is a summary based on microelectrode recordings from the cortex of monkeys, combining determinations of (1) the adequate peripheral stimuli that drive the cortical neurons with (2) their motor outflow established by the electrical stimulation or by their task-related discharges when observed in behaviorally trained animals that were carrying out specified motor tasks. Figure 11.11 thus adds another aspect, the information contents, to the connections shown previously in Figs. 11.3 and 11.5. What is communicated to the motor cortex? The rostral (anterior) part of area 4 contains many neurons that are responsive to central commands but unresponsive to somatosensory stimuli. These neurons, like their counterparts in area 5, probably

deal with preparatory, "premotor" information rather than with movement instructions related to external conditions. Other rostral neurons in area 4 receive mostly deep inputs (from muscle, tendon, and joints) and visual input, more so that neurons located more caudally, which are mostly sensitive to superficial inputs (i.e., from the skin). These points are explored further in Chap. 12.2.

The area categories marked in Fig. 11.11 are meant to indicate the great likelihood of cells having certain properties, not their absolute separations. Many "cytoarchitectonic" delineations of brain areas (by their histological appearance) contain several distinct functional areas. Area 4 belongs to this group, and so does the premotor cortex (area 6 L, PM in Fig. 11.7). Figure 11.11 shows that visual input is added to the sensory mix in area 4 through connections from the premotor area 6, which likely receives important processed inputs from association area 7 (see Fig. 11.2 and 11.5) The numerous cross-connections between the areas of sensorimotor cortex presumably serve for selective summations to activate particular outputs in relation to a selected range of inputs (Fig. 11.5). How these selections are made is still unknown, but studies of the response properties of neurons, combined with those of results of local lesions, reveal *progressive processing of peripheral afferent information in the sensorimotor areas*. Area 3a receives information from "deep" receptors located in joints and muscle spindles, particularly group I muscle afferents, and area 2 responds to input from joints and perhaps from spindles as well (Fig. 11.11). Area 3b is activated by "superficial," slowly adapting cutaneous (skin) receptors, and area 1 from rapidly adapting skin receptors.

The lemniscal system's projections to precentral cortex are not as massive as those to postcentral cortex, but there is a direct thalamocortical input to area 4 through the border of VPLo. This presumably enables precentral CSNs to react quickly and accurately to somatosensory feedback of the lemniscal type, particularly to the all-important proprioceptive input. The normal responsiveness of monkey's motor cortex is the balance between this input (mostly concerned with deep modalities), specific input relayed from the primary sensory area (mostly concerned with superficial modalities), and spinothalamic inputs relayed through VPLo. Which sensory inputs can facilitate an output from area 4 depends on the additional influences of the transcortical connections, the cerebellum, and the basal ganglia. Area 3b receives the densest projection from thalamocortical afferents. Its information is not forwarded directly to area 4, however, but instead is directed to areas 1 and 2, which, in turn, project to areas 4, 5, and rostral 7. This directional flow of information to motor cortex is apparent, without indication of content, in Fig. 11.3. These are largely one-way, nonreciprocal connections, originating from "supragranular" layers near the cortical surface (see Fig. 12.1). Although all sensory areas are granular ("konio") cortex, the relative densities of their internal granular layers correlate with the density of their thalamocortical projections and they relate inversely to the density of their corticocortical connections. (Areas 1 and 2, for example, have thin internal granular layers.)

The main point to grasp is the multiple, parallel, spatial representation of the body in adjacent cortical areas (with the feet medially and the hands and face laterally). Each area, or subsector of it, highlights a

Fig. 11.11. Summary of corticocortical connections and of the sensory information processed in the sensorimotor cortex (of the monkey). **V, J,** and **C** represent connections over which inputs from visual, joint, or cutaneous receptors could be relayed transcortically to area 4 or to the SMA (medial area 6). *Interrupted arrows* denote connections between areas dealing with different modalities. Central inputs reach the SMA and the premotor cortex (6 L, lateral area 6; APA in Fig. 11.8), which in turn project to area 4. Compare to Fig. 11.5 (which also shows connections of area 5) and Fig. 11.7. (Modified from Humphrey, 1983; based on Jones and Porter, 1980; also see Jones, 1983)

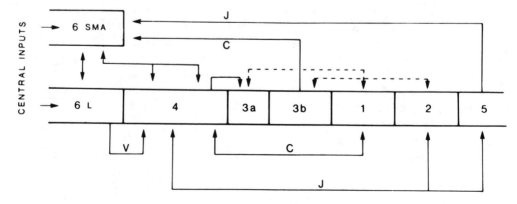

particular input, which, as we will see, is used in local input–output relations for participating in certain stereotyped motor responses as well as in voluntary, intended movements. All sensorimotor areas of the cerebral cortex are organized as "representing" similar spatial (somatotopic) input fields in multiple, parallel fashion. Recall that each area receives convergent ascending inputs dealing with various afferent modalities concerning the same somatotopy. The areas of the sensorimotor cortex link these afferent inputs to their own special efferent ("topographic") output connections (e.g., Fig. 5.9). This entails multiple combinations of inputs and outputs, which accounts for the "patchy" appearance of the projections between information-processing centers. Afferent inputs include messages from sensory centers as well as commands that modulate them. This is the special input–output transformation that occurs in the cortex and, in fact, at all levels of the sensorimotor system: the spinal cord, the cerebellum, the basal ganglia, the thalamus, and the higher association areas as well. The sensorimotor cortex reassembles inputs from their

thalamic nuclei, the cerebellum, and the putamen loop of the basal ganglia in a particular spatial (topographic) framework ready for output to the next stage. *The recombination of relevant inputs from various sources into common, shared topographic output units is the basis for processing the spatial aspects of motor learning and of motor execution.*

Modular Structure

An important advance in understanding cortical function was the recognition that all cortical tissue has definite inputs and outputs restricted (1) to certain horizontal layers, and (2) to vertical columns of cells. This arrangement, illustrated diagrammatically in Fig. 11.12, has been demonstrated for visual, somesthethic, and motor cortex. A better name for the vertical orientation is "radial," which means vertical with respect to the (curving) cortical surface. Each column, of about 0.3 mm diameter, contains neurons with individual inputs from closely overlapping peripheral receptive fields. Mountcastle discovered that in the

Fig. 11.12.   The somatosensory cortex is organized radially and horizontally. Each radial column is specific for a submodality (e.g., **J** joint; **P**, pressure; **H**, hair stimulation). The horizontal layers receive inputs from certain regions of the brain and project to other regions. Layer **II** also projects across the corpus callosum to the equivalent area on the opposite hemisphere; layer **V** also projects to the brain stem and spinal cord. Outputs from equivalent layers in motor cortex are marked in Fig. 12.6. (From Kandel, 1981).

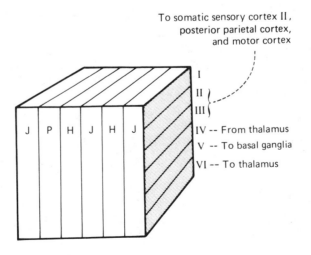

To somatic sensory cortex II, posterior parietal cortex, and motor cortex

I
II
III
IV -- From thalamus
V -- To basal ganglia
VI -- To thalamus

J   P   H   J   H   J

postcentral sensory cortex, all neurons in a column are activated by the same adequate stimuli. These postcentral columns are "modality-pure" either for deep or for superficial inputs, that is, deep pressure or joint movements as opposed to hair-bending or light touch. This is shown diagrammatically in Fig. 11.12. Small fields (like those in Fig. 11.10) afford extensive "shifted overlap" within and between columns, which yields accurate localization of the stimulus and fine two-point discrimination, including the mapping of the direction of a moving contact.

The sharp borders of the small receptive field in the medial lemniscal system are enhanced by progressive processing of the afferent information in successive nuclei of the system. In the dorsal column this is achieved by presynaptic inhibition, and by descending effects from the corticobulbar tract (Chap. 5.2). In the thalamic relay nu-

clei (e.g., VPLc in Fig. 11.9), field size is restricted by postsynaptic ("afferent") inhibition fed forward from the dorsal column nuclei. In the primary sensory cortex, feedforward inhibition cooperates with feedback inhibition mediated by recurrent axon collaterals of cortical pyramidal cells. An example of the resultant "surround" inhibition for a postcentral neuron is illustrated in Fig. 11.13. The excitatory and inhibitory areas on a monkey's arm are delineated on the left, and a measure of their concurrent activation is conveyed on the right by plots of the change in discharge rate of the neuron. Reduction of neural discharge rate indicates that the excitatory field shrinks—that is, that it covers a smaller part of the arm—during stimulation of its inhibitory surround.

The preceding pages have offered some general rules about integration at the higher and middle levels. Corticocortical

Fig. 11.13. Interaction of excitatory and inhibitory effects on a postcentral neuron of a monkey that was produced by cutaneous stimulation in a field on the arm and inhibited by stimuli in the large surrounding area. Graph plots discharge frequency versus time, implying that the excitatory field shrinks during excitatory–inhibitory interactions. Compare to Fig. 12.7. (From Mountcastle and Powell, 1959; in Mountcastle, 1980)

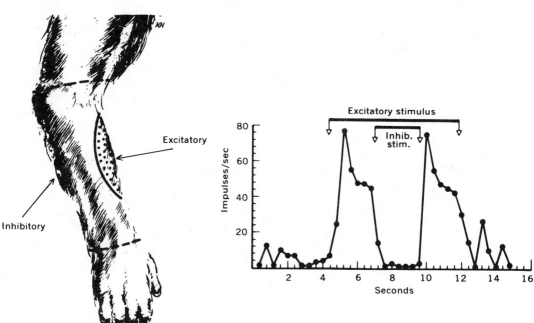

connections have been outlined for both levels, and thalamocortical projections once more for the middle level. We now compare these projections with those of the higher level. The sensorimotor cortex (of the monkey) and its afferent projections, singled out in Fig. 11.9, are contrasted in Fig. 11.14A(2), with association cortex in Fig. 11.14A(1). The *thalamic connections* are drawn in Fig. 11-14B, identified by equivalent markings for connected thalamic nuclei and cerebral areas. The prefrontal cortex is hatched vertically, and the posterior parietal as well as the temporal cortex are dotted. Between them lies the precentral and postcentral sensorimotor cortex, which is marked separately in Fig. 11.14A(2). The identifying markings of the cortical areas, drawn in Fig. 11.14A, correspond to those entered in the transverse sections of their thalamic projection nuclei in Fig. 11.14B. To help in visualizing the locations of the nuclei from the transverse sections, Fig. 11.14C present a three-dimensional diagram of the (human) thalamus.

A simple rule is immediately apparent in the pattern of connections: *"higher order" association cortex and "middle-level" sensorimotor cortex have separate thalamic projections.* This separation is understandable in view of the different codes used for communication in the higher and lower levels. Remember that middle-level codes translate into muscle function, while abstract codes of the higher level are still impenetrable. As explained in Chap. 11.2, information processing in the higher level cortex is controlled by the caudate loop of the basal ganglia, and that in the middle level by the putamen loop and by the two cerebellar loops (cf. Fig. 2.7). Their particular functions are taken up in Chaps. 13 and 14. The importance of the separate projections lies in the assembly of appropriate cortical input–output functions as explained in relation to Fig. 11.11.

It is not important to worry unduly about the names of the numerous thalamic nuclei. They are retained in Fig. 11.14 be-cause lumping them together would falsify the pattern too much. The scheme is incomplete anyway: the most dorsal nuclei (the "epithalamus") are not marked, nor are the projections to the limbic cortex illustrated. Another reason for showing the nuclei separately is their property of processing their information without connecting to other thalamic nuclei. They safeguard the identities of their contributions to the crucial reassemblies of cortical input–output functions. There are, however, two coordinating sets of connectivities at work. The first is the intrathalamic distribution of the influence of the ascending reticular formation through the "intralaminar" nuclei, of which CM is the largest in the human. Their location in the lamina internal to the thalamus is best seen in Fig. 11.14C. They are the conduit through which reticular arousal reaches the entire cerebral cortex. The second intrathalamic connectivity is organized around the integrative action of the reticular nucleus of the (ventral) thalamus, which is a thin shell of tissue wrapped around the dorsal thalamus (R in Fig. 11.14B,C). The reticular nucleus of the thalamus gates the inputs to and outputs from dorsal thalamic nuclei through its connections with the thalamocortical and corticothalamic fibers that all pass through this stategically located shell of tissue (which makes it look "reticular"). This complex set of connections serves thalamocortical integration and is controlled selectively by the prefrontal cortex.

One important difference between the two groups of thalamic nuclei was mentioned above: the nuclei projecting to association cortex—such as medialis dorsalis (MD), lateralis dorsalis (LD), and anterior nuclei (AD, AM, AV), and the pulvinar (P)—receive heavier limbic inputs than the nuclei projecting to the sensorimotor cortex, such as the ventrolateral and ventrobasal groups of the dorsal thalamus (VL, VA, VPL, VPM, VPI). The alignments of the projections to association cortex from thalamic nuclei under limbic (hypotha-

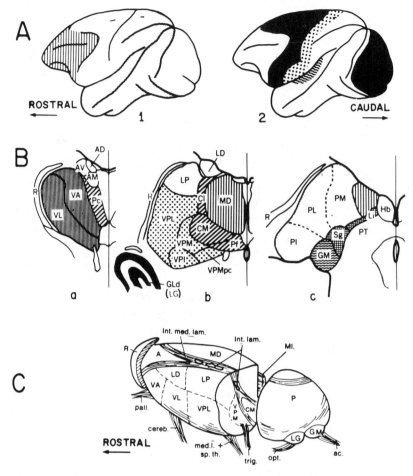

Fig. 11.14. Diagram of thalamocortical systems. (A, **1**) Projections to cortical association regions (compare to Fig. 11.8A). (A, **2**) shows projections to pericentral cortex (compare to Fig. 11.9). (B) Outlines of monkey thalamic nuclei, as coronal sections in frontocaudal sequence from **a** to **c**. Areas similarly marked indicate thalamic nuclear groups and cortical regions to which they project. (C) Reconstruction of human thalamus. Abbreviations for nuclei of *dorsal thalamus* shown: VL, VA, ventralis lateralis and ventralis anterior; VPL, VPM, VPMpc, VPI, ventroposterolateralis, -medialis, and pars compacta, -inferior (ventrolateral group); A, AV, AD, AM, anteroventralis, -dorsalis, -medialis (anteromedial group); CL, CM, centrum lateralis, medianum; Pc, paracentral; Pf, parafascicularis; int. lam. (intralaminar group); GLd, LG, geniculatus lateralis dorsalis; GM, LG, geniculatis medialis and lateralis; Li, nucleus limitans; Sg, suprageniculate; (caudal group); LD, lateralis dorsalis; LP, lateralis posterior; MD, medialis dorsalis; P, PM, PL, PI, pulvinar medialis, lateralis, inferior (dorsolateral group); R, reticular nucleus of *ventral thalamus*; Hb, habenula; PT, pretectal region of *epithalamus*; MI, midline; int. med. lam., internal medullary lamina; ac., accessory optic nerve; opt., optic nerve; trig., trigeminal nerve; med. l. + sp. th., medial lemniscus and spinothalamic tract; pall., pallidum. Also see Fig. 11.9. [(A, B) From Poggio and Mountcastle, 1980; (C) adapted from Brodal, 1981]

lamic and amygdaloid) influence coincide with the projections from the caudal cingulate cortex to those areas shown in Fig. 11.8 as well as the projections from the rostral cingulate area 24. Thus the thalamocingulate complex may contain meeting places for the ascending limbic drives and descending limbic cortical controls.

These meeting places may be loci for the creation of set-points of limbic actions on the sensorimotor system whose cortex does not receive cingulate projections. Other meeting places of ascending and descending limbic projections may be in the basal ganglia and perhaps the cerebellum. (This thought is expressed in condensed form in Fig. 2.7.) It would seem there should be tiers of such set-points: for instance, the hypothalamus can control some aspects of feeding within its own confines, but some of the associated behavior depends on loops reaching out of this extraordinary center of nuclei. Similarly, the integration of autonomic controls depends on hypothalamic loops of various lengths and complexities. The autonomic system is influenced by the hypothalamus through descending paths to the central grey matter, for instance the locus ceruleus, and the parabrachial nucleus, which project to the intermediolateral column of the spinal cord where they innervate sympathetic preganglionic nuclei.

Having reviewed the corticothalamic system, we need to take a final, quick look at some limbic connections that have only been described schematically (Fig. 2.3). The *hypothalamus* influences the sensorimotor system through many paths: two of the most relevant to this study are indicated in Fig. 11.15A. The hypothalamus (H) projects to its most posterior nucleus, the mammillary body (M) and to the amygdala (BL, basolateral amygdaloid nucleus). Both connections are reciprocal. The mammillary body projects to the anteroventral (AV) nucleus of the thalamus and the amygdala to the dorsomedial (MD) nucleus. Both these nuclei also receive projections from the septum, which is connected reciprocally with the hypothalamus (see Fig. 2.3B). The AV nucleus projects to the cingulate cortex (mostly its caudal area 23), and the MD to the rostral cingulate and the prefrontal cortex (Fig. 11.8A,B). The caudal cingulate (area 24) receives a heavy projection from the medial pulvinar (PM in Fig. 11.14B,c; cf. Fig. 11.8B). The cortical areas are interconnected, as are indeed all association areas. The limbic connections to the basal ganglia and the cerebellum, indicated in Fig. 2.7, run respectively through reciprocal connections with the substantia nigra (SN, Fig. 14.1), as well as through the amygdala, and via M to a pontine nucleus (n. reticularis tegmentum pontis, NRTP), which receives a return connection from the cingulate gyrus. Potentially important connections for modulating motor programs run from the anterior cingulate gyrus to the pontine nuclei, which receive inputs from the main sensorimotor areas (Fig. 13.7, later). Thus we have a rough outline of how the limbic loops influence the sensorimotor system.

Another structure with great influence on the sensorimotor system whose connections we should know something about is the memory-encoding *hippocampus*. Figure 11.15B outlines broadly these connections. The hippocampus receives hypothalamic influences through its reciprocal connection with the septum and through the medial forebrain bundle with the amygdala, mediated in great part through the ancient (allo)cortex that adjoins the hippocampus and forms part of the medial wall of the temporal lobe (dentate gyrus, subiculum, and entorhinal cortex; cf Fig. 2.8). All fibers to the hypothalamus arise from the subiculum, travelling through the fornix. The hippocampus reaches the neocortex through its projection via the septum (S), which is reciprocally connected with the entorhinal cortex and subiculum and through corticocortical connections of the cingulate cortex. The subiculum (Sub.) also projects to the septum and the cingulate, but in addition also to AV and M.

All these connections are very important for motor learning since the entorhinal cortex, as well as the amygdala, receive the output of the highest association areas. As we have seen, learning is facilitated greatly by emotional factors, motivation is

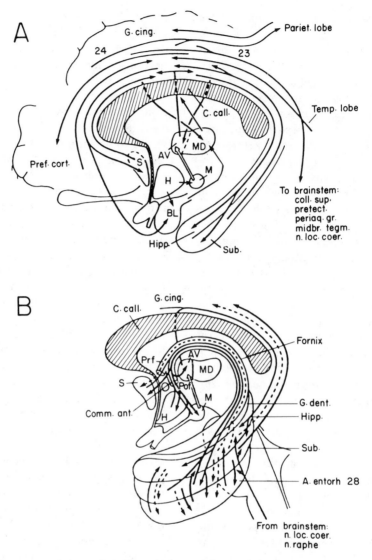

Fig. 11.15. Some connections of the hypothalamus (A) and of the hippocampus (B). Efferent and afferent paths of hippocampus (Hipp.), *broken and light lines;* efferent paths of subiculum (Sub.), *heavy lines; white arrow,* mammillothalamic bundle. Abbreviations: C. call., Corpus callosum; G. cing, cingulate gyrus, areas 23, 24; Pariet. (parietal) lobe; Temp. (temporal) lobe; Prefr. cort., prefrontal cortex; H, hypothalamus; S, septum; M, mammillary body; BL, basolateral amygdaloid nucleus; AV, antero ventral thalamic nucleus; MD, dorsomedial nucleus of thalamus; G. dent., dentate gyrus; A. entorh. (entorhinal) area 28; Pof, primary olfactory area; Prf, perforating bundle; Comm. ant., commissure anterior. (Adapted from Brodal, 1983)

all-important (Chap. 1.3), and bilateral disconnection of the hippocampus and of the amygdala deprives humans and monkeys of their abilities for "insightful" learning (Fig. 1.5 and Chap. 2.3).

Neurotransmitters

Knowledge about neurotransmitters, which were last taken up at the end of Chap. 5.1, is an aspect of physiology and pharmacology of great and rapidly growing clinical importance. "Replacement therapy" has become commonplace since the introduction of L-dopa for treatment of patients with Parkinson's disease, but this is only one of a growing number of applications of this knowledge.

Functioning synapses are a prerequisite for installing motor capabilities. Figure 11.14 presents differences between the conventional projection systems to association (Fig. 11.14,1) and to sensorimotor cortices (Fig. 11.14A,2). The "conventional" transmitters are glutamate for excitation and gamma-amino butyric acid (GABA) for inhibition. Another system to be added here is the "modulatory" ascending projection of catecholamine-releasing fibers to association cortex. Only the frontal and limbic lobes receive dopaminergic (DA) projections from the mesencephalic, ventral tegmental area (Fig. 2.3; located medially and superior to the substantia nigra), and noradrenergic (NA) input from the locus ceruleus. This "mesocortical" system is paralleled by projections from the mesencephalic raphe nuclei that release serotonin (5-hydroxytryptamine, 5-HT; see Figs. 5.8 and 5.11 for anatomical orientation). Both sets of fibers synapse between cortical layers II and VI, with the serotoninergic one particularly in layer IV (see Fig. 12.6). The layered termination is mentioned because layers II and IV are missing from precentral cortex (including areas 4 and 6, some part of 8, and the rostral cingulate area 24), giving them an "agranular" appearance caused by the dispersed, rather than packed, distribution of "stellate" interneurons. They form a dense "internal granular" layer IV in granular cortex, typical of postcentral sensory cortex, as related above. Some ascending brain-stem projections reach both granular and agranular cortex. For example, virtually the entire neuraxis is reached by the arousal- and vigilance-related projections from the locus ceruleus (whose surprisingly small number of neurons are located in the pons; Fig. 11.4). This slowly acting,

noradrenergic (NA) system synapses in the superficial layer I of the cerebral cortex (Fig. 12.6). Replacement therapy of failing NA systems by implantation of subjects' adrenal tissue has attracted much recent attention.

The nucleus basalis of the forebrain (Fig. 11.2) is part of the ventral basal ganglia. Its projection to the cerebral cortex releases acetylcholine (ACh), which provides a tonic, nonspecific, facilitation of pyramidal cells. Loss of this facilitation contributes to the onset of Alzheimer's disease. The substantia innominata, also a part of the ventral basal ganglia, influences initiation of motor responses to emotionally or motivationally powerful stimuli. The cholinergic projection from the nucleus basalis to the cortex is not unique but instead is one of at least six subcortical centers that provide such cholinergic supportive projections to various target nuclei. Those from the septal nuclei reach the hippocampus (Fig. 2.3), which may explain why memory is enhanced by ACh agonists and depressed by ACh antagonists. Cholinergic projections from the ascending reticular activating system (of Magoun, Fig. 5.8) reach the intralaminar and midline nuclei of the thalamus and cause cortical arousal.

4. Summary

This chapter stresses the main anatomical connections that support the functions of the middle level of the motor hierarchy. Transcortical and thalamocortical mechanisms combine to impose task orientation on the motor cortex by grouping its output neurons into appropriate input–output units. Premotor selection of *what* to do are made in high-level association cortex, when it has been put in a "need"-related task mode by the limbic system. High-level instructions reach the premotor and supplementary motor cortex (lateral and medial areas 6) through transcortical connections. From area 6 onwards, instructions largely deal with *how* to carry out intended motor acts.

The transition from "what" to "how" is paralleled by decreased input from the limbic lobe (of which the cingulate cortex forms the central keystone), which steers the motor cortex mostly indirectly. Its rostral part, area 24, projects to intermediate-level association areas that are related to motor control (including areas 6 and 7) as well as to motor cortex. The caudal part, area 23, projects to high-level association cortex (temporal, prefrontal, and parietal). Lesions of the anteriorventral (AV) thalamic nuclei exaggerate the limbically mediated emotional component of postural attitudes, making them persistent and resistant to external change (dystonia). It is suggested that the limbic system checks the achievements of motor behavior with reference to their fulfillment of biological and emotional urges. Such checks are probably made by "comparison" of inputs to neuronal colonies that receive both limbic projections ascending from the hypothalamus through the mediodorsal and anteroventral (MD and AV) thalamic nuclei and the amygdala as well as descending limbic projections from the cingulate gyrus. These comparisons are similar in principle to those made in relation to other functions of the sensorimotor system. The middle level determines the balance between exploratory and avoiding behavior. Both have limbic components that influence the frontal (precentral) and parietal cortex, of which the former facilitates subcortical extensor-oriented movements and the latter flexor-oriented movements.

All sensorimotor areas of the cerebral cortex are organized as "representing" similar spatial ("somatotopic") input fields in multiple, parallel fashion. Each area receives convergent ascending inputs dealing with various afferent modalities concerning the same somatotopy. The areas of the sensorimotor cortex link these afferent inputs to their own special efferent ("topographic") output connections. This entails multiple combinations of inputs and outputs, which accounts for the "patchy" appearance of the projections between information-processing centers. Afferent inputs include messages from sensory centers as well as commands that modulate them. This is the special input–output transformation that occurs in the cortex and, in fact, at all levels of the sensorimotor system: the spinal cord, the cerebellum, the basal ganglia, the thalamus, and in the higher association areas as well. The sensorimotor cortex reassembles inputs from their thalamic nuclei, the cerebellum, and the putamen loop of the basal ganglia, in a particular spatial (topographic) framework ready for output to the next stage. The recombination of relevant inputs from various sources into common, shared topographic output units is the basis for processing the spatial aspects of motor learning and of motor execution.

The primary motor area of the cerebral cortex (area 4) receives instructions from lateral and medial areas 6, all of which are connected reciprocally. These connections permit flexible information flow through a variety of alternate cortical stations, each of which has its own thalamic connections. Subcortical input reaches the supplementary motor area (SMA) from the putamen loop of the basal ganglia via VLo, and the rostral motor cortex from the lateral cerebellum via VLc. Caudal motor cortex receives feedback via VPLo about ongoing movements from the intermediate cerebellum. Sensory afferent information projects from the border of VPLo to the primary motor cortex, which combines this with processed sensory information and commands received through transcortical links from other sensorimotor areas and feedback loops from cerebellum and the putamen loop of the basal ganglia.

The high-level, "selective" functions of association cortex are the consequence of successive outward-converging projections from the primary somatosensory, visual, and auditory cortex. What is lost in somatotopy is gained in the ability to select significant categories of general concern.

Selective actions can be triggered in higher association cortex by a variety of inputs, including "emotional" ones from the limbic projections. Conversely, cortico-subcortical loops can presumably channel limbic drives into actions more concerned with social conditions of the individual (sublimation). The progressive sensory-processing projections converge in the prefrontal and temporal cortices, from where they project to the limbic amygdaloid nuclei and thence to the mainspring of limbic function, the hypothalamus. The amygdala project to the basal ganglia whose thalamocortical projections presumably contribute to mergers of limbic and non-limbic functions.

The caudate loop of the basal ganglia receives input from all high-level areas of cortex and projects its output to the prefrontal cortex. It thus parallels corticocortical processing, which it presumably controls with regard to forming overall motor plans. The prefrontal cortex forms motor plans, for complex motor acts, to be fed forward to the premotor cortex (area 6). The putamen loop of the basal ganglia receives its input from middle-level cortex and returns its output to the supplementary motor cortex (SMA, medial area 6). Presumably it acts as a control circuit for scaling the amplitudes of motor patterns in the context of the required task. The lateral cerebellum receives its input from the premotor cortex and returns its output to it and the primary motor cortex as well as to subcortical targets. It is involved in establishing, optimizing, and triggering programs for complex and simple movements. The intermediate cerebellum receives peripheral input and returns its output to the motor cortex (for updating central programs) as well as to subcortical motor centers.

An example of high-level motor action is described in terms of successive neural "gating" activities in the inferior parietal cortex (area 7, part PG), leading from task motivation and reward recognition to visual attention and to generally appropriate motor-related actions. The loss of these neural events can account for the "contralateral neglect" (a form of apraxia) exhibited by patients with lesions in the inferior parietal lobule. It is still unknown, however, how these selections are finally transferred to the sensorimotor cortex (including the superior parietal lobule, area 5) for specicic motor execution.

The dysfunctions described in this chapter show what can be learned from the study of lesions. Lesions reveal what the brain can still do without an excised part; that is, they reveal residual functions after loss of specific information or commands, or of a previously maintained functional balance. "Release" of abnormal functions can teach us about the controls exerted by the excised tissue. Neurotransmitter replacement may become a potent support for therapies designed to assist acquisition of new motor capabilities.

References

Allen, G. I., and Tsukahara, N. 1974. Cerebrocerebellar communication systems. *Physiol. Rev.* 54:957–1006.

Arbib, M. A. 1981. Perceptual structures and distributed motor control. In *Motor control.* Sect. 1, vol. 2. *Handbook of physiology,* ed. V. B. Brooks, pp. 1449–1480. Bethesda, Md.: American Physiological Society.

Asanuma, C., Thach, W. T., and Jones, E. G. 1983. Distribution of cerebellar terminations and their relation to other afferent terminations in the ventral lateral thalamic region of the monkey. *Brain Res. Rev.* 5:237–265.

Baleydier, C., and Mauguiere, F. 1980. The duality of the cingulate gyrus in monkey. *Brain* 103:525–554. [Fig. 11.8B]

Barr, M. L., and Kiernan, J. A. 1983. *The human nervous system.* 4th ed. Philadelphia: Harper & Row. [Fig. 11.1]

Brodal, A. 1981. *Neurological anatomy.* 3rd ed. Oxford: Oxford University Press. [Figs. 11.14C and 11.15]

Bruce, C. J., and Goldberg, M. E. 1984. Physiology of the frontal eye fields. *Trends Neurosci.* 7:436–441.

Calaresu, F. R., Faiers, A. A., and Mogenson, G. J. 1975. Central neural regulation of heart and blood vessels in mammals. *Prog. Neurobiol.* 5:1–35.

DeLong, M. R., Georgopoulos, A. P., and Crutcher, M. D. 1983. Cortico-basal ganglia relations and coding of motor performance. In *Neural coding of motor performance,* eds. J. Massion, J. Paillard, W. Schultz, and M. Wiesendanger. *Exp. Brain Res.* Suppl. 7, pp. 30–40. [Fig. 11.2]

Denny-Brown, D. 1966. *The cerebral control of movement.* Springfield, Ill.: Charles C. Thomas.

Emson, P. C. 1983. *Chemical neuroanatomy.* New York: Raven Press.

Foote, S. L., Bloom, F. E., and Aston-Jones, G. 1983. Nucleus locus ceruleus: new evidence of anatomical and physiological specificity. *Physiol. Rev.* 63:844–914.

Fuster, J. M. 1984. Behavioral electrophysiology of the prefrontal cortex. *Trends Neurosci.* 7:408–414.

Fuster, J. M. 1981. Prefrontal cortex in motor control. In *Motor control.* Sect. 1, Vol. 2. *Handbook of physiology,* ed. V. B. Brooks, pp. 1149–1178. Bethesda, Md.: American Physiological Society.

Goldman-Rakic, P. S. 1984. The frontal lobes: uncharted provinces of the brain. *Trends Neurosci.* 7:425–429.

Goodale, M. A. 1983. Vision as a sensorimotor system. In *Behavioral approaches to brain research,* ed. T. E. Robinson, pp. 41–61. New York: Oxford University Press.

Heimer, L., Switzer, R. D., and Van Hoesen, G. W. 1982. Ventral striatum and ventral pallidum, components of the motor system? *Trends Neurosci.* 5:83–87.

Humphrey, D. R. 1983. Corticospinal systems and their control by premotor cortex, basal ganglia and cerebellum. In *Neurobiology.* Vol. 5. *The clinical neurosciences,* ed. W. D. Willis, pp. 547–587. New York: Churchill Livingston [Figs. 11.2, 11.9, and 11.11]

Humphrey, D. R. 1979. On the cortical control of visually directed reaching: contributions by nonprecentral motor areas. In *Posture and movements,* eds, R. E. Talbott and D. R. Humphrey, pp. 51–112. New York: Raven Press.

Jasper, H. H. and Bertrand, G. 1966. Thalamic units involved in somatic sensation and voluntary and involuntary movements in man. In *The thalamus,* eds. D. P. Purpura and M. D. Yahr, pp. 365–390. New York: Columbia University Press. [Fig. 11.10]

Jones, E. G. 1981. Anatomy of cerebral cortex: columnar input–output organization. In *The cerebral cortex, eds. F. O. Schmitt, F. G. Worden, G. Adelman, and M. Dennis, pp. 199–235. Cambridge, Mass.: The M.I.T. Press.

Jones, E. G. 1983. The nature of the afferent pathways conveying short-latency inputs to primate motor cortex. In *Motor control mechanisms in health and disease,* ed. J. E. Desmedt. *Adv. Neurol.* 39:263–285. [Fig. 11.9]

Jones, E. G. 1984. Organization of the thalamocortical complex and its relation to sensory processes. In *Sensory processes.* Sect. 1, vol. 3. *Handbook of physiology,* ed. I. Darian-Smith, pp. 149–212, Bethesda, Md.: American Physiological Society.

Jones. E. G., and Porter, R. 1980. What is area 3A? *Brain Res. Rev.* 2:1–143. [Figs. 11.9 and 11.11]

Jones, E. G. and Powell, T. P. S. 1970. An anatomical study of converging sensory pathways within the cerebral cortex of the monkey. *Brain* 93:793–820. [Fig. 11.15]

Kandel, E. R. 1981. Central representation of touch. In *Principles of neural science,* eds. E. R. Kandel and J. H. Schwartz. New York: Elsevier/North-Holland. [Fig. 11.12]

Keele, S. W. 1981. Behavioral analysis of movement. In *Motor control.* Sect. 1, vol. 2. *Handbook of physiology,* ed. V. B. Brooks, pp. 1391–1414. Bethesda, Md.: American Physiological Society.

Lynch, J. C. 1980. The functional organization of posterior parietal association cortex. *Behav. Brain Sci.* 3:485–534.

MacLean, P. G. 1980. Role of transhypothalamic pathways in social communication. In *Behavioral studies of the hypothalamus.* Vol. 3. *Handbook of the Thalamus,* eds. P. J. Morgane and J. Panksepp, pp. 259–287. New York: Marcel Dekker, Inc.

Mesulam, M. M. 1983. The functional anatomy and hemispheric specialization for directed attention. *Trends Neurosci.* 6:384–387. [Fig. 11.4]

Mesulam, M. M., Mufson, E. J., Wainer, B. H., and Levey, A. I. 1983. Central cholinergic pathways in the rat: an overview based on an alternative nomenclature (Ch1–Ch6). *Neuroscience* 10:1185–1201.

Mogenson, G. J., Jones, D. L., and Yim, C. Y. 1980. From motivation to action: functional interface between the limbic system and the motor system. *Prog. Neurobiol.* 14:69–97.

Mountcastle, V. B. 1981. Functional properties of the light-sensitive neurons of the posterior parietal cortex and their regulation by state controls: influence on excitability of interested fixation and the angle of gaze. In *Brain mechanisms of perceptual awareness and purposeful behavior.* Vol. 8. *IBRO Monograph Series,* eds. O. Pompeiano and C. A. Marsan, pp. 67–99, New York: Raven Press.

Mountcastle, V. B. 1980. Neural mechanisms in somesthesis. In *Medical physiology,* ed. V. B. Mountcastle, pp. 348–390. St. Louis: C. V. Mosby Co. [Figs. 11.10 and 11.13]

Mountcastle, V. B. 1976. The world around us: neural command functions for selective attention. *Neurosci. Res. Prog. Bull.* (Suppl.) 14:1–47.

Mountcastle, V. B., and Powell, T. P. S. 1959. Neural mechanisms subserving cutaneous sensibility, with special reference to the role of afferent inhibition in sensory perception and discrimination. *Bull. Johns Hopkins Hosp.* 105:201–232. [Fig. 11.13]

Nauta, W. J. H., and Feirtag, M. 1979. The organization of the brain. *Sci. Am.* 241:88–111 (special issue on "The Brain").

Oomura, Y. and Aou, S. 1984. Catecholaminergic and cholinergic involvement in reward related responses in monkey orbitofrontal cortex. In *Modulations of sensorimotor activity during alterations in behavioral states.* ed. R. Bantler, pp. 269–290. New York: Alan R. Liss, Inc.

Paillard, J. 1983. The functional labelling of neural codes. In *Neural coding of motor performance,* eds. J. Massion, J. Paillard, W. Schultz and M. Wiesendanger. *Exp. Brain Res.* Suppl. 7, pp. 1–19.

Pandya, D. N., Van Hoesen, G. W., and Mesulam, M. -M. 1981. Efferent connections of the cingulate gyrus in the rhesus monkey. *Exp. Brain Res.* 42:319–330. [Fig. 11.8A]

Poggio, G. F., and Mountcastle, V. B. 1980. Functional organization of thalamus and cortex. In *Medical physiology,* ed. V. B. Mountcastle, pp. 271–298. St. Louis: C. V. Mosby Co. [Fig. 11.14]

Popper, K. R., and Eccles, J. C. 1977. *The self and its brain.* Berlin: Springer Verlag. [Fig. 11.5]

Roland, P. E. 1984. Metabolic measurements of the working frontal cortex in man. *Trends Neurosci.* 7:430–435.

Roland, P. E. 1984. Organization of motor control by the normal human brain. *Hum. Neurobiol.* 2:205–216. [Fig. 11.6]

Rolls, E. T. 1983. The initiation of movements. In *Neural coding of motor performance,* eds. J. Massion, J. Paillard, W. Schultz, and M. Wiesendanger. *Exp. Brain Res.* Suppl. 7, pp. 97–113.

Rolls, E. T. 1981. Processing beyond the inferior temporal visual cortex related to feeding, memory, and striatal function. In *Brain mechanisms of sensation,* eds. Y. Katsuki, R. Norgren, and M. Ito, pp. 241–269. New York: John Wiley & Sons.

Schell, G. R. and Strick, P. L. 1984. The origin and thalamic inputs to the arcuate premotor and supplementary motor areas. *J. Neurosci.* 4:539–560.

Seal, J., Gross, C., and Bioulac, B. 1982. Activity of neurons in area 5 during a simple arm movement in monkeys before and after deafferentation of the trained limb. *Brain Res.* 250:229–243.

Shepherd, G. M. 1983. *Neurobiology.* New York: Oxford University Press. (Chap. 29, "Emotion," pp. 528–544).

Somjen, G. G. 1983. *Neurophysiology: the essentials.* Baltimore: Williams & Wilkins. [Fig. 11.3] (Chap. 18, "Control of Movement by the Brain.")

Stein, D. G., Finger, S., and Hart, T. 1983. Brain damage and recovery: problems and perspectives. *Behav. Neurol. Biol.* 37:185–222.

Wiesendanger, M. 1981. Organization of secondary motor areas of cerebral cortex. In *Motor control.* Sect. 1, vol. 2. *Handbook of physiology,* ed. V. B. Brooks, pp. 1121–1147. Bethesda, Md.: American Physiological Society.

Wise, S. P., and Strick, P. L. 1984. Anatomical and physiological organization of the nonprimary motor cortex. *Trends Neurosci.* 7:442–446. [Fig. 11.7]

Wurtz, R. H. Goldberg, M. E., and Robinson, D. L. 1982. Brain mechanisms of visual attention. *Sci. Am.* 246(6):124–135.

12

The Motor Cortex

This chapter focuses on the primary motor cortex (MI in Figs. 11.6 and 11.7, PMA in Fig. 11.2, area 4 in Figs. 11.1, 11.3, 11.5, 11.9 and 11.11). The sensorimotor cortex instructs the spinal cord about how to implement intended movements and postures. Our purpose here is to understand these instructions with particular reference to area 4, to see how the necessary cortical actions are brought about and how they engage the spinal mechanisms that were described in Chapt. 5.2. The chapter begins by relating the functions of motor cortex to those of other sensorimotor areas and, after a brief review of cortical structure, goes on to its input–output relations. We will follow the trail of how cortical responses are integrated into voluntary actions (Chaps. 6.2 and 9.6), which leads to the roles of motor cortex *neurons* in the control of posture and movements. The chapter traces many of the arguments presented in the reviews by Evarts and by Fetz, and concludes by showing how motor set assigns the output neurons of area 4 to special aspects of natural motor tasks. The main lesson is that neurons in primary motor cortex tend to act as specialists when motor set has assigned them their parts in the total repertoire. Motor action is the product of a whole company of players, not of individ-

ual performers. Management of intended movements amounts to bringing motor set to bear on special parts of the sensorimotor cortex, including the neurons in area 4.

Distinct populations of sensorimotor neurons make distinct contributions to the beginnings of movements, to their ongoing modulations, and to their endings (Chaps. 6.1–6.3, 7.3, 11.1, and 11.2). The motor cortex is not a simple keyboard that merely calls forth the actions of particular muscles, as was once thought; it is not a stereotyped mosaic of output keys. Instead, it reacts to central and peripheral influences according to the functional needs of the individual through variable participation of its input–output columns. The motor cortex moves and holds joints in response to central commands and sensory inflow, and it adjusts its own input.

Loss of corticospinal projection does not paralyze muscles but eliminates their use for *skilled* movements. The motor cortex, through the pyramidal tract, in particular manages skilled tasks that depend on finely "fractionated" hand and finger movements (Chap. 5.2). For example, pyramidal control over intercostal muscles is used for speech and song but is not essential for breathing any more than pyramidal control of leg muscles is essential for walking. For another example, precentral neurons discharge in accord with learned jaw movements but not with the more automatic task of chewing. In brief, the motor cortex is of special importance for the execution of learned, programmed movements.

1. Specialized Areas

Cortical instructions are forwarded to the spinal cord by three main couriers (Fig. 12.1). The first carries *preparatory messages,* from areas 2 and 5, and some neurons in area 4, for adjusting the sensory inflow at supraspinal and spinal levels and also the excitability of interneurons (INs) in the spinal dorsal horn. These messages are transmitted directly by corticospinal endings as well as indirectly through the extrapyramidal systems. They reach the spinal cord within 0.1 second before movement onset (i.e., they follow the anticipatory input from the SMA by another 0.1–0.2 second or even more, because SMA can lead movement onset by as much as 1 second). These delays accrue from central calculation times, since conduction from cortex to cord takes only 2–3 msec.

The second courier is the precentral, predominantly slow corticospinal tract, which *starts* and *stops* movements by setting the activity levels of spinal motoneurons (MNs) and interneurons (INs). The third courier, from areas 3a, 3b, and 1, as well as partly from area 4, *guides* ongoing movements. These areas are activated late by feedback from central corollary discharge loops or from somatosensory receptors in the moving body part, or both.

Corticospinal neurons (CSNs) in areas 4 and 3a synapse with spinal MNs either monosynaptically or through INs in the spinal intermediate zone. Postcentral CSNs connect primarily in the basal part of the dorsal horn with INs that serve segmental reflex arcs or somatosensory pathways (Chap. 5.1). An overall scheme of sequential actions is presented in Fig. 12.1, taken from Humphrey's review, which gives the *time relations* to movement onset. (These were not contained in the display of connections in Figs. 5.10 and 5.11 or in that of the peripheral inputs in Fig. 11.11.) We have already traced the relevant pathways in Figs. 5.9–5.12. Timing is determined by records from single neurons in the brain and can therefore be detailed in units of milliseconds (fractions of one one-thousandth of 1 second) instead of fractions of minutes as afforded by the method of regional cerebral blood flow (Fig. 11.6).

Figure 12.1 stresses the division of labor between adjacent cortical areas. The most rostral part of area 4 contains CSNs with strong central drive, which suggests that they are more involved in advance calculations for movements than in their actual initiation. Each area sends messages that have a special role in composing the intended response. The contributions by sensory area 5 (and premotor area 6) are the most centrally driven and least concerned with the peripheral details of the action.

Fig. 12.1. Timing of discharge of corticospinal projections from areas of the sensorimotor cortex of the monkey. Projections drawn as *solid lines* become active before movement onset, and affect spinal MNs and INs. Projections drawn as *broken lines* become active at movement onset or later. Compare to pathways in Figs. 5.9–5.12. (From Humphrey, 1983)

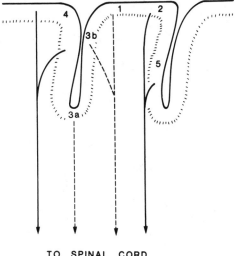

TO SPINAL CORD

Those neurons discharge in relation to planned movements and their general direction in space. Starting movements and guiding them by means of proprioceptive information is the task of CSNs in area 3a and in the middle rostral part of area 4, where neurons receive strong central drives as well as topographically precise feedback about the movement of joints. These neurons send commands to spinal alpha MNs and INs, whereas those from areas 2 and 5 bias segmental reflexes and ascending somatosensory information before and during movement. About one-third of the neurons in area 5 receive advance information on how to bias their target cells, through "corollary" projections (internal to the brain, cf. Fig. 2.7). About one-tenth of the connections from area 4 to MNs are monosynaptic (see Fig. 5.13B) and give specific instructions for MN activation. CSNs in areas 3b, 1, and the caudal third of area 4 (which is located in the anterior bank of the central sulcus) receive cutaneous input that is used by the precentral CSNs in the starting of move-

ments and by postcentral CSNs in their guidance thereafter.

The two solid lines extending from the rostral and caudal parts of area 4 in Fig. 12.1 indicate two separate descending systems, although they are drawn as converging into one line. Peripheral stimuli from moving joints are adequate to drive CSNs in the rostral part of area 4 (located in the exposed precentral gyrus), while stimuli from the skin are effective in the caudal part, which in humans and higher monkeys is buried in the anterior wall of the central sulcus (see Figs. 11.9 and 11.11). This discovery by Strick and Preston, illustrated in Fig. 12.2, led them to propose that the double representation reflects two motor control systems within area 4 that deal with different components of motor behavior. On the one hand, the rostral area with deep inputs could serve movements that use kinesthetic feedback for their execution and guidance, as in Phillips' "long-loop" stretch responses to loads on the joints, for instance (Chap. 6.2). On the other hand, the caudal area with superfi-

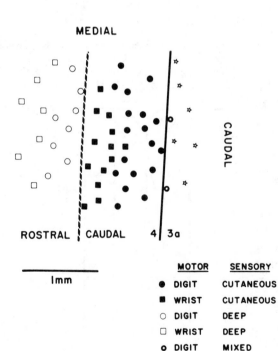

Fig. 12.2. Dual motor representations serve separate deep and cutaneous inputs in the rostral and caudal parts of the motor cortex, respectively. *Broken line* separates these parts in the forelimb map in area 4 of a squirrel monkey. Symbols indicate sites of penetration for intracortical microstimulation in areas 4 and 3a, and the movements evoked at each site. *, no response to stimulation up to about five times threshold strength: 30 μA. (From Strick and Preston, 1983)

cial inputs could serve movements that use tactile feedback for their execution and guidance, such as exploratory "active touch" and Denny-Brown's "tactile grasping" responses (Chap. 11.1). A similar observation to that of Strick and Preston was made by Murphy's group, who reported, however, that the two representations are concentric ring-shaped areas. The discovery of double representation in motor cortex resurrects Denny-Brown's proposal that this cortex determines the balance between exploratory and avoidance behavior (Chap. 11.1). Cutaneous input is of overriding importance for use of the fingers, because its loss abridges sense of movement and leads to gross movement errors. This clinical result has been substantiated by Moberg with use of local anesthesia. It seems reasonable to assign a role in exploratory movements to the cutaneous input to motor cortex (which is not essential for sensing).

Chapter 11.3 stressed that various inputs are directed to input–output modules with common output targets (afferent convergence), and that particular inputs are distributed to modules with diverse targets (efferent divergence). The motor cortex presents examples of these somatotopic-topographic transformations, of which one example can be given for adjustments of joint stiffness through coordinated outputs to antagonistic muscles (Figs. 3.4–3.6 and 4.6). The patchy distribution of input-output modules is revealed by electrical stimulation of the cerebral cortex, which shows that the same muscles can be activated from points several millimeters apart. Comparison of maps of motor representation shows that effective zones for activation of antagonistic muscles overlap most in the rostral part of area 4. Figure 12.3A demonstrates this point from trials with electrical stimulation of the cortical surface in anesthetized animals in which intracellular records could be made from the activated spinal MNs. Figure 12.3B makes the same point based on electro-myographic (EMG) recording in alert

monkeys where muscles were activated by intracellular stimulation of cortical neurons. The hindlimb maps in Fig. 12.3A show that antagonists can be made to co-contract by intense activation of the rostral part of cortex. The forelimb maps in Fig. 12.3B show that co-contraction of antagonists is elicited more often in rostral than in caudal motor cortex. In the rostral transition zone between areas 6 and 4, voluntary joint stiffening is accompanied by central activation of a population of neurons that respond only to central commands but not to sensory stimulation of the limb.

How neurons in the rostral part of area 4 are functionally engaged recalls Denny-Brown's finding on the integrative action of that area with regard to the hand and its supporting arm. Excision of the hand area in primary motor cortex of the chimpanzee (our closest subhuman primate relative) leads to spastic finger flexion and a paralyzed hand for about a month; this is exacerbated to include the proximal joints if the lesion encompasses the anterior part of area 4. Conversely, if only the anterior edge of area 4 is ablated, a situation resembling that of hemiplegic patients results: instinctive grasping remains intact, but proximal spasticity is released and tone of the flexors of the elbow, wrist, and fingers is increased in response to stretch of adductors and retractors of the shoulder (the "traction reaction").

Intracortical Microstimulation

The method of stimulating through a microelectrode was adapted from spinal physiology to cortical studies by Asanuma, who named it "intracortical microstimulation" (ICMS). It is a very useful electroanatomical method, because it applies current pulses to a small volume of neurons and their branches. (Surprisingly, the branches are more excitable than the neuronal cell bodies.) ICMS reveals the most probable connections between neurons near the site of electrical stimulation and

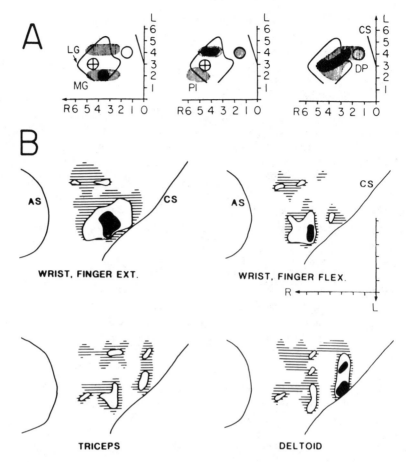

Fig. 12.3. Co-contraction of antagonist muscles is most likely to be facilitated in the most rostral part of the motor cortex. Maps of sites for activation of spinal MNs (and muscles) by electrical stimulation of monkey cortex. Note patchy distributions for each muscle (cf. Fig. 11.4). (A) Projection sites to lateral gastrocnemius (LG, *open lines*) superimposed, by *hatched and filled areas,* on total and optimal sites for synergistic medial gastrocnemius (MG) and plantaris (Pl), and antagonist deep peroneal (DP). Weak cortical surface stimulation and intracellular recording of EPSPs from spinal MNs in an anesthetized monkey. (B) Maps for threshold intracortical microstimulation for extension of the contralateral wrist of an alert monkey. Stimulation also activated synergistic arm extensor (triceps) and antagonistic wrist and finger flexors as well as shoulder abductor, measured by EMG. Lowest, medium, and highest thresholds indicated by *filled, shaded, and open areas,* respectively. Scales for (A) and (B) (mm) indicate lateral (L) and rostral (R) map coordinates on cortical surface. CS, AS, Central and arcuate sulci (see Fig. 11.8). [(A) From Jankowska, Padel, and Tanaka, 1975; in Phillips and Porter, 1977; also in Asanuma, 1981; (B) from Humphrey, 1983]

their putative outputs. ICMS cannot, however, reveal what additional connections are made and unmade during natural activity. The patchy texture of the cortex, demonstrated in Fig. 12.3, shows that several muscles are activated by local, minimal stimulation of cortex, and also that the same muscles can be activated from cortical points several millimeters apart. There is thus both convergence from distinct cortical foci onto the same spinal MN nuclei and divergence from any one focus to spinal targets. This result has been obtained through stimulating output neurons by passing current pulses from the cortical surface as well as through stimulation

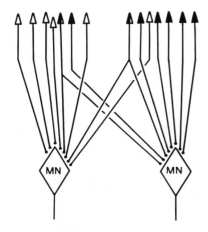

Fig. 12.4. Schematic drawing of the organization of output units in motor cortex that would yield the observed convergence from cortical sites and divergence from single corticospinal neurons (see Fig. 5.13). The CSNs from two colonies (or "efferent zones") are intermingled, and some send axon branches to two different MNs. Clusters of cells, distributed in patches, yield points of lowest threshold for activation of particular spinal MNs by electrical stimulation of motor cortex. (From Asanuma, 1981; Modified from Andersen, Hagan, Phillips, and Powell, 1975.)

within the cortex with weak (micro) pulses. Both surface and intracortical stimulation reveals an overlapping patchwork of neural "colonies" (or "efferent zones") with common spinal targets, spread through the cortical gray matter beneath several millimeters of cortical surface. This confirms the histological evidence for afferent and efferent divergence in the cortex, presented in Fig. 5.13A. The patchy maps in Fig. 12.3 also reconfirm that there is no ready provision for independent cortical activation of single muscles (cf. Chap. 9.6). A stylized projection pattern from two colonies of CSNs to two spinal MNs is shown in the diagram of Fig. 12.4.

2. Input–Output Modules

Natural conditions are approached more closely by recording muscular activity in relation to natural *task-related discharges* of single CSNs recorded from monkeys while they perform a motor task. Such recording was developed by Jasper and, 10 years later, was applied to the study of motor cortex by Evarts. It has been an extremely useful method. The closest approach to making causal links between CSNs recorded in this manner and muscles has been made by cortical "spike-triggered averaging" of the EMG, which was adapted from spinal to cerebral physiology by Fetz (see Fig. 4.4A). Figure 12.5 provides examples of records from a cortical unit in the top row, EMGs from various finger and wrist muscles in the next six rows, and at the bottom of Fig. 12.5A, the torque and position traces of a handle moved by a monkey by alternate flexions, holds, and extensions of its wrist. Figure 12.5A shows that the cortical unit is clearly task-related, because it discharges with an intense burst when the wrist is held in the extended position, as do most of the muscles shown below. But is the discharge of the CSN unit related to any or all of these muscles?

The method provides a closer look at possible causal relations by recording EMG responses when triggered by the first unit spike in a burst, as in Fig. 12.5B. Averages of many thousands of trials reveal, on a time scale 100 times faster than in Fig. 12.5A, postspike facilitation in the lower two traces of muscle records. Spike-triggered averaging (Fig. 12.5B) discloses detail of natural activity that is hidden from view in ordinary EMG records (Fig. 12.5A). In this example, it reveals that the extensor of the fingers (ED IV,V) and even more so an extensor of the wrist (ECU) constitute the main "muscle field" of the unit CSN studied. The short response latency ($<$10 msec) suggests that the corticospinal connections are made through direct, monosynaptic synapses (called corticomotoneuronal (CM) synapses: Fig. 5.13B).

Cortical Columns

The layers in motor cortex are organized much like those in sensory cortex (Fig.

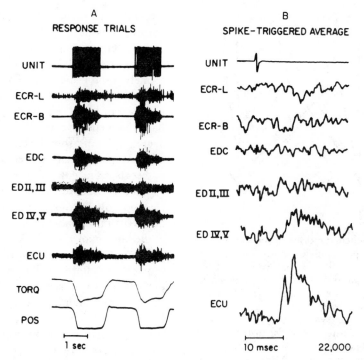

Fig. 12.5. Corticospinal preferred connections can be visualized with "spike-triggered averaging" of EMG activity. The two lowermost traces in (B) show transient postspike facilitation of two fore-limb muscles coactivated in relation to the task-related discharge of a CSN of a monkey ("unit" traces in the top rows of A and B). The animal alternately flexed and extended the wrist against an elastic load, which requires active torque proportional to wrist displacement [lowest two traces in (A)]. (A) Six rows of ordinary EMGs, on slow time scale, of extensors of the wrist (ECR-L, ECR-B, ECU) and digits (EDC, EDII, III, EDIV, V). (B) Traces are spike-triggered averages of mean rectified EMGs of the coactivated muscles, triggered by the first action potential (top line) of each of 22,000 bursts of the unit. Abbreviations: ECR-L, ECR-B, extensor carpi radialis longus and brevis; ECU, extensor carpi ulnaris; EDC, extensor digitorum communis; EDII, III, ED IV, V, extensor digitorum II–III, IV–V. (Simplified from Fetz and Cheney, 1980; in Fetz, 1981)

11.12), except that the granular layer IV of packed stellate INs is missing because they are dispersed in other layers. The space is taken up by intracortical fibers whose presense makes area 4 thicker than other cortical areas. The motor cortex, like the sensory cortex, is organized radially by the connections of its afferent branches, which encompass a cortical volume with a diameter of about 0.3 mm. Since excitatory INs are also oriented radially, afferent inputs link the neurons in radial "columns" of that diameter. These columns, each of which contains about 10^4 neurons with some common inputs, can surround themselves with a shell of inhibition that is dis-tributed by recurrent axon collaterals of CSNs ending on inhibitory INs (like spinal motor nuclei, Fig. 5.4).

About two-thirds of the neurons in a column are output neurons, with axons that leave the cortex for one of the eight targets named at the bottom of Fig. 12.6. The histologically defined columns have physiological meaning because of the functional relations between their adequate inputs and their output targets. Neurons within columns share much the same inputs and outputs, but there is progressive processing from input to output. *The basic organization in motor cortex is such that the peripheral afferent inflow to radial col-*

umns of CSNs comes from parts of the body that are moved by their motor outflow. Just how they are moved depends on the task-related columns that grade the influence of central commands in relation to those more influenced by peripheral inputs. Which sensory or central input is successful in dominating a column may simply be a matter of competition through daily usage. Busy lines occupy the neural territories and, in addition, shape the columns by putting up inhibitory fences around them (see Chap. 2.3). The coordinated mobilization of cortical columns, together with their associated structures in the thalamus, cerebellum, and putamen loop of the basal ganglia, is ensured by their shared, common topographic features (Chap. 11.3).

Histological Structure

Let us now examine the columnar "wiring," which in its consistent details conjures up vision of a modular chip for cortical computation. Area 4 is particularly well fitted for extensive switching of signals: it bulges with an extra thick "neuropil" of synapses between axon terminals and dendritic spines, in addition to housing the same cell complement as other cortical areas. Figure 12.6 indicates that each layer in motor cortex is used for particular inputs and outputs, much like the arrangement in sensory cortex (Fig. 11.12). Thalamocortical projections from VPLc relay lemniscal information from specific sensory afferents to postcentral sensorimotor cortex, but not to the precentral motor cortex, which is reached instead in layers III and Va by some lemniscal fibers from the border of VPLo, by sensory afferents from the spinothalamic tract (via VLc; Fig. 11.9), and from the cerebellum (via VPLo; Fig. 11.7).

Afferent fibers may branch more widely than Fig. 12.6 suggests, widely enough to permit contact with the dendrites of about five pyramidal output neurons. This offers flexibility of CSN participation. Area 4 re-

ceives no projections from the dorsal basal ganglia or the cortical limbic system (Fig. 11.9). Incoming fibers connect with whatever is in their way: pyramidal dendrites, inhibitory INs (not illustrated), and excitatory INs whose axons make spiny contacts on the apical shafts of pyramidal tract neurons (PTNs). One such "spiny stellate" IN is drawn next to the specific afferent on the left in Fig. 12.6. These INs present opportunities for the radial distribution of incoming excitatory information and for its inhibitory restriction to the columns (squatters' occupation and installation of picket fences, according to Edelman's theory; Chap. 2.3). Transcortical afferents end on the outer apical dendrites of PTNs in layers I and II, conveying information, for instance, about "deep" and visual inputs from areas 2 and 5 (Fig. 11.11).

It was mentioned in relation to Fig. 11.2 that CSNs are driven tonically by projections from the basal forebrain through release of acetylcholine (ACh). We add here that phasically active afferents transmit to CSNs by releasing glutamate, which is also the (efferent) neurotransmitter of CSNs to their target neurons, as well as that of cortical excitatory INs. Most cortical inhibitory INs release gamma-aminobutyric acid (GABA); they are "GABA-ergic." Their bursting pattern of discharge is most active during sleep, when they inhibit cortical output cells. Conversely, during arousal to wakefulness by the mesencephalic reticular formation, cortical INs are suppressed and cortical output cells become activated. Furthermore, during arousal from inattention to attending a novel stimulus, phasic CSNs are made more responsive for the forthcoming action by clearing of otherwise busy input lines (disfacilitation).

Corticocortical fibers leaving area 4 originate in layer III. This includes the transcallosal ones to symmetrical locations in the opposite hemisphere, with the exception of the hand representation. Corticostriate projections (to the putamen loop of the basal ganglia; Chap. 14) come from the upper part of layer Va, while corticopontine connections (destined for the cerebellum) arise from the transition between Va and Vb. The cells of origin for the corticorubral tract (connecting with the main descending motor tract of group **B**; Fig. 5.7) lie in layer Va, while those of the corticospinal tract lie in Vb. We have already seen that the properties of the corticorubrospinal route resemble those of the corticospinal one (Chap. 5.2). Here we note similarities for their neural participation in intended movements. Neurons in the (magnocellular) red nucleus and precentral corticorubral projection in the monkey fire in task-related manner before starts or stops. These rubral neurons are an impor-

tant link for cerebellar influence (Chap. 13).

The corticospinal cell in Vb of Fig. 12.6 is shown with a recurrent axon collateral (branching toward the left). Such collaterals from large CSNs innervate inhibitory INs that reduce the discharge of other neurons nearby (analogous to Renshaw cells in the spinal cord; Fig. 5.4). Recurrent collaterals of small CSNs, in contrast, facilitate their neighbors. (In postcentral sensorimotor cortex, layer Vb also contains corticobulbar neurons, whose importance to locomotion was emphasized in Chap. 10.) Finally, it should be noted in passing that the thalamocortical afferents reaching

Fig. 12.6. Internal organization of motor cortex. "Specific" afferents from cerebellar and vestibular nuclei and the spinothalamic tract end largely on cortical interneurons. Note laminar separation of afferent and efferent connections. Compare to other diagrams of projections in Figs. 5.9–5.12, and 11.12 (From Porter, 1981; based on Jones and Wise, 1977, and on Jones, Coulter, Burton and Porter 1977)

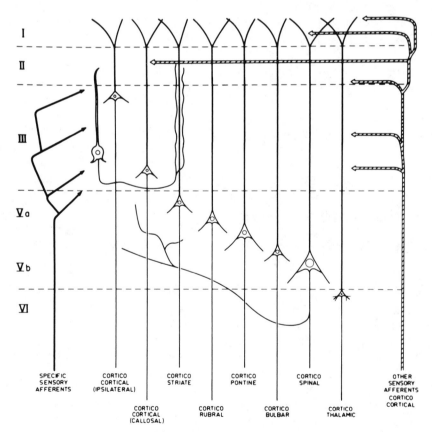

layer III and the corticothalamic efferents leaving layer VI are the cortical ends of those myelinated fibers that enter the reticular nucleus of the thalamus to integrate thalamic responses (Chap. 11.3; Fig. 11.13).

Inhibition mediated by recurrent axon collaterals of CSNs is illustrated in Fig. 12.7. The normal peripheral receptive field of a neuron in the cat motor cortex is drawn in Fig. 12.7A. It contains a focus on the left forearm, where cutaneous stimulation produces the most intense discharge, but responses could also be obtained from a wide area over most of the body. This wide-field neuron signals information about a particular spot on the forearm in relation to the rest of the body. The signals may concern changing interrelations between parts of the wide receptive field, as was discussed for some spinal INs in Chap. 5.1. Figure 12.7B shows that activation of recurrent axon collaterals (through antidromic stimulation of the pyramidal tract) shrinks the focus and accentuates the contrast between it and the nonfocal excitatory surround. The same effects can be observed for neurons with local, rather than wide, receptive fields. The recurrent INs shrink receptive fields by means of GABA release, a system like the one operating in postcentral somatosensory cortex.

At this point an interim summary of cortical function may be helpful. The sensorimotor cortex is organized somatotopically to process information concerning particular parts of the body. Both the sensory and the motor areas contain multiple representations for special purposes. The uses to which these areas can be put are steered by higher levels, conveyed through the premotor cortex, and are coordinated by the cerebellum and the putamen loop of the basal ganglia (Figs. 11.2, 11.3, 11.9 and 11.11). The operational units of the cortex are task-related cell assemblies that occupy cortical columns, or parts of several of them. Each assembly has its own reciprocal set of links to the thalamus as well as

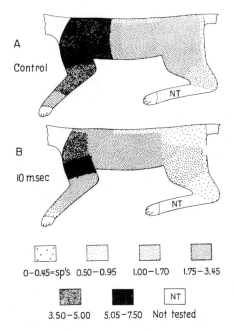

Fig. 12.7. Recurrent inhibition shrinks the focus of the peripheral receptive field of a CSN in the cat motor cortex and accentuates the contrast between it and the excitatory surround. (A) Diagram displays normal intensities of maximal discharges (see key) in response to stimuli applied to skin areas shown. (B) Equivalent responses during peak of recurrent inhibition produced by antidromic stimulation of the medullary pyramid 10 msec before skin stimulation. sp's, Spontaneous discharge level (average impulses per second). NT, not tested. Compare to Fig. 11.13. (From Brooks and Asanuma, 1965)

to the premotor and supplementary motor areas (Figs. 11.7, 11.9, and 12.6). This system can therefore be pictured as a number of special-purpose computers, each of which can be set to perform a variety of tasks. The system is made more flexible by allowing separate access to parts of the special-purpose computers. The parts are, in fact, physically distributed in the sensorimotor cortex. In essence, this cortex works by having its specific functions assigned by controllers from the higher level of the motor hierarchy and amended by two assistants, the cerebellum and the basal ganglia.

3. Input-Output Stereotypes

The output of middle-level structures is modulated by projections from higher levels and the limbic system (e.g., motor set; Chap. 6). In addition, the output of the motor cortex is molded by other middle-level components: the premotor areas, the cerebellum, and the putamen circuit of the basal ganglia. Such influences are mostly feedforward, and they, together with feedback from lower levels, play upon the basic input–output relations of the motor cortex, which they may amend, enhance, or attenuate. These basic relations vary according to cortical location. The most rostrally located CSNs tend to be linked to central but not peripheral commands. Those activated for co-contraction of opposing muscles during willed stiffening of a limb are an example of this. Another rostral group is under peripheral influence and receives input from moving limbs. A third group is located caudally and receives input from the skin.

The somatotopic, columnar organization of peripheral inputs to motor cortex was defined by Brooks, at the same time as topographically organized columnar output to muscles was defined by Asanuma. (The separation of deep and superficial inputs into two spatially separate systems had to await the work of Strick and Preston, described in Fig. 12.2.) Explorations of the combined inputs and outputs of columns in motor cortex by Asanuma soon revealed input–output stereotypes. Precentral zones that control a particular set of muscles receive input principally from joint movements caused by these muscles or from cutaneous regions that would be stimulated by the resulting movement. Close correspondence between the motor fields of a set of precentral neurons and their somatosensory receptive fields is called "tight input–output coupling." The existence of such coupling has been taken to indicate that the motor cortex is arranged as a sheet of radially oriented cell columns, each controlling a small set of contralateral muscles and receiving somatosensory feedback from body regions closely affected by those muscles.

Tightly coupled input–output relations represent events linked with high probability or, put in another way, connections operating with high synaptic security. The lack of versatility of these stereotyped responses is not surprising, since they typically are demonstrated in animals that are not engaged in a purposeful motor task, that is, when the modulating influences of the brain are least active. The responses can be regarded, however, as "building blocks" of sensorimotor behavior. CSNs with cutaneous input can be discharged by ICMS to make the limb move in the direction of the skin contact. This *positive feedback* is shown in Fig. 12.8 by the receptive skin fields and the movements evoked by ICMS (identified by symbols along the microelectrode tracks). Such a relation could promote exploratory touching movements and some aspects of tactile placing and grasping (see Chap. 9.5).

The basic stereotyped relations shown above have been demonstrated under strictly defined conditions, but other reactions besides positive feedback to skin contact also occur. Figure 12.9 illustrates such exceptions and shows that the details of motor actions evoked by ICMS cannot be predicted from either the cutaneous receptive fields of CSNs or their kinesthetic input. The variability is grounded in the subtleties of cortical activation that modulate the most securely linked connections activated by ICMS. Yet the input–output stereotypes might serve consecutive phases of touch through transcortical activation of CSN assemblies.

CSNs with *kinesthetic input,* that is, from passive joint movement, can be discharged by ICMS to move the joint in the opposite direction to that which led to their sensory excitation (not illustrated in Fig. 12.9). This relates the ICMS-evoked motor responses to kinesthetic input as a *negative feedback* (the opposite to positive feedback responses to skin input). Kines-

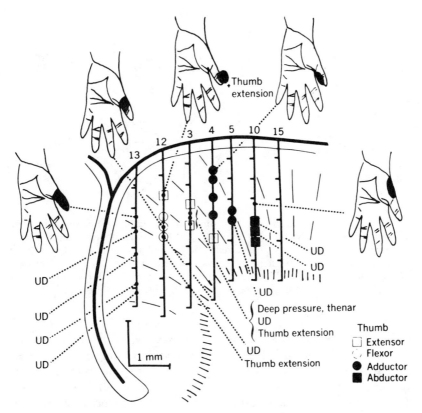

Fig. 12.8. Stereotyped, positive feedback input–output relations of skin driven cells in thumb area of monkey motor cortex. Intracortical microstimulation (ICMS) can move the limb in the direction of the cutaneous input, which itself excites CSNs in that volume of cortex. Reconstruction of electrode tracks and cell locations (*solid lines,* identified by numbers) in efferent zones to various thumb muscles. Symbols identify effects of ICMS. UD, Undriven cells. (From Rosén and Asanuma, 1972; in Asanuma, 1981)

thetic negative feedback may be part of transcortical responses to stabilize joint positions. (Once more, exceptions appear in Fig. 12.9.) Transcortical kinesthetic responses could serve "load compensation," which would assist voluntary joint movements in a servolike manner by increasing CSN discharge when a joint is moved by external forces in a direction opposite to that which was intended. Dependence of load compensation on intact cerebral connections was shown in Fig. 6.9. Experimental proof for this idea has been obtained from animals that are carrying out willed, intended motor acts, of which examples are presented below.

The participation of a precentral neuron in *load compensation* is illustrated in Fig. 12.10 with records from the motor cortex of a monkey engaged in a motor task. The task requires the monkey to turn a handle in the direction of either elbow flexion or extension, and to hold it in specified end zones before making the return movement to the alternate target zone according to visual instructions (Figs. 1.5A and 12.12A). The trace in Fig. 12.10A demonstrates how *central* influences make a CSN highly task-related: it discharges briskly before each flexion and during its acceleration, and then pauses until the next flexion. This task-related enhancement of discharge reflects the cortical influence of the animal's motor set.

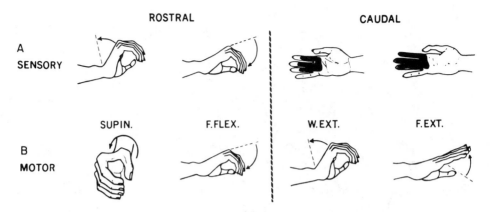

Fig. 12.9. Stereotyped cortical responses (like those in Fig. 12.8) are fine-tuned by set-dependent influences. In awake monkeys, sensory responses of CSNs to passive manipulation of limb (A) cannot predict active motor responses evoked by electrical microstimulation near those CSNs (B). (A) Sensory kinesthetic and cutaneous receptive fields of CSNs in rostral and caudal parts of motor cortex of monkey separated by broken line; (B) motor responses evoked by ICMS near those CSNs. *Arrows* indicate directions of imposed or evoked movements. (From Strick and Preston, 1979)

Figure 12.10B helps explain the relation between central and peripheral influences through displays in each column on a time scale about 10 times faster than that in Fig. 12.10A. The two top rows show superimposed elbow flexions and their velocities, followed below by EMGs of the agonist (biceps) and antagonist (triceps). In the lowest rows are displays of the CSN ("unit") discharge, which normally begins about 100 msec before movement onset (left column: normal, "no load" movements). CSN responses are displayed as histogram averages of many trials, and as successive discharges in individual trials, line by line, in the "rasters" shown above the histograms. Each method of display has its virtues: histograms stress the main events as gathered by average discharge rates (per bar or "bin" in the graph), while the dot display in the rasters describes the variability of the timing of individual responses that make up the average.

The middle and right columns in Fig. 12.10B illustrate how the CSN responds to *peripheral* influences. When the movement is opposed temporarily by a load that the arm has to overcome (just after movement onset), CSN discharge increases above normal with an "early" response.

Conversely, when the movement is assisted by brief unloading of the arm, neural firing in that time slot decreases below the voluntary (no load) level. The stereotyped CSN responses occur at the right time to support the long-loop functional stretch responses that occur a few milliseconds later (EMG within 50 msec of the perturbation for the monkey arm. Human examples were illustrated in Figs. 6.5, 6.7, 6.8, and 6.9). The consequences of long-loop action in Fig. 12.10 include joint stabilization through co-contraction of biceps and triceps muscles (cf. Fig. 6.7). The CSN responds to changes of task conditions (perturbations of the task), as would be expected of the stretch reflex; the CSN discharge reduces mismatch between intended and actual movements.

The findings fulfill Phillips' prediction that the cortical consequence of muscle spindle input (to area 3a) may serve a transcortical stretch response (Chap. 6.2). What sort of a response is it? Our previous considerations of the modest gain of spindle-based servo-responses (Chap. 4.2) suggests that this application of Matthews' theory of spindle action might normally function with small, internal adjustments but not with large, externally applied loads. The primary significance of the kinesthetic transcortical loop may be for adjustments of internal disturbances arising from the natural interactions of joints, rather than for external disturbances arising from the environment. External disturbances are corrected by voluntary, programmed actions (Figs. 4.12, 6.3 and 6.10) and by lower level reflexes.

CSNs participating in transcortical responses to muscle stretch include those with monosynaptic spinal (CM) connections, as confirmed by Cheney and Fetz with spike-triggered averaging as diagrammed in Fig. 12.11. CM neurons respond to passive joint movements that stretch their target muscles, like other CSNs (e.g., Fig. 12.10). The neural loop is sketched on the left, and the anatomical antecedents, as well as the timing, of the cortical responses appear on the right. The relation to spindle function, established by

Fig. 12.10. Corticospinal neurons (CSNs) can assist "load compensation" with transcortical long-loop responses. (A) and (B, left column) Normal, task-related discharges of a CSN "unit" preceding normal flexions without load. [(B) Flexions in superimposed top traces; unit histogram and raster in bottom two rows. Time scale 10 times faster than in A.] Same task situation as in Figs. 1.5A and 12.12. (B, middle column) Long-loop CSN response to a brief load pulse, delivered at vertical line, that had temporarily halted and reversed ongoing flexions. EMG traces show M1, M2, and later responses to load, restoring trajectory (cf. Figs. 6.2 and 6.6). (B, right column) Unloading the intended flexions reduces CSN discharge below normal ("no load") levels. Abbreviations: F, flexion; X, extension. See Fig. 12.11. [(A) Recorded at time of experiment of B but previously unpublished; (B) from Conrad, Matsunami, Meyer-Lohmann, Wiesendanger, and Brooks, 1974; in Evarts, 1981; and in Fetz, 1981]

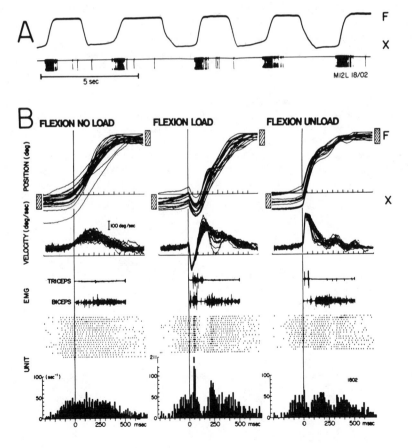

Phillips, is such that the largest inputs from neurons in motor cortex go to those spinal alpha MNs that also receive the largest spindle inputs.

The figure also summarizes another aspect of task-related cortical discharges that was established by concurrent work in the laboratories of Brooks and of Evarts. CSN responses to perturbations consist of two successive phases with different properties: the first is a stereotyped "reflex" response, occurring 20–50 msec after the perturbation to whose properties it is tightly coupled. Later discharges, and particularly the second cortical response occurring 50–100 msec after a perturbation, are more under central than peripheral control. The first response is tightly coupled to muscle stretch and contributes to the medium-latency muscular (M2) response. In contrast, the second and the late cortical responses are activated by the intent of the animal, that is by central *motor set*, and contribute to M3 and voluntary muscle discharges (this was identified by Evarts). All responses increase when the central set for that neuron calls for an extra effort. Stereo-

typed and voluntary responses may vary together or in opposition to each other, depending on what loads are applied, and when, in relation to the central set. Thus, the effects of kinesthetic (load) pulses on intended movements can be used to distinguish "reflex" from "intended" neural discharges.

Most precentral units show increased discharge for a given direction of voluntary movement, and decreased discharge when that same direction of movement is imposed passively. This reciprocal relation, which would be expected for the spinal stretch reflex, makes such CSNs good candidates for driving spinal alpha MNs. Figure 12.12 presents examples by Brooks and by Evarts, showing how the same perturbations can evoke different CSN responses depending on the preexisting motor set. In both cases the animals were instructed before the movements, through light signals, about what kind of arm movements to make, and were rewarded with juice through a dispensing tube situated within reach of their mouths. In Fig. 12.12A, alternate arm flexions and

Fig. 12.11. Response sequence initiated by muscle stretch in a subject prepared and set to make a voluntary contraction of that muscle. *Arrows* indicate conduction of neural activity through spinal segmental stretch reflex loop (mediating M1 response) and stereotyped transcortical loop (contributing to M2, the functional stretch response). Circled numbers (**1**) and (**2**), identifying first and second precentral response to stretch perturbation, have been added to original illustration, as well as "M3" designation. Compare to Fig. 12.10. (From Fetz, 1981; based on Cheney and Fetz, 1984)

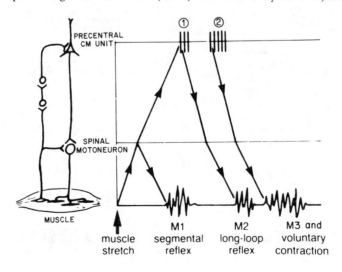

extensions were called for after hold periods in the respective target zones. In Fig. 12.12B, alternate push and pull arm movements were required, after hold periods in a central target zone. The trials in Fig. 12.12A involved a perturbation shortly after elbow movements had begun in response to a visual "start" signal (thus testing motor set early in the movements, as in Fig. 12.10), while in Fig. 12.12B shoulder movements moved the lever in response to a perturbation that served as the "start" signal (and thus tested motor set before movement onset created by an earlier visual signal). The records in the top row depict CSNs firing in their respective task-related modes, "flex" (Fig. 12.12A) and "push" (Fig. 12.12B). The histogram (Fig. 12.12A) and the raster (Fig. 12.12B) both show that the CSNs responded to perturbations that opposed the intended movements with successive first (reflex) responses and second (intended) discharges. The lower row shows the sequences when the same perturbations were applied to the opposite movements, to which the CSNs were not task-related. In both Fig. 12.12A and B (lower row), the first (reflex) response to peripheral feedback about muscle stretch was followed by silence imposed by a central inhibitory program (because the CSNs were not task-related to the movement) in the time slot for the set-related second response.

The intensities of first and second precentral responses depend on their timing in relation of the task set of individual CSNs. In Fig. 12.10B, for example, most of the early response is reflex (0–50 msec). The CSN did not emit a second, intended response (50–100 msec), probably because is was challenged by the perturbation after it had already reached the peak of its programmed brief, phasic contribution to movement onset (compare the slow and fast traces in Fig. 12.10A and B). In contrast, the CSN in Fig. 12.12A fired brief bursts whenever quick application of flexion force was called for (apparently to stabilize the joint through co-contraction as

in Fig. 12.10, not illustrated). The rasters in Fig. 12.12B show that the CSN discharged when the monkey pushed on the lever and stopped discharging when it pulled it. The transition from one movement to the other is marked by a heavy dot in each row, which indicates when the lever has reached the prescribed central target zone. In the top raster, dots mark the completion of "push" movements, followed by CSN silence as the monkey pulls the lever back into the central hold zone. In the bottom raster, the dots occur during CSN silence as the monkey pulls, and discharge recommences during the push back to the central target zone.

The firing patterns of both CSNs, in Fig. 12.12A and B, demonstrate how arrival of the central program abruptly changes the stereotyped responses (near 40 msec). This discussion shows how precentral contributions to "voluntary" actions depend on central programs as well as on sensory feedback and long-loop transcortical responses. We are now well into the transition from consideration of stereotyped to voluntary actions.

4. Voluntary Actions

How are pyramidal messages encoded so that they may be useful to spinal motoneurons, interneurons, and other targets? We saw in the preceding section that the discharge of some CSNs is related to central commands and that of others to peripheral input as well. Some CSNs react to peripheral input that signals limb position or its rate of change. Some others discharge in proportion to the magnitude of muscular contraction underlying the force exerted against an external object. Some CSNs relate to force, some to its rate of change, and some to both. Responsiveness of many CSNs changes according to the prevalent motor set. Cortical control of the momentary values of muscular force is important for the fine gradation of slow, precise movements, and cortical control of how fast muscular force can change is impor-

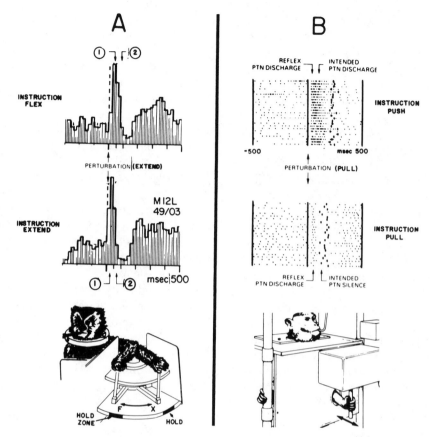

Fig. 12.12. Central programs (motor set) for voluntary actions override initial transcortical loop responses. Comparison of CSN responses when perturbations are applied just after movement onset (A) as in Fig. 12.10, or before (B), shown as histograms and rasters, respectively. Similar task situations are pictured at the bottom, showing also the delivery tubes for fluid rewards in front of monkeys mouths. (upper row) CSN responses when loads oppose intended movements ["flex" in (A) and "push" in (B)]; (lower row) CSN responses when loads assist intended movements ("extend" and "pull"). *The first precentral [(1), "reflex"] response is linked to the stimulus, and the second [(2), "intended"] response to the instruction.* Heavy dots in rasters indicate when handle has reached intended push or pull end zones. Identification of instructions given to monkeys has been added to original illustrations. [(A) From Conrad, Meyer-Lohmann, Matsunami, and Brooks, 1975. Circled numbers (1) and (2) have been added for first and second precentral responses to perturbations, as identified in Vilis, Hore, Meyer-Lohmann and Brooks, 1976. (B) From Evarts and Tanji, 1976; Evarts, 1979]

tant for grading of acceleratory transients in movement starts and stops (cf. Fig. 7.9).

CSNs function as task-related specialists under the influence of motor set. They discharge phasically ahead of the movement (about half of all precentral neurons change activity more than 80 msec before movement onset), and they also fire tonically during particular joint postures. Small CSNs are never completely silent for long, while larger ones are recruited for their contributions to larger efforts. Thach has studied tonic responsiveness by dissociating the responses of cortical neurons to force, position, and intended direction of movement, using an elaboration of the method of Fig. 12.12B. Monkeys were trained to hold and move a handle, on visual command signals, in the sequence 1 to 8 shown in Fig. 12.13. Motor cortex neurons were classified by the task relation of their steady (tonic) discharge rates to overcoming steady loads (not brief perturbations, as before). Moving the handle from positions 1 to 8 correlates cell properties in different ways. In positions 1, 2, 3, 4 versus 5, 6, 7, 8 the same muscle patterns are employed to steady the handle against either wrist flexions or extensions. About one-third of the CSNs studied are related to muscle patterns. Task relation to joint position is distinguished for that to loads by comparing steady discharges in positions A (1, 5), B (2, 4, 6, 8), and C (3, 7). Another third of the sample is related to joint position regardless of loads. The final third of the cell sample is related not to any aspect of the ongoing movement, but instead to the motor set for the direction of the *next* movement in the light-triggered, learned sequence. Such neurons are distinguished from the other two groups, relating to loads or joint positions, by comparing steady discharge levels in positions that precede flexions (3, 4, 7, 8) or extensions (1, 2, 5, 6).

Most force-related CSNs respond to perturbations (loads on a limb) in opposite manner to the task-related exertion of voluntary force. This reciprocal manner of CSN discharge (active force is opposite to the imposed, passive one) is appropriate for modulating spinal alpha MNs, like the examples in Figs. 12.10 and 12.12. The discharge rates of most of these neurons use the whole range available to the cells, whether they are firing with intended

small or large movements. The motor set for anticipated movement rescales the cellular input–output relations by resetting the cellular firing mechanisms of membrane depolarization and repolarization (the output) to the appropriate range of inputs.

This kind of "takeover" by the central effects of set, described by Evarts, recalls the sudden changes of excitability between the first and second responses to loads, illustrated in Fig. 12.12. For force-related neurons, the change of discharge rates from spontaneous to task-engaged levels is greatest when the limb exerts little force. This implies that these CSNs, which form the majority and are mostly small, affect spinal MNs that are recruited early in a task, that is, tonic MNs that are used in the fine gradations of force (cf. Fig. 4.5). About half of these CSNs can participate in small, feedback-dependent movements as well as in large movements. Large CSNs, in contrast, are more likely to be related to large movements, implying that they tend to modulate large spinal MNs that are recruited late in the build-up of muscle force. A fraction of force-related CSNs respond uniformly, instead of reciprocally, to active movements as opposed to passively imposed loads. Such CSNs may innervate spinal gamma MNs, according to a suggestion by Evarts. It is an attractive possibility because gamma MNs receive monosynaptic connections from motor

Fig. 12.13. A method to distinguish three alternate task relations of central neurons by combining various forces exerted by a torque motor with different positions of the handle and directions of its movements. A monkey was trained to move a handle sequentially from position A to B to C holding it in each for a prescribed time, and then to reverse the sequence, and so on. Steady, tonic discharge rates of motor cortex neurons relate to muscle patterns used (extensors versus flexors), or to the joint position maintained (A, B, or C), or to motor set for the next intended movement (direction of next movement). (From Thach, 1978)

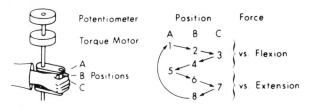

cortex and can respond to passive as well as to active tension. Furthermore pyramidal tract section decreases tonic fusimotor bias of muscle spindles, but the possibility still awaits experimental proof.

Behavioral tests to classify task relations of cortical neurons described so far have been based on movements restricted to one joint, a useful but unnatural condition, as noted before. New aspects of cortical organization are revealed when the monkey is allowed to use two joints to move its arm. This has been studied by Georgopoulos with a task and a two-jointed lever arrangement similar to that illustrated in Fig. 7.4. Allowing a wide range of movements on a horizontal plane reveals more subtle cellular accomplishments instead of all-or-none linkages to all-or-none choices such as flex versus extend. Precentral motor cortex neurons were found to discharge with hand movements aimed over a wide range, but they are "tuned" to some preferred angle. The *population* as a whole encodes the intended movement direction of the object of greatest CSN attention, which in this task is that of the hand guiding the lever. Response ranges could be as wide as 300 deg of arc, with discharge intensities distributed in bell-shaped fashion, the upper half of which covers about half the bell range. Cellular peak discharge is reached reproducibly at a narrow range of about 10 deg, marking the most task-related direction for that cortical neuron.

Figure 12.14 shows the relative contributions of one large sample of precentral neurons for eight movement directions, displayed as lines representing intensities at their preferred directions. (Intensities are displayed as the excess over the average of the peak values in the other directions.) The net task relation of the whole population is drawn for each of the eight directions as the sum of these vectors (heavy broken-line arrows), and we see that each turns out to coincide with the direction of movement. Thus the population of cortical neurons encodes the direction of the path

of the object of greatest attention for the central nervous system, a neural embodiment of the processes described in Chap. 7.1.

The importance of the pyramidal tract for making fractionated movements has been stressed in this chapter and in Chap. 5.2. The most important contribution is the stabilization of the fingers to accomplish precisely graded apposition of the thumb and forefinger. This uniquely primate property is accomplished by planned co-contractions of opposing muscles (for instance the first dorsal interosseus muscle to move the index finger; see Figs. 4.4 and 12.3). This "precision grip" is used to hold and pick up objects (Figs. 12.15 and 12.16B), or even to hold on to a support surface if we are in danger of toppling (Fig. 9.11, right). Swift accomplishment of the grip depends on corticospinal function. After section of the pyramidal tract, motor programs for cortical modulation of spinal MNs are degraded, resulting in prolonged buildup of the intended force (ΔF increases by an extra 50 msec). Neurons in motor cortex that are related to this programmed activity appear to code for force and its rate of change, much like others described above.

The co-contractions of the precision grip are an extreme form, a model, for other programmed movements requiring controlled postural maintenance. As related in Chaps. 3.2, 6.3, and 7.2, Bizzi has shown that trained monkeys remember previously learned arm movements after section of the afferent, dorsal roots and that they can position their arms in previously learned targets according to the length–tension properties of the muscles involved. It is significant in the current context that those deafferented monkeys could carry out these "open-loop" movements more easily by co-contracting the opposing muscles that move the arm. Normally, the precision grip is modulated by long-loop actions based on proprioceptive as well as cutaneous input. Without cutaneous discrimination of the kind of sur-

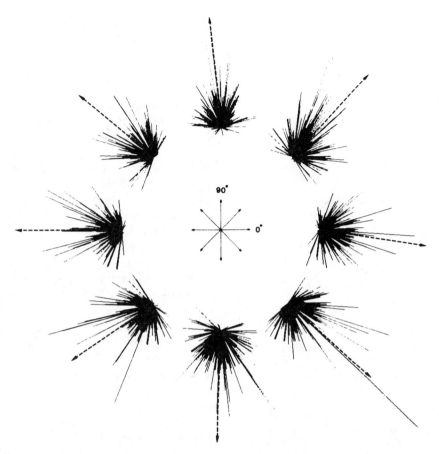

Fig. 12.14. Direction of the intended hand path is encoded by the whole population of task-related, participating neurons in primary motor cortex. Monkeys moved a two-jointed lever in a horizontal plane, using an arrangement similar to that in Fig. 7.4. The diagram shows the contributions of 241 precentral neurons to arm movements guiding the hand in eight different directions. Each "burst" represents the relative contributions made by the peak phasic discharges of each neuron ("vectors" incorporating intensities and directions). Note how the sum of the vectors in each burst *(heavy broken lines with arrowheads)* coincides with one of the eight movement directions indicated in the center of the diagram. (From Georgopoulos, Caminiti, Kalaska, and Massey, 1983; also in Brooks, 1985)

face to be gripped (e.g., silk vs. sandpaper), the precision of the force applied between the fingers is degraded; in fact the applied force becomes excessive by a factor of three times normal. Adjustment of the grip for small slippages is made by long-loop responses involving cutaneous receptors in the glabrous (nonhairy) skin of the gripping fingers. This observation, which is based on experiments with regional anesthesia in humans (made by Johansson and Westling), opens another window through which to observe establishment and updat-

ing of human motor programs. Proprioception seems to suffice for the exertion of steady force, but not for integrated, fine adjustments of finger pressure, since prescribed pressure can be exerted by one finger when sensations from the skin and joints have been blocked (as shown by Marsden). Recall that loss of proprioceptive as well as cutaneous sensations prevents a person from maintaining constant muscular contractions (Fig. 9.6) and, as a consequence, disables subtle, manipulatory motor acts even when they are under vi-

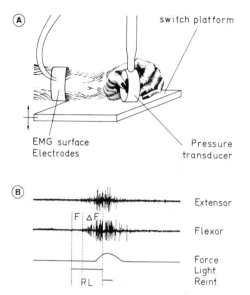

Fig. 12.15. A method to make quantitative measurements of the "precision grip", a programmed movement/posture that depends on the corticospinal tract. (A) The monkey compresses a pressure transducer between thumb and forefinger. (B) Typical recordings from one trial showing co-contraction of opposing muscles and curve of the resultant, intended force for which the animal was rewarded (reinforcement of operant training). Abbreviations: RL, response latency; F, onset latency of EMG; ΔF, duration of force buildup to intended level. (From Hepp-Reymond, Trouche, and Wiesendanger, 1974; in Wiesendanger, 1981)

sual control. We need feedback from our fingers to beat clumsiness, and the motor cortex is a vital instrument for this motor skill.

It is hard to overestimate the importance of peripheral feedback for voluntary actions. Monkeys can be trained, for instance, to control the firing frequency of individual CSNs, provided they are given some indication of their success. How do they control individual neurons? Control is exerted with the aid of somatosensory feedback. Normally, biofeedback control over cortical discharge appears to be mediated through peripheral movements that are small enough to escape detection and that discharge mechanoreceptors that, in turn, drive those cortical neurons. Section

of the ventral, motor roots abolishes accurate "operant" control of precentral neurons that receive proprioceptive feedback from the flaccid arm regions. This experiment (made by Wyler in Fetz's laboratory) speaks to the question of how we learn to make movements only by active motor trials (Chap. 1), using our sense of effort (Chap. 7.4). As pointed out by Porter, the precise peripheral information furnished by the dorsal columns (of the medial lemniscal system) is most needed during the *learning* of movements. After section of the dorsal columns and a period of retraining, monkeys could execute even discrete movements of the fingers. These animals could retrieve a raisin from a slot-shaped foodwell (as in Fig. 12.16B), which requires apposition of the thumb and index finger while keeping all other fingers out of the way. Recovery is aided by sprouting of nerve fibers that form new connections from other cortical areas which provides less precise, but adequate, sensory information.

We have now progressed from simple movements to complex tasks in exploring the cortical correlates of motor actions. The analysis of human movements reveals that the brain simplifies motor complexity by steering the object requiring its greatest attention, which often is the hand (Chap. 7.1; e.g., Fig. 7.4). This is accomplished by the hierarchical function of the cortical areas sending axons to the spinal cord (Fig. 12.1), as demonstrated in the laboratories of Porter and of Kuypers. A method, developed by Porter, is illustrated in Fig. 12.16, which shows that records can be obtained from single cortical neurons while a monkey operates a food-vending machine. The animal is trained to make first a free reaching movement toward a handle, which it has to grasp and pull forward into a target zone, followed by a completely different movement, namely to extract a raisin from a slot-shaped foodwell that requires apposition of thumb and forefinger in a prescision grip (Fig. 12.16A,B). Cinematography was used to document the command-controlled behavior at the exact time of neural recording with pictures of the animals' posture that relate to single-unit discharge. This approach illuminates how motor set guides the action of precentral neurons.

Arm movements that transport the hand (as the object of attention of the brain) towards the lever-pull task are supported by groups of specialized neurons in area 4. Lemon has shown that in this natural, complex task situation, CSNs related to arm movements are distinct from those related to the subsequent hand movements, which remain silent while the arm transports the hand. The *power grip* used to pull the handle (with all digits) tends to engage a different population of neurons from that which is activated thereafter for the *precision grip* to pick up the raisin. The operation of programs was revealed further by the ability of the experimenters to test sensory inputs to these neurons because the animals had been gentled to permit touching and exploration of their arms and hands. During task performance, responses of task-related neurons to relevant afferent input are heightened and those to irrelevant inputs are suppressed. This is a striking demonstration of a change of state, of sensory editing in relation to the motor purposes (Chap. 11.1). It recalls the suppression of unwanted reflex responses during intended movements (Fig. 12.12).

Participation of the premotor and supplementary motor areas in this task has been described by Brinkman and Porter. The arcuate premotor area (APA in Fig. 11.8) serves visuomotor integration: the largest group of its task-related neurons are driven by task-related visual events and discharge in relation to the movements before their onset. Very few are driven by peripheral input from the limbs (see Figs. 11.11 and 12.1). The discharge of some neurons is modulated throughout the successive phases of the task. Unlike CSNs for area 4, premotor CSN output is related to movements of either limb—that is, to the task movement plan—before specification regarding how to carry it out. Neurons in the supplementary motor area (SMA) are important mediators of the output from the putamen loop of the basal ganglia to the motor cortex. SMA cells share the properties of premotor cells, except that many react to peripheral afferent input, albeit with little influence on their task-related discharges (see the schematics of the connections in Figs. 11.3 and 11.11).

Fig. 12.16. Corticospinal neurons are specialized during voluntary actions, which is best revealed by recording during complex tasks. (A) Monkey makes free reaching movements of the arm to guide the hand to a handle, which it has to grasp and pull into a "target zone." In some experiments this yields a reward; in others (B) it permits access to a slot-shaped food well from which the animal can extract a raisin if it uses the precision grip (as in Fig. 12.15). Most CSNs relate to only one phase of this complex tast. [(A) From Brinkman and Porter, 1979, 1983; (B) from Haaxma and Kuypers, 1974; cf. Lemon, 1981]

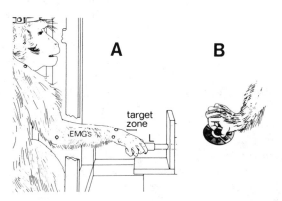

Tasks such as those in Figs. 12.10–12.13 and 12.16 raise the question of how the cortex reassigns the responsibilities for action to various cell groups during changes of resistance to joint movements, that is, changes calling for altered ratios of isometric and isotonic muscle contractions. Such changes need to be sensed in order to let the fusimotor-spindle system readjust (Chap. 3.1; Fig. 4.12), and to prepare the way for changes in recruitment of spinal MNs because of the nonlinear properties of muscle tissue (Chap. 3.2). When the joint is allowed to rotate, the agonist shortens rapidly and its force output falls (Figs. 3.5B and 3.6B) owing to its length–velocity properties (Fig. 4.6). Since this occurs despite continued motor nerve signals to the muscle, more muscular discharge is required to exert a given force against an external object when the muscle is short than when it is long. These are changes that the spinal motor servo can adjust for (Figs. 4.9 and 5.1), but afferent signals must call forth long-loop responses to sustain the intended action.

At present little can be done to reactivate motor cortex that has been devastated, for instance by a stroke. We know, however, that exercise leads to sprouting of task-related fibers (cf. Chap. 11.3). It is therefore conceivable that connections between various areas of sensorimotor cortex (Fig. 11.11) might one day be harnessed. What would be required is cortical reorganization by combined pharmacological and physical therapies that might create supportive, new uses for related healthy cortex with functioning ascending and descending connections.

5. Summary

All parts of the sensorimotor cortex (with its specialized areas) participate in motor acts. Messages preparatory to movement onset are dispatched from areas 2, 5, and 4, followed by onset commands from area 4. Ongoing movements are guided from areas 3a, 3b, and 1. The motor cortex, area 4, is made up of specialized parts. The rostra part contains corticospinal neurons (CSNs) with strong central inputs as well as others with peripheral (kinesthetic) input from moving limbs, while caudal CSNs are responsive to skin input.

Neurons in primary motor cortex are specialists; they are assigned particular roles by motor set emanating from higher centers. Motor action is the result of their cooperation with each other and with other parts of the brain; it is the result of the action of large populations of such neurons. Cortical motor outflow arises from small colonies of CSNs projecting to one or two muscles. Each spinal MN pool for a particular muscle receives input from several colonies that may be several millimeters apart in area 4. Cortical representation of muscles is thus interlaced in cortical patches, with the likelihood of obtaining antagonist co-contraction being greatest in rostral area 4. Output colonies are located in radially oriented columns of about 0.3 mm diameter that contain about 10^4 neurons. Each cortical layer makes connections for particular inputs or outputs. CSNs, located mostly in layer V, project to one or two spinal MN nuclei. Columns in motor cortex process information from higher and lower levels of the motor hierarchy, but not from the limbic system.

Two basic peripheral input–output stereotypes can be observed in nonalert animals whose motor cortex is modulated only minimally by other brain areas. Columns in caudal area 4 contain CSNs that respond to skin input and that can be activated by intracortical microstimulation (ICMS) to facilitate muscles that move the limb into the path of skin contact. This positive feedback pattern may serve exploratory "active" touch as well as the cortical tactile and grasping responses. Columns in rostral area 4 contain CSNs that respond to kinesthetic input and that can be activated by ICMs to move the limb in the opposite direction of the input-effective limb movements. This negative feedback pattern may serve limb stabilization and load compensation, particularly for small (internal) loads generated by the interaction of muscles and joints. Cortical neurons in alert animals respond in this stereotyped fashion to perturbations of a motor task. Such feedback-dependent responses, however, are followed and overwhelmed by feedforward responses to the animal's intent, or motor set.

In alert, task-engaged brains, CSNs in area 4 are used as specialists. Motor set assigns them to particular aspects of natural motor tasks. Their phasic discharge mostly precedes movement onset and, for many, it is related to the force to be exerted or to its rate of change. Others relate to joint position or only to central commands. Whatever the relation, motor set scales the cellular responsiveness so that the entire frequency range of discharge is available for the task-related action. During maintained limb postures, CSNs discharge tonically in relation to muscle patterns used, to the joint position, or to the direction of the next movement. In natural movements (using two or more joints), movement direction is encoded by the relative contributions of all task-related CSNs in area 4. Yet CSNs function as specialists under the influence of motor set in the participation of complex tasks. For instance, if related to hand use, they fire either when it is used for major force application as in the power grip, or for fine finger work such as the precision grip.

Knowledge of cortical physiology is likely to lead to new forms of rehabilitation in which biochemical, pharmacological, and physical therapies might bring about a reorganization of related cortical areas to reinnervate and activate disabled cortical tissue.

References

Andersen, P., Hagan, P. J., Phillips, C. G., and Powell, T. P. S. 1975. Mapping by microstimulation of overlapping projections from area 4 to motor units of the baboon's. *Proc. Roy. Soc.* (London) *B*, 188:31–60.

Asanuma, H. 1981. The pyramidal tract. In *Motor control*. Sect. 1, vol. 2. *Handbook of physiology*, ed. V. B. Brooks, pp. 703–733. Bethesda, Md.: American Physiological Society. [Figs. 12.3A, 12.4, and 12.8]

Asanuma, H. and Arissian, K. 1984. Experiments on functional role of peripheral input to motor cortex during voluntary movements in the monkey. *J. Neurophysiol.* 52:212–227.

Brinkman, C., and Porter, R. 1983. Supplementary motor area and premotor area of the monkey cerebral cortex: functional organization and activites of single neurons during performance of a learned movement. In *Motor control mechanisms in health and disease*, ed. J. E. Desmedt. *Adv. Neurol.* 39:393–420. [Fig. 12.16A]

Brinkman, C., and Porter, R. 1979. Supplementary motor area in the monkey: activity of neurons during performance of a learned motor task. *J. Neurophysiol.* 42:681–709. [Fig. 12.16A]

Brooks, V. B. 1985. How are "move" and "hold" programs matched? In *Cerebellar Functions.* eds., J. R. Bloedel, J. Dichgans, and W. Precht. pp. 1–23. Berlin: Springer Verlag.

Brooks, V. B. 1981. Task-related cell assemblies. In *Brain mechanisms and perceptual awareness*, eds. O. Pompeiano and C. Ajmone-Marsan, pp. 295–309. New York: Raven Press.

Brooks, V. B. 1971. Tight input–output coupling. In *Central control of movement*, eds. E. V. Evarts, E. Bizzi, R. E. Burke, M. DeLong, and W. T. Thach. *Neurosci. Res. Prog. Bull.* 9:51–56.

Brooks, V. B., and Asanuma, H. 1965. Recurrent cortical effects following stimulation of medullary pyramid. *Arch. Ital. Biol.* 103:247–278. [Fig. 12.7]

Brooks, V. B., and Stoney, S. D. 1971. Motor mechanisms: the role of the pyramidal system in motor control. *Ann. Rev. Physiol.* 33:337–392.

Cheney, P. D., and Fetz, E. E. 1984. Corticomotoneuronal cells contribute to long-latency stretch reflexes in the rhesus monkey. *J. Physiol.* (London) 349:249–272. [Fig. 12.11]

Conrad, B., Matsunami, K., Meyer-Lohmann, J., Wiesendanger, M., and Brooks, V. B. 1974. Cortical load compensation during voluntary elbow movements. *Brain Res.* 71:507–514. [Fig. 12.10]

Conrad, B., Meyer-Lohmann, J., Matsunami, K., and Brooks, V. B. 1975. Precentral unit activity following torque pulse injections into elbow movements. *Brain Res.* 94:219–236. [Fig. 12.12A]

Darian-Smith, I., Goodwin, A., Sugitania, M., and Heywood, J. 1984. The tangible features of textured surfaces: their representation in the monkey's somatosensory cortex. In *Dynamic aspects of neocortical function*, eds. G. M. Edelman, W. E. Gall, and W. M. Cowan, pp. 475–500. New York: John Wiley & Sons.

Dykes, R. W., Landry, P., Metherate, R., and Hicks, T. P. 1984. The functional role of GABA in cat primary somatosensory cortex: shaping the receptive fields of cortical neurons. *J. Neurophysiol.* 52:1066–1093.

Evarts, E. V. 1970. Brain mechanisms in movement. *Sci. Am.* 229:96–103. [Fig. 12.12B]

Evarts, E. V. 1981. Role of motor cortex in voluntary movements. In *Motor control.* Sect. 1, vol. 2. *Handbook of physiology*, ed. V. B. Brooks, pp. 1083–1120. [Fig. 12.10]

Evarts, E. V., and Tanji, J. 1976. Reflex and intended responses in motor cortex pyramidal tract neurons of monkey. *J. Neurophysiol.* 39:1069–1108. [Fig. 12.12B]

Evarts, E. V., and Fromm, C. 1981. Transcortical reflexes and servo control of movement. *Can. J. Physiol. Pharmacol.* 59:757–775.

Fetz, E. E. 1984. Functional organization of motor and sensory cortex: symmetries and parallels. In *Dynamic aspects of neocortical function*, eds. G. M. Edelman, W. E. Gall, and W. M. Cowan, pp. 453–473. New York: John Wiley & Sons.

Fetz, E. E. 1981. Neuronal activity associated with conditioned limb movements. In *Motor coordination.* Vol. 5. *Handbook of behavioral neurobiology*, eds. A. L. Towe and E. S. Luschei, pp. 493–526. New York: Plenum Press. [Figs. 12.5, 12.10, and 12.11]

Fetz, E. E., and Cheney, P. D. 1980. Postspike facilitation of forelimb muscle activity by primate corticomotoneuronal cells. *J. Neurophysiol.* 44:751–772. [Fig. 12.5]

Georgopoulos, A. P., Caminiti, R., Kalaska, J. F., and Massey, J. T. 1983. Spatial coding of movement direction by motor cortical populations. In *Neural coding of motor performance*, eds. J. Massion, J. Paillard, W. Schultz, and M. Wiesendanger. *Exp. Brain Res.* Suppl. 7, pp. 327–336. [Fig. 12.14]

Georgopoulos, A. P., Kalaska, J. F., Crutcher, M. D., Caminiti, R., and Massey, J. T. 1984. The representation of movement direction in

the motor cortex: single cell and population studies. In *Dynamic aspects of neocortical function*, eds. G. M. Edelman, W. E. Gall, and W. M. Cowan, pp. 501–524. New York: John Wiley & Sons.

Ghez, C., Vicario, D., Martin, J. H., and Yumiya, H. 1983. Sensory motor processing of target movements in motor cortex. In *Motor control mechanisms in health and disease*, ed. J. E. Desmedt. *Adv. Neurol.* 39:61–92.

Gilman, S., Marco, L. A., and Ebel, H. C. 1971. Effects of medullary pyramidotomy in the monkey. II. Abnormalities of spindle afferent responses. *Brain* 94:515–530.

Haaxma, R., and Kuypers, H. 1974. Role of occipito-frontal cortico-cortical connections in visual guidance of relatively independent hand and finger movements in rhesus monkeys. *Brain Res.* 71:361–366. [Fig. 12.16B]

Hepp-Reymond, M. C., Trouche, E., and Wiesendanger, M. 1974. Effects of unilateral and bilateral pyramidotomy on a conditioned rapid precision grip in monkeys. *Exp. Brain Res.* 21:519–527. [Fig. 12.15]

Humphrey, D. R. 1983. Corticospinal systems and their control by premotor cortex, basal ganglia and cerebellum. In *Neurobiology.* Vol. 5. *The clinical neurosciences*, ed. W. D. Willis, pp. 547–587. New York: Churchill Livingstone. [Fig. 12.1]

Humphrey, D. R. and Reed, D. J. 1983. Separate cortical systems for control of joint movement and joint stiffness: reciprocal activation and coactivation of antagonist muscles. In *Motor control mechanisms in health and disease*, ed. J. E. Desmedt. *Adv. Neurol.* 39:347–372. [Fig. 12.3B]

Jankowska, E., Padel, Y., and Tanaka, R. 1975. Projections of pyramidal tract cells to alpha motoneurones innervating hindlimb muscles in the monkey. *J. Physiol. (Lond.)* 249:637–667. [Fig. 12.3A]

Johansson, R. S., and Westling, G. 1984. Roles of glabrous skin receptors and sensorimotor memory in automatic control of precision grip when lifting rougher or more slippery subjects. *Exp. Brain Res.* 56:550–564.

Jones, E. G. 1983. The columnar basis of cortical circuitry. In *Neurobiology.* Vol. 5. *The clinical neurosciences*, ed. W. D. Willis, pp. 357–383. New York: Churchill Livingstone. [Fig. 12.2]

Jones, E. G., Coulter, J. D., Burton, H., and

Porter, R. 1977. Cells of origin and terminal distribution of corticostriatal fibers arising in the sensory-motor cortex of monkeys. *J. Comp. Neurol.* 173:53–80. [Fig. 12.6]

Jones, E. G., and Wise, S. P. 1977. Size, laminar and columnar distribution of efferent cells in the sensory-motor cortex of monkeys. *J. Comp. Neurol.* 175:391–438. [Fig. 12.6]

Lamarre, Y., Bioulac, B., and Jacks, B. 1978. Activity of precentral neurones in conscious monkeys: effects of deafferentation and cerebellar ablation. *J. Physiol. (Paris)* 74:253–264.

Lemon, R. 1981. Functional properties of monkey motor cortex neurones receiving afferent input from the hand and fingers. *J. Physiol. (Lond.)* 311:497–519. [Fig. 12.16]

Marsden, C. D., Rothwell, J. C., and Day, B. L. 1984. The use of peripheral feedback in the control of movement. *Trends Neurosci.* 7:253–257.

Moberg, E. 1983. The role of cutaneous afferents in position sense, kinaesthesia, and motor function of the hand. *Brain* 106:1–19.

Murphy, J. T., Kwan, H. C., MacKay, W. A., and Wong, Y. C. 1978. Spatial organization of precentral cortex in awake primates. III. Input-output coupling. *J. Neurophysiol.* 41:1132–1139.

Phillips, C. G., and Porter, R. 1977. *Corticospinal neurones: their role in movement.* New York: Academic Press. [Fig. 12.3A]

Porter, R. 1981. Internal organization of the motor cortex for input–output arrangements. In *Motor control.* Sect 1, vol. 2. *Handbook of physiology,* ed. V. B. Brooks, pp. 1063–1081. Bethesda, Md.: American Physiological Society. [Fig. 12.6]

Rosén, I., and Asanuma, H. 1972. Peripheral afferent inputs to the forelimb area of the monkey motor cortex: input–output relations. *Exp. Brain Res.* 14:257–273. [Fig. 12.8]

Seal, J., Gross, C., and Bioulac, B. 1982. Activity of neurons in area 5 during a simple arm movement in monkeys before and after deafferentation of the trained limb. *Brain Res.* 250:229–243.

Smith, A. M. 1981. The coactivation of antagonist muscles. *Can. J. Physiol. Pharmacol.* 59:733–747.

Steriade, M. 1978. Cortical long-axoned cells and putative interneurons during the sleep-wake cycle. *Behav. Brain Sci.* 3.465–514.

Strick, P. L., and Preston, J. B. 1983. Input-output organization of the primate motor cortex. In *Motor control in health and disease,* ed. J. E. Desmedt. *Adv. Neurol.* 39:321–327. [Fig. 12.2]

Strick, P. L., and Preston, J. B. 1979. Multiple representation in the motor cortex: a new concept of input–output organization for the forearm representation. In *Integration in the nervous system,* eds. H. Asanuma and V. J. Wilson, pp. 205–221. Tokyo: Igaku-Shoin. [Fig. 12.9]

Thach, W. T. 1978. Correlation of neural discharge with pattern and force of muscular activity, joint position, and direction of the intended movement in motor cortex and cerebellum. *J. Neurophysiol.* 41:654–676. [Fig. 12.13]

Tsukahara, N., and Murakami, F. 1983. Axonal sprouting and recovery of function after brain damage. In *Motor control mechanisms in health and disease,* ed. J. E. Desmedt. *Adv. Neurol.* 39:1073–1084.

Vilis, T., Hore, J., Meyer-Lohmann, J., and Brooks, V. B. 1976. Dual nature of the precentral responses to limb perturbations revealed by cerebellar cooling. *Brain Res.* 117:336–340. [Fig. 12.12A]

Wiesendanger, M. 1981. The pyramidal tract: its structure and function. In *Motor coordination.* Vol. 5. *Handbook of behavioral neurobiology,* eds. A. L. Towe and E. S. Luschei, pp. 401–491. New York: Plenum Press. [Fig. 12.15]

13

The Cerebellum

The cerebellum is essential for the adaptation, learning, and execution of motor actions in a skillful manner. It comes into play after the overall motor plans have been communicated to premotor cortex by the prefrontal and parietal cortex and have been "enabled" by the limbic system and the basal ganglia (Fig. 2.7). The lateral cerebellum programs goal-directed motor activities and optimizes their component postures and movements. This is achieved with the aid of the intermediate, medial, and vestibular cerebellum by coordinating and adapting the necessary actions of muscles (Chaps. 2.2; 7.1 and 11.3). The cerebellum receives its inputs from the middle and lower levels of the motor hierarchy. The targets of cerebellar adjustments and adaptations are the sensorimotor cortex and related subcortical systems. Cerebrocerebellar programming confers motor skill, that is, the maximal ability to use programmed movements with optimal trajectories. In this chapter we consider how the cerebellum performs these functions.

What makes the cerebellum such a special part of the middle hierarchy? Its unique construction equips it to adapt, and thus to optimize, the coordinated execution of the motor intent. With this process it also completes the translation of the coordinates of the external world into those of the internal world of the body, suitable for use by the motor cortex and subcortical motor centers. Although many cerebellar functions and their neural mechanisms resemble those found in the cerebral cortex, the cerebellum is set apart by its adaptive ability for the guidance of postures and movements of the head, eyes, body, and limbs. Cerebellar control of motor acts depends on comparisons of motor commands and their execution. This comparator function is made possible by the fact that cerebellar inputs and outputs form side loops of the transcortical projections in the middle level of the motor hierarchy and of those to the lower level (Figs. 2.7 and 13.1). The cerebellar cortex can govern large numbers of events at the same time by means of its very many small efferent zones ("microzones"), that are task-related, specialized cell assemblies.

The connections in the cerebellar cortex are so uncommonly uniform that Eccles was moved to compare their appearance to the wiring of a computer. Reports about motor commands and their execution reach the cerebellar cortex through an orderly array of many ("parallel") fibers that reflect the usual neural message traffic in their high discharge rates. In addition, however, each microzone receives a small number of special ("climbing") fibers. Their infrequent discharges do not report about neural representations of the world or the body. Instead, they sound an alarm that the motor action is not being controlled optimally, and then they adapt the output (Purkinje) cells of the microzones to make long-lasting improvements in the control. The cerebellum performs a regulatory role for the middle level as it functions not only to coordinate but also to control its own quality of function.

To begin this study of the cerebellum it is instructive to summarize the effects of its dysfunction. Understanding what the brain can and cannot do without certain cerebellar parts tells us something about their contributions to the control exerted by the middle level. This summary is followed by an overview of cerebellar connections and their neural actions (Chap. 13.2). The findings gleaned from lesions and from neuronal records match well for the cerebellum, and this enhances our confidence in their interpretation. Subsequent sections consider cerebellar contributions to posture and movements in the light of its outputs (Chap. 13.3), its mossy fiber inputs (Chap. 13.4), cortical organization (Chap. 13.5), and climbing fiber inputs as related to the cortical microzones (Chap. 13.6). The chapter concludes with a consideration of the adaptive properties of cerebellar control and motor learning (Chap. 13.7).

1. Cerebellar Dysfunctions

When the cerebellum is damaged, muscles acting on joints that normally move together lose their synergies (Chap. 9.6). Intended movements are decomposed into sequential constituents and are made with errors of direction, force, velocity, and amplitude, all associated with delayed movement starts and stops (e.g., Fig. 1.2B). These errors were deduced by Gordon Holmes from his examination of patients with cerebellar lesions inflicted by gunshot wounds. We can now think of cerebellar symptoms as the consequences of the subject having lost control over movement "trajectories." (Recall that *trajectories*

were defined as the programmed use of muscular force in relation to its rate of change; see Fig. 7.5. If the limb can move in response to the force, then the trajectory is the directional path in relation to the velocity with which it is traversed; see Fig. 6.6.) The errors are most pronounced with lesions of the lateral cerebellum, particularly if its output nucleus (the dentate) is also damaged. Intended movements are guided along their reference trajectories with the aid of long-loop paths through the motor cortex (Chap. 6.2). Patients with cerebellar lesions know what movements they want to make, but they cannot carry them out accurately and they cannot maintain intended postures because long-loop responses are degraded or fail altogether during cerebellar dysfunction (Chaps. 6.2, 7.1, 9.6, and 12.4). Furthermore, cerebellar dysfunctions cause "intention" tremor during purposeful maintenance of steady postures, but not at rest when muscles are relaxed. Intention tremor is brought about by decomposition of intended postural cocontractions of opposing muscles, and consists of inaccurate corrective movements toward intended positions of a limb or of the whole body ("sway"). As Tanaka has shown for patients with cerebellar disorders, corrective movements suffer the same errors as "ordinary" voluntary movements, because they are made toward an *intended* goal.

Use of muscle synergies is lost in cerebellar dysfunctions, because the brain cannot implement the motor programs that ordinariliy come into play. For instance, patients with cerebellar lesions cannot control the appropriate timing and tensions of the muscles acting on the ankle and the thigh, and thus lose the synergies for postural, compound movements (muscle patterns, Figs. 6.4C and 9.9). Postural adjustments of the body (and of the eyes, in cerebellar nystagmus) are degraded by the loss of programmed responses of long-loop, transcortical "functional stretch" responses (Fig. 6.9) or of the vestibular system (e.g. Fig. 9.12). (Programs for intended simple movements are also degraded, as we will see below). Moreover, intended postures and movements are no longer *adapted* to the realities of a given situation. It is a crippling loss not to be able to adapt—to optimize—motor performance in the face of changing circumstances. We observe the loss of adaptive, predictive programming as inappropriately scaled intensities and timing of muscles, forming unsuitable and nonadaptive patterns with resultant errors of task execution (Fig. 6.4C,D).

Yet, patients with cerebellar lesions have normal cognitive abilities: they know their predicament, they can report on their ataxia, and they can work out strategies to accomplish their aim despite "unwilling limbs" (Fig. 1.2B). Trained animals similarly give every sign of knowing what is required of them despite cerebellar dysfunction, and they too perform previously learned tasks by substituting actions that they can manage for those impaired by cerebellar deficit. Cerebellar dysfunctions degrade but do not abolish movements, and cerebellar stimulation evokes only a narrow repertoire of movements. These facts indicate that the cerebellum performs a *regulatory* role. It coordinates and adjusts the responses of middle- and lower-level structures to the commands received from the higher levels (Figs. 2.7, 11.2, and 11.3).

Programming functions of the type described above are carried out with the aid of the lateral cerebellum, as evidenced by lesions of the lateral cerebellar cortex and its output through the dentate nucleus. (The functional anatomy is taken up below.) Dysfunctions of the medial and intermediate cerebellum do not cause as drastic a loss of program use, but rather a degraded use, because programs are not "updated" in the usual way by peripheral, as well as processed, afferent information. This loss of updating is important, because ordinary movements are never run entirely according to preformed programs but instead their course is modified by feedback

(Chap. 1.1 and 1.2). Updating of programs by the cerebellum make it part of an adaptive control system (Fig. 4.14). Cerebellar programming helps to convey motor set to the premotor and primary motor cortices, the reticular formation, and the vestibulospinal system. The cortical and reticular routes deal mainly with movements for which fusimotor adjustments are only partially useful, leaving much of that control to be exerted primarily on alpha MNs, with secondary adjustments of gamma MNs (Chap. 4.2).

Dysfunctions of the vestibulocerebellum produce disequilibration characterized by falling oscillations of the head and trunk, staggering gait on a broad base, and reluctance to move about without support of the body against gravity. Actions in which vestibular control is not involved remain unimpaired; for example, voluntary and postural reflex movements of the extremities are well performed if the trunk is supported. Eye movements are also abnormal in that they exhibit nystagmus, that is, corrections against incorrect gaze control, with the quick phase toward the side of the lesion. There are neither impairments of awareness of gravity or of movement in space, nor are there vertigo or hallucinations of movement. We know that postures of the head, eyes, and trunk are regulated by the vestibulospinal system, which exerts bilateral facilitatory control of antigravity extensors, taking full advantage of segmental reflex mechanisms. Slow and small, or mostly isometric, interactions of muscles can be adjusted through modulation of the coactivation of alpha MNs and static gamma MNs. This might be important while motor acts are being learned (Chaps. 4.2 and 13.7). In sum, the cerebellum *coordinates* the acquisition and smooth use of movements in motor performance, that is, of motor skill (Chap. 1.3). It "packages" programs and subprograms (Chap. 2.3), helps to establish and maintain "models" of expected muscular actions by programming alpha as well as gamma MNs, and in the process also makes task-oriented adjustments of spinal and vestibular reflexes (Chaps. 4.2, 5.1, and 9.1).

2. Overview of Cerebellar Connections

The cerebellum is attached to the brain stem by three pairs of peduncles (Fig. 5.8) that contain its afferent and efferent fibers. It is folded under the posterior aspect of the cerebral hemispheres (Fig. 2.1B,C). The main cerebellar inputs come from the cerebral sensorimotor and visual cortex, the vestibular system, and the spinal cord (Figs. 2.2, 11.2, and 11.3). The cerebellar functions outlined in the preceding section are based on *comparisons* of central motor commands with somatosensory, vestibular, and visual reports reaching the cerebellum from the periphery and the central nervous system. As pointed out previously, intended and ongoing motor activity, intent and reality, what should be and what actually is: these critical entities were identified by Bernstein as the cornerstones for the calculations of motor control. Sperry and von Holst recognized independently that these entities could be compared in the CSN by internal corollary discharge (Chaps. 2.2, 3.1, and 7.4).

The main pathways carrying detailed information about somatosensory peripheral events to the cerebellum are the dorsal spinocerebellar tract (DSCT, and its forelimb equivalent) and the vestibulocerebellar afferents (arising as branches of the primary afferents and as fibers from the vestibular nuclei). The detailed, local information conveyed by the DSCT about receptors in muscles, joints, and skin resembles that ascending in the medial lemniscal system to the somatosensory cerebral cortex. In contrast, other spinocerebellar paths carry information about activity signaling the internal state of lower motor centers (Fig. 13.8, later). Visual information reaches the cerebellum as detailed descriptions of the visual field from the geniculostriate system, and as processed information about

the control of eye movements from the accessory optic tract. The latter indicates when the gaze is slipping from its intended fixation point, and just how the visual field is slipping as a consequence. In addition, there is an autonomic projection to the vermal cerebellum from the nucleus of the solitary tract, which deals with gustatory, cardiovascular, and respiratory reflexes.

An overall scheme of connections, highlighting the somatosensorimotor aspect of the cerebellar circuit, is presented in Fig. 13.1. The cerebellum is shown as consisting of lateral, intermediate, and medial rostrocaudal ("sagittal") zones, each of which is reciprocally connected with its own output nucleus (the dentate, interposed, and fastigial). The diagram is partial and oversimplified, nuclear groups have been combined, connections of particular parts omitted, and laterality ignored. The open downward arrows indicate higher centers convey intent to premotor cortex. The connections of afferents and efferents of all the zones are stressed as forming *side loops suitable for functioning as comparators*. Cerebellar outputs descend, indirectly, to the spinal cord and ascend to areas 4 and 6 by way of the ventrolateral (VL) nucleus of the thalamus. The diagram is meant to convey the idea of the flow of motor commands and the important corollary monitoring of those commands. The path of the "evolving movement" (Eccles' felicitous term that implies initial planning as well as the accommodations to momentary circumstances) runs from spinal motor centers to muscles back to receptors and relay nuclei.

Figure 13.1 indicates how the cerebellum corrects the consequences of erroneous motor commands from the cerebral cortex by monitoring those commands with the help of the precerebellar nuclei (inferior olive and pontine and reticular nuclei). Signals about the activity in lower and higher motor centers and the evolving movement are fed back internally, and through loops that include the external world. (Note that the direct spinocerebellar connections are omitted in the figure.) Cerebellar input paths thus provide for comparison of these events with commands from the cerebellum and the precerebellar nuclei to generate corrections. Comparison through internal loops (i.e., monitoring of the corollary motor commands) allows corrections to begin before movements are initiated, an important saving of time because it prevents corrections from lagging behind ("phase lag"), which

causes unwanted oscillations (i.e., tremor). The power of "phase advance" in forestalling ("transport") delays due to the slow time course of electromechanical coupling has already been introduced (Fig. 7.5). The internal loops through programmed neurons, including those in areas 4 and 6, provide internal "models" of the intended activity, which can be used to estimate and produce early corrections of their anticipated performance. These models—that is,

Fig. 13.1. The "cerebellar circuit," stressing its position in a side loop between higher centers and spinal cord, suitable for a comparator function, which could initiate corrections before movements have begun. This grossly oversimplified scheme omits all intervening nuclei and ignores laterality. Descending efferent lines and ascending afferent lines from the cerebral cortex: open, *hatched filled arrows;* cerebellum and its output nuclei: fastigial (F), interposed (IP), and dentate (D). Cerebellar inputs: *checkered arrows.* Cerebellocerebral route is drawn through ventrolateral (VL) thalamus (see Fig. 11.7). Outputs from motor cortex are indicated by one *black arrow,* corticocortical loops by *small horizontal arrows.* Compare to Figs. 2.2 and 11.3. (From Brooks and Thach, 1981; also in Brooks, 1984)

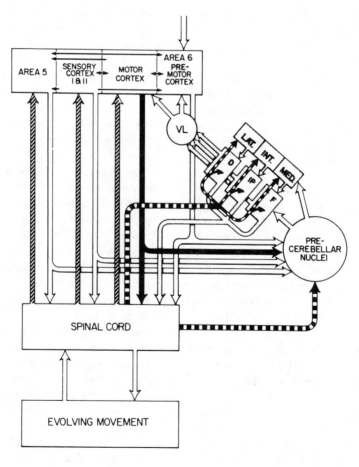

subprograms for reference trajectories—engage spinal alpha MNs (and gamma MNs if it benefits spindle feedback within the confines of the task context; cf. Fig. 4.12).

A more realistic description of information flow is presented in Fig. 13.2, specifying how cerebellar inputs from the ipsilateral side of the body are channeled to contralateral (or bilateral) output targets. Here we again see the three sagittal zones (introduced by Jansen and Brodal), shown superimposed at right angles on the transverse cerebellar lobes. The anterior and posterior lobes are folded into five and four lobules, respectively. The most caudal (flocculonodular, FN) lobe is drawn separated from the others because of its deep separating fissure. This lobe is called the vestibulocerebellum, because its predominant, labyrinthine input comes from the vestibular nuclei (Figs. 5.8, 9.1, and 9.2).

The input–output relations of the rest of the cerebellum align it sagittally rather than by lobes. The difference between the peripherally connected intermediate zone and the centrally connected lateral zone has already been referred to (Fig. 2.7). Spinocerebellar input reaches the medial and intermediate parts (spinocerebellum) that also project back to the spinal cord, the medial one exclusively so. The "spinocerebellum," however, also receives inputs from the cerebral sensorimotor cortex, by way of the pontine nuclei which project to the intermediate and lateral cerebellum. The lateral zone, which is the newest part of the cerebellum (hence "neocerebellum") is called the "pontocerebellum" because its input is exclusively from the pontine nuclei, but pontocerebellar as well as vestibular projections also reach the medial part of the cerebellar cortex (the vermis). The lateral and intermediate parts make up the hemispheres. The lateral part projects to the premotor and primary motor cortices, and the intermediate part projects mainly to the brain stem and primary motor cortex. The medial part projects to the spinal cord and brain stem, but not to the cerebral cortex. These connections are shown in Figs. 13.2 and (in a different way) Fig. 13.6.

3. Cerebellar Outputs

The connections of the sagittal zones make it clear that the lateral zone is connected with central structures appropriate for giving movements feedforward commands, while the intermediate zone is connected better for feedback guidance of ongoing movements. This scheme, proposed first by Eccles, was elaborated by Allen and Tsukahara whose summary diagram appears, variously modified, in Figs. 2.7 and 11.2. The timing and the correlates of discharge of neurons in the output nuclei of the lateral and intermediate zones fit the distinction between their anatomical connections. Thach showed (with the method illustrated in Fig. 12.13) that *dentate discharge is related to movement intent and not to somatosensory reflexes.* Dentate cells tend to discharge before movement onset and slightly before precentral neurons that are related to the same task. Half of the dentate neurons discharge in relation to muscle patterns used, one-quarter in relation to joint position, and another quarter in relation to directional set for the next movement. In contrast, *neurons of interpositus (anterior) tend to discharge after onset of movements and in relation to their properties.* One of their main correlates is movement velocity, which largely reflects that of lengthening antagonists. This measure is important for the comparison of the intended and actual movement trajectories (cf. Chap. 7.1). *Fastigial neurons* also fire after movement onset, some in relation to force and others to movement onset. Neurons of the flocculonodular lobe send their output to the vestibular nuclei, some of which fire ahead of intended eye movements.

Anticipatory timing of dentate discharge for intended movements is illus-

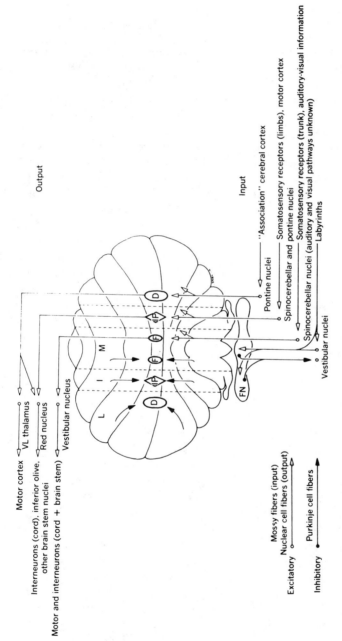

Output

Motor cortex
VL thalamus
Red nucleus
Interneurons (cord), inferior olive,
other brain stem nuclei
Vestibular nucleus
Motor and interneurons (cord + brain stem)

Input

"Association" cerebral cortex
Somatosensory receptors (limbs). motor cortex
Pontine nuclei
Spinocerebellar and pontine nuclei
Spinocerebellar nuclei (auditory and visual pathways unknown)
Somatosensory receptors (trunk), auditory-visual information
Vestibular nuclei
Labyrinths

Mossy fibers (input)
Excitatory   Nuclear cell fibers (output)

Inhibitory   Purkinje cell fibers

Fig. 13.2. Overall cerebellar organization, stressing sagittal input–output relations, superimposed on the medial vermis and the lateral hemispheres, which are folded into transverse lobes. VL, Ventrolateral nucleus of thalamus; lateral (L), intermediate (I), and medial (M) cerebellar cortex. Output nuclei: D, dentate; IP, interpositus; F, fastigial; FN, flocculo nodular lobe. (From Thach, 1980; in Brooks and Thach, 1981; Brooks, 1984)

262

trated in Fig. 13.3A, which was obtained in a task situation like that of Fig. 12.12A. The raster of individual trials describes the brisk discharge of dentate neurons in responses to visual or auditory cues (marked by the vertical line), well before movement onset (marked by the curving line). The trials have been reordered in the raster according to their reaction times, and are summarized in the histogram. Figure 13.3B shows that intense dentate action precedes shortened reaction times of movement onset. Conversely, Fig. 13.4 reflects the depression of dentate activity by local anesthesia, produced by local dentate cooling, in the delayed discharge of a neuron in the motor cortex and of the prolonged reaction time accordingly (in the same task situation as in Fig. 12.12A). The trials are shown in their natural sequence in Fig. 13.4A, and reordered according to their reaction times in Fig. 13.4B. Dentate neurons thus provide a trigger signal for the motor cortex to start intended movements. (They also provide such a trigger for their stops as shown by Hore and Vilis, not illustrated here.)

The dentate trigger signal is elaborated in the nucleus from a general "go" signal to one cued to particular movements. Specifications are imposed probably through processing in the multiple body "representations" in the caudal and rostral parts of the cerebellar output nuclei, which hint at separate coding functions of the sort we saw in the motor cortex (e.g., Figs. 12.1–12.3). The discharging dentate neuron illustrated in Fig. 13.3 was chosen (by Lamarre) for its responsiveness to the cue signal to move, which reflects recognition of the significance of the signal to get set for an impending movement.

Many dentate neurons discharge equally before flexions or extensions; that is, they do not encode the subprogram for the intended movement direction. These neurons are located in the caudal part of the nucleus, which is connected to arcuate premotor cortex (APA, Fig. 11.8). Their nondirectional discharges resemble those of some neurons in sensorimotor association cortex (Chap. 11.1). In contrast, the properties of neurons in the rostral dentate resemble those of motor cortex neurons to which they project (MI, Fig. 11.7).

Some dentate neurons do encode the intended direction, as witnessed by their response to a perturbation reflecting that aspect of motor set. This result (obtained by Strick with the task situation of Fig. 12.12B) is illustrated in Fig. 13.5. It shows that the neuron responds strongly to a small imposed displacement away from the intended push (upper rasters and histogram), while the same stimulus fails to elicit any reaction if the intended movement is a pull, that is in the same direction as the stimulus (lower records). The directionally set reaction to the perturbation occurs during the same time slot as that in the motor cortex that is triggered by it: 50–100 msec after the stimulus. (That reaction is called the "second response" in Fig. 12.12A, and the "intended discharge" in Fig. 12.12B.) Cerebellar nuclear dysfunction depresses this set-related, second precentral response that causes long-loop muscular contractions. In contrast, the first precentral response, which is tightly coupled to the peripheral input, is not affected by cerebellar dysfunction (not illustrated here; see Figs. 12.10 and 12.11 for examples).

Dentate neurons thus provide a trigger for intended movements in response to a relevant stimulus and some can also specify movement direction. The motor cortex follows dentate instructions from which it derives its predictive code for movement direction (Fig. 12.14) as well as for timing and intensity of movement starts, stops, and corrections (Figs. 12.10–12.13). These properties are essential for making skilled movements at optimal velocities—that is with optimal reference trajectories— whether the movements are simple or compound (Chap. 7.1; Figs. 1.3, 1.5, and 7.9). These essential properties are lost during cerebellar dysfunction. They are *implemented* with the help of the lateral

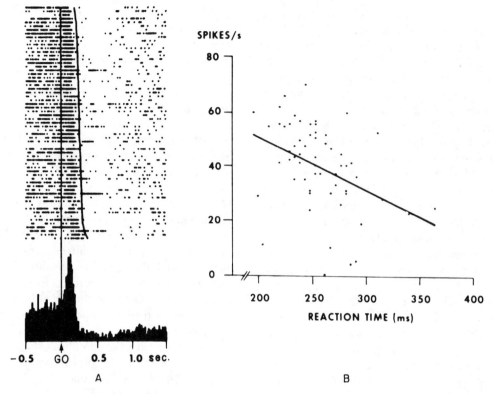

Fig. 13.3 Dentate discharge encodes the timing for movement onset. (A) Raster and histogram of movements in one work session (trial) of a monkey performing the flex–extend task illustrated in Fig. 12.12A. The monkey's motor set was created by instruction to alternate elbow flexions and extensions. Rasters are aligned with the "go" stimulus (visual or auditory cues) and have been reordered according to reaction time of movement onset *(heavy dots)*. (B) The intensities of dentate discharges obtained in trial (A) are correlated to the reaction times of the movements. (From Lamarre, Spidalieri, and Chapman, 1983)

cerebellum and are *updated* by the intermediate cerebellum. Updating programs (i.e., updating the model) amounts to adapting the control device that governs the movement. (A general diagram for adaptive control was presented in Fig. 4.14). Use of continuous movements, for instance, is abandoned during dysfunction of the lateral cerebellum unless the task is such that it can still be carried out successfully with movements of less than optimal properties (i.e., with degraded programs). The symptoms of cerebellar dysfunction described by Holmes—decomposition and tremor of intended movements, decreased tone and tremor of intended postures, errors of movement direction, force, speed,

amplitude, and regularity—are reproduced by temporary reduction or inactivation of lateral (neo)cerebellar function. Programmed movements are operated by muscle actions for starts and stops with the right intensity and with sufficiently early timing to accelerate and decelerate smoothly (e.g., Fig. 7.5). Loss of the predictive start signals leads to use of nonprogrammed movements and, as shown by Hore and Vilis, loss of predictive stop signals leads to inadequate reflex damping (i.e., tremor).

When movements are run by predictive timing, corrections arriving too late because of long latencies through the peripheral loop are unnecessary. When predictive

CONTROL   COOL DENTATE

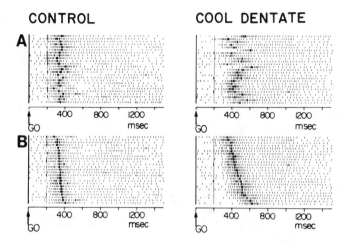

Fig. 13.4. Dentate discharge predictively encodes the time of movement onset and transmits that to the motor cortex. Dentate dysfunction delays the discharge of task-related neurons in the motor cortex and, correspondingly, of movement onset *(heavy dots)*. Rasters of normal function (left) of a task-related neuron in precentral cortex of a monkey are aligned with the "go" stimulus, and are shown in their natural sequence in (A) and reordered according to reaction time in (B). Rasters obtained during cooling of the dentate nucleus (right) are displayed in the same way. Flex–extend task as in Figs. 12.12A and 13.3; animal had to move the arm as soon as possible after the "go" stimulus, which was a light cue when the target stepped from one position to another. (From Meyer-Lohmann, Hore, and Brooks, 1977; also in Brooks and Thach, 1981; and Brooks 1984).

controls fail, the fast, internal "long-loop" messages (efference copies) for starts or stops are replaced by cumbersome, slow ones through peripheral loops, with the evident result of degraded performance. Faults of either planned starts or stops prevent the learned, smooth matching of move and hold programs (e.g., Fig. 1.5), that is, they lead to decomposition of compound as well as simple movements. The same fault operates, whether it concerns the "continuous" trajectory for the object of greatest attention for the CNS in a multi-joint movement, or the trajectory of a single-joint movement (Chap. 7.1).

The cerebellum organizes all kinds of movements, as evidenced by the properties of the dentate nucleus. Stimulation of its rostral part (magnocellular in the human) yields complex movements involving muscle synergies, while that of the caudal part yields simple movements (parvicellular in the human). The complex movements produced by dentate stimulation are composed in the pericentral cortex from divergent dentate projections, as judged by their similarity to the sum of the movements induced by stimulation of each cortical point that receives excitatory projections from that same dentate focus. It is relevant that there is a group of dentate neurons that discharge in relation to a compound (reaching and pointing) movement but not to its details, which are more common with interpositus neurons. The lateral cerebellum is known to influence the motor cortex through the use of learned, preferred connections, because motor learning is retained in trained monkeys whose operant arm was subsequently deafferented (e.g., Fig. 7.7). These special connections are considered further in Chap. 13.7.

The programs of the middle level of the motor hierarchy do not reside in one particular part of the brain, such as the cerebellum or the motor cortex; instead they are *distributed* in the middle level, linked by preferred synaptic paths. [We will see that the adaptive properties of climbing fiber synapses make participation by the cerebellum mandatory (Fig. 13.11)]. The quickest route for *updating* the part of a

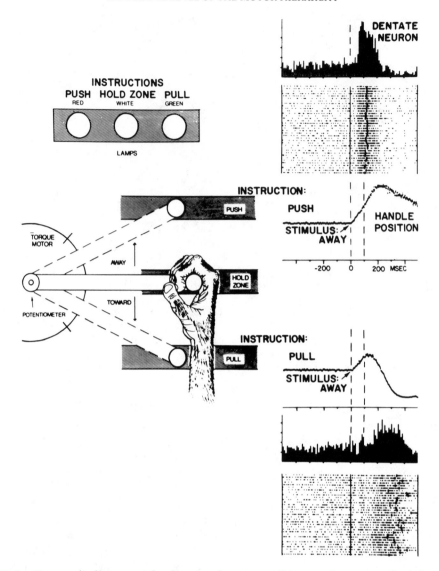

Fig. 13.5. Dentate discharge encodes directional motor set. Diagram shows a monkey's hand performing the push–pull task illustrated in Fig. 12.12B. Rasters and histograms of dentate discharge are aligned with the "go" stimulus, which is a small perturbation of the handle. Handle paths on right side compare responses to the same stimulus, but with different motor sets created by "instruction" lights. During the truly comparable periods (between the *broken vertical lines*), dentate discharge increased (above) and decreased (below). (From Strick, 1983; also in Brooks, 1985)

program that is resident in motor cortex is through convergent projections from the rostral parts of the interpositus nucleus to the motor cortex, and from the dentate nucleus to the thalamic nuclei (VL, Fig. 13.1) and thence to the motor cortex. Figure 13.6 indicates the convergence of projections from the dentate and interposed nu-

clei; in fact they converge even on individual corticofugal neurons (e.g., CSNs). The intermediate cerebellum, in contrast to the lateral part, receives information about the progress of movements from peripheral receptors as well as from spinal INs (Fig. 13.2). Both the lateral and intermediate parts are also connected with a variety of nuclei in the brain stem and midbrain, which can add to the updating through more circuitous paths (Chap. 13.4).

So far, only cerebellar outputs to the cerebral cortex have been mentioned. Outputs to subcortical targets such as the red nucleus have been well studied in cats and monkeys, but little is known about the human equivalent (Chap. 5.2). The interpositus sends an excitatory projection to the contralateral red nucleus (RN), which is also facilitated by tonically active, smaller corticofugal neurons and inhibited by phasically active, larger neurons (not illustrated). The effects on the RN are exerted mostly by corticorubral neurons in the primate, but more so by axon collaterals of corticospinal neurons in the cat. Either way, during slow movements the influence of feedback through the intermediate cerebellum is greatest, presumably to adjust the kinematic task groups of alpha MNs (Chap. 4.2). Cerebellar projections to the reticular and vestibular systems (Chaps. 5.2 and 13.1) are taken up in their functional contexts later in Chap. 13.4, and the connections with the inferior olive in Chap. 13.6.

4. Mossy Fibers

The cerebellar cortex receives two main types of afferent fibers from subcerebellar sites. The first type, the "mossy" fibers (MFs), come from reticular and pontine brain-stem nuclei as well as from the spinal cord and the cerebellar output nuclei. MFs innervate the granular layer of the cerebellar cortex, whose functions are considered in Chap. 13.5. The second cerebellar input type, the "climbing" fibers (CFs), arise from the inferior olivary brain-stem nuclei and innervate the dendritic tree of Purkinje cells in the cerebellar cortex. They are considered in the contexts of the cortex (Chap. 13.5) and its functional input–output units, the "microzones" (Chap. 13.6).

Mossy fibers of *central origin* reach the cerebellum indirectly after relay in the precerebellar nuclei, which are located in the brain-stem close to the connecting cerebellar peduncles (Fig. 5.8). The precerebellar pontine and reticular nuclei forward processed information via mossy fibers. In the human, the pontine nuclei give rise to the main mossy fiber input, especially to the lateral cerebellum. Most precerebellar nuclei process information ascending from the spinal cord in addition to their more massive inputs from the cerebral cortex. More direct mossy fiber connections are made, without brain-stem relay, by the spinocerebellar tracts ending in the spinocerebellum.

The cerebellum is here described as part of the middle level of the motor hierarchy, because direct cerebrocerebellar connections, contrary to previous impressions, originate almost exclusively from middle-level areas (Figs. 2.7, 11.2, and 11.3). The phylogenetically newest (lateral) part of the cerebellum and its output nucleus (the dentate) have evolved to great size together with the expansion of the association cortex, particularly the prefrontal cortex. This implies that they require each other's mutual services but not that they are necessarily connected by direct projection fibers. Cerebrocerebellar connections through the pontine nuclei (PN) are shown semidiagrammatically in Fig. 13.6. Their origins are similar to those of the corticospinal tracts. Figure 13.6 shows that cerebral and cerebellar parts are connected reciprocally, returning to the cerebellum through the PN with mossy fibers and through the inferior olive (IO) with climbing fibers.

The main direct cerebrocerebellar projections come from the motor, supplementary and premotor, somatosensory, and visual cortices, and a limbic connection from the cingulate gyrus to PN also exists (cf. Fig. 2.7). Direct higher order connections to the cerebellum are very sparse: a little from area 7 (cf. Fig. 11.4) and from prefrontal cortex (areas 9 and 10; Fig. 11.1). The overwhelming importance of

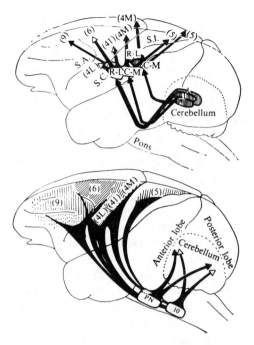

Fig. 13.6. Cerebrocerebellar connections (established by evoked potentials in the monkey) have reciprocal, topographical components, but there is also convergence in area 4 from the lateral and intermediate–medial cerebellum (dentate, interpositus, and fastigial nuclei). Numbers indicate cortical areas (as in Fig. 11.1). Abbreviations: L, I, M, lateral, interpositus, and medial cerebellar output nuclei; 4L, 4I, 4M, lateral, intermediate, and medial parts of area 4; R-L, C-M, rostrolateral and caudomedial nuclear groups of the thalamus; PN, IO, pontine and inferior olivary (precerebellar) nuclei; S.A., S.C., S.I., arcuate, central, and intraparietal sulci. (From Sasaki, 1979; also in Sasaki and Gemba 1983; Ito, 1984)

the direct projections from the middle level to the cerebellum (by way of the PN) is indicated in Figs. 13.6 and 13.7. The pontine nuclei are connected appropriately for middle-level functions such as triggering or restructuring movement programs. Visual information reaches the PN both as detailed factual representation from the visual geniculostriate system, and in processed form relevant for directed visual attention from the superior colliculus (Chap. 11.1; Fig. 11.4). Vision, however, does not help patients with cerebellar disorders to make accurate intended movements (cf.

Fig. 1.2). On the contrary, they can become more undulating, presumably because of more time-consuming corrections. (Normal suppression of unwanted sensory inputs to optimize motor control was discussed in Chap. 9.6.) Localization of sound is brought to the pontine nuclei through the inferior colliculus. The spinal input to the PN ascends as spinopontine fibers (in the dorsolateral funiculus). The PN is a complex coordinating center with much local convergence from different cortical areas and from patches of functionally related cell groups in the sensorimotor cortex (cf. Figs. 12.3 and 12.4).

Other integration centers are located in three *reticular nuclei* with inputs that are suitable for updating ongoing movements. The cerebral input to these nuclei comes only from the sensorimotor cortex. The lateral reticular nucleus (LRN; Fig. 5.8) projects to all parts of the cerebellum. It receives inputs from cortical areas 4 and 6, the red nucleus, and a number of ascend-

Fig. 13.7. The pontine nuclei (PN) receive direct inputs (established histologically in the monkey) from various cerebral areas (including sensorimotor, visual, and cingulate, but excluding higher association areas), superior and inferior colliculi, and the spinal cord. The relative intensities of the direct cerebral connections are indicated by the heaviness of the arrows. The PN are reciprocally connected with the cerebellum, shown on the right (F, IP, D, fastigial, interpositus, and dentate nuclei). Compare to Fig. 13.6. (From Wiesendanger, 1983)

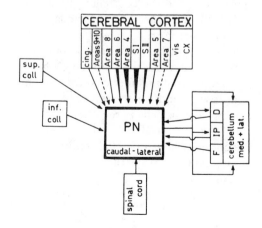

ing spinal pathways including spinoreticular fibers and collateral branches from ongoing spinocerebellar paths (cf. Chap. 9.1). We have already met some spinoreticular neurons, under the name of their spinal classification as "propriospinal" neurons (Fig. 5.5B) and also as INs on the flexor reflex afferent chain (FRA; Fig. 5.6A).

The LRN combines reports about spinal INs (received from the FRA) with corollary discharges from three central motor-related structures, including midbrain locomotor pattern generators (Chap. 10). The LRN thus functions as a comparator of these inputs and forwards its output to the anterior lobe of the cerebellum, which facilitates quick corrections. Integrative INs such as those in LRN give flexible service. For instance, LRN neurons forward detailed reports about peripheral events that cease, however, when locomotion begins and are replaced by discharges that fluctuate in rhythm with the central locomotor program. We are already familiar with programs taking over neural control, from our discussion of the cerebral cortex (Chap. 12.3; Figs. 12.10 and 12.12), and from the description of the input-switching capabilities of INs in the FRA chain (Fig. 5.6). The response of neurons to different input is a little like our response to the weather. We might be sitting outside in the sunshine, doing this or that, when a heavy cloud comes over. We look up, attend, and sprint for cover just before the downpour begins. There you have a tightly coupled input–output relation that triggers a highly programmed operation that cancels whatever we were interacting with before!

Another reticular nucleus, the paramedian reticular nucleus, combines peripheral and cerebral inputs and projects to the medial and intermediate (paramedian) cerebellar cortex. Fastigial and vestibular inputs are coordinated with that from the medial lemniscal system (Chap. 11.1; Fig. 11.4), and with descending projections from the premotor and sensorimotor cortex (Figs. 5.9–5.12). The third reticular nucleus, n. reticularis tegmenti pontis (NRTP), is the only precerebellar nucleus without peripheral inputs. It produces early corrections entirely by coordination of central, corollary discharges. Like the other two reticular nuclei, its cerebral connections are with the sensorimotor cortex and its cerebellar connections with the medial and intermediate cerebellum. It is important for coordinating visual and vestibular inputs for the control of eye movements exerted by the vestibular nuclei (Chap. 9.1) and also participates in locomotor functions (to the extent that it reflects inputs from cerebellar afferents and the rhythms of mesencephalic locomotor pattern generators; Chap. 10). NRTP may also regulate hypothalamic drives to the cerebellum, since it receives inputs from the mamillary body and from the cingulate cortex. They could serve for comparisons of hypothalamic commands with their cortically processed form (Chap. 11.2).

Mossy fibers of *peripheral origin* arise from the dorsal and ventral spinocerebellar tracts. These tracts project in somatotopic fashion to overlapping areas, in both the anterior and posterior lobes, creating two convergent body representations, one anteriorly and the other posteriorly, that together make up the medial and intermediate sagittal strips. Autonomic and vestibular projections to the cerebellum have already been mentioned (Fig. 13.2).

The dorsal spinocerebellar tract (DSCT) conveys the only cerebellar input concerned with precise peripheral information. It originates in a long spinal nucleus in the base of the dorsal horn (Clarke's column) and ascends ipsilaterally to the medial and intermediate "spinocerebellar" cortex (Fig. 13.8A). Like other afferents reaching the cortex, collateral branches of the main fibers innervate the cerebellar output nuclei. Exteroceptive (skin and joint) fibers report about small, lemniscal-sized, peripheral receptive fields. Proprioceptive fibers report about groups of interrelated muscles acting on a particular joint by combining inputs about stretch of one muscle with the responses of opposing

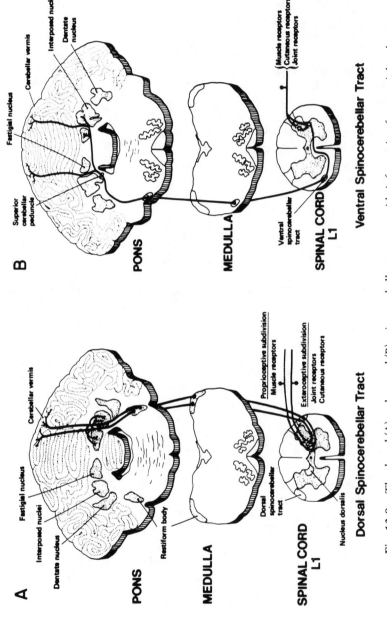

Fig. 13.8. The dorsal (A) and ventral (B) spinocerebellar tracts provide information from peripheral receptors, and in the ventral tract also from spinal interneurons. They project to the medial and intermediate (but not to the lateral) cerebellum. (From Gilman, Bloedel, and Lechtenberg, 1981)

muscles. This afferent cerebellar information thus concerns the torque exerted on a joint, which corresponds to efferent messages from some neurons in motor cortex (Chap. 12.4). Integration begins in Clarke's column with interactions of afferents from opposing muscles and also with convergence of various other inputs, including flexor reflex afferents. We already know that the FRA are under the influence of corticospinal fibers (Fig. 5.6B) and other tracts descending from the brain stem, similar to those modulating impulse traffic destined for the cerebral cortex (Fig. 5.11).

The ventral spinocerebellar tract (VSCT) arises from the lateral ventral horn and ascends contralaterally. Most fibers recross to the ipsilateral medial and intermediate cerebellum (Fig. 13.8B), where their somatotopic projection overlaps that of the DSCT. Proprioceptive and exteroceptive inputs interact on the cells of origin of the VSCT ("spinal border cells") in the same way as they do on spinal MNs; that is, they play out the same sequences of excitation and inhibition. As we know from studying this spinal interaction (Fig. 5.5C), it provides the VSCT with a copy of the activity of spinal inhibitory INs, which it forwards to the cerebellum. Furthermore, the VSCT also reflects the influence exerted on spinal INs by descending cortical and subcortical control paths (Fig. 5.5D). This arrangement prompted Lundberg's suggestion that the VSCT monitors transmission in the segmental inhibitory pathways to spinal MNs. Such monitoring is also well documented for the centrally induced rhythmic activity of spinal INs for locomotion (or rhythmic scratching).

5. Cerebellar Cortex

How is the cerebellar cortex organized and how does it function? Figure 13.9 illustrates a slice through a transverse folium (of a lobule, Fig. 13.2). The main elements are the sole output (Purkinje) cells, which all lie in the same layer, in contrast to the distribution of eight types of corti-

cofugal cells in layers III–VI of the sensorimotor cerebral cortex (Fig. 12.6). The mossy fibers branch in the granular layer where they synapse with granule cells whose axons ascend to the molecular layer. Each axon forms branches that extend for about 2 to 5 mm parallel to the direction of the folium. These are the "parallel" fibers, which distribute mossy fiber input in such a remarkably uniform manner. They intersect the dendritic trees of successive Purkinje (P) cells at right angles, because P cells are aligned one next to the other, like opened, flat Japanese fans. In Fig. 13.9, one is drawn in full view and two others, to its left, in profile. Each parallel fiber contacts the dendritic spines of about 125 P cells/mm of fiber length, or about 250 to 750 total. (Each P cell thus receives input from about 80,000 parallel fibers.) The high discharge rates of MFs produce a high level of tonic activity in the cerebellar cortex as well as in the cerebellar output nuclei, which all receive collateral afferent branches (not illustrated). Cerebellar cortical activity is supported and modulated by the "reverberating circuits" formed by the reciprocal connections between the cortex and its subcortical nuclear sources of MFs (Figs. 13.6 and 13.7).

Climbing fibers (CFs), in contrast to the mossy fibers (MFs), ascend to the molecular layer where they branch in a profuse, fanlike pattern that matches and entwines the dendrites of about 10 P cells. (Each P cell receives the branches of only one CF.) All climbing fibers originate in the inferior olive, a complex of nuclei lying beneath the brain-stem reticular formation. Collateral branches of climbing fibers, like those of mossy fibers, innervate the cerebellar output nuclei.

The influence of MFs and CFs can be distinguished, because CFs cause an almost simultaneous depolarization of the whole dendritic P-cell tree, producing a more complex response than the "simple" ones caused by MF discharges. The "complex spike" (CS) consists of an initial discharge followed by several, smaller (dendritic)

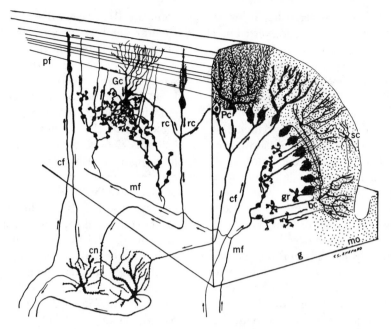

Fig. 13.9. The cerebellar cortex is organized to channel mossy and climbing fibers (mf, cf) to the only type of output neuron, the Purkinje cells (Pc). Mossy fibers synapse with granule cells (gr) in the granular layer (g), whose axons branch into parallel fibers (pf). Parallel fibers intersect the fan of dendrites of Purkinje cells, and dendrites of Golgi cells (Gc), basket cells (bc) and stellate cells (sc) in the molecular layer (mo). The cerebellar nuclei (cn) receive the efferent axons from Purkinje-cells and collateral afferent axons from mossy and climbing fibers. Recurrent collaterals (rc) of Purkinje cells branch in granular layer. (From Fox, 1962; in Eccles, 1967, 1973)

spikes riding on a plateau of depolarization that can last from 25 msec to 1 second. This makes complex spikes appear larger than simple spikes (SSs). The difference in amplitudes allows investigators to distinguish the influences of MFs and CFs by microelectrode recording. The high discharge rates of simple spikes (50–100 per second) can reflect and transmit rapid transient changes of MF input and can also sustain tonic influences. CSs, in contrast, occur "spontaneously" at irregular intervals of only about 1 second! (Figs. 13.10C, 13.12A, and 13.13A). This extraordinary, slow rate is not the fast cadence of neurons transmitting peripheral or central information of the kind we have discussed in this book so far (e.g., Figs. 12.10 and 12.12). Instead, this is the cadence of movements in their entirety.

Climbing fibers are discussed in Chap. 13.6, but we need to ask here: what do CFs

signal? The exact answer is not certain. Whatever it is, we know that their signals are crucial for cerebellar function because the consequences of olivary lesions mimick those of cerebellar lesions. We will follow Ito's argument that CFs provide feedback about errors in the *central control* (rather than in the peripheral, actual execution) of movements. The facts are that CFs in awake animals can respond to isolated inputs, such as moving a joint or pulling on a muscle. These responses are still unsuitable, however, to transmit time-varying functions, because at best they reach 4 per second (e.g., Fig. 13.10C). Olivary cells with proprioceptive input, for instance, can be discharged by externally produced interference with an intended posture that the animal is trying to maintain, such as rotation of a joint or a small displacement of the surface on which the animal is standing. Other olivary neurons are sensitive to light tactile stimuli and/or displacements of the limbs supporting the body weight. Yet, olivary neurons are not driven by the *intentional* consequences of the animal's movements, that is, when there is no deviation from the intended control.

CF responses (CSs) seem to be activated only when a change from the expected outcome has occurred. This recalls our description of neurons in motor cortex during long-loop corrective functions (Chap. 6.2; and Figs. 12.10 and 12.12), but CS action clearly differs from that of motor cortex neurons: it occurs only infrequently and not during routine adjustments. Could olivary action be related to *adaptive* changes? That would fit their extraordinary pattern best (see below). In order to alter cerebellar input–output relations, CSs should be followed by alterations in SS responses to external stimuli. This is indeed the case: CFs modulate the sensitivity of P cells to subsequent MF signals. Depending on the circumstances, "spontaneous" CSs may enhance or depress the responsiveness of MFs to natural, adequate peripheral stimulation for up to about 1 second (i.e., the duration of plateau depolarization of P cells mentioned above).

A link between adaptation of movements to unexpected circumstances and cerebellar olivary function has been reported as a component of motor learning by Thach. Figure 13.10A illustrates the corrective arm movements made by monkeys when a load displaces the arm from an intended posture. The left column shows that this is accomplished easily if the arm is displaced by a perturbation of known, expected intensity. The right column illustrates how the monkey learns to steady its wrist against a new load (against extension, at the arrow). The important point is that the progressive improvement of motor performance is accompanied by task-related discharge of the inferior olive, as shown in Fig. 13.10B for the same trials. (CSs are indicated by heavy dots.) The effects are summarized in Fig. 13.10C, which

also shows that SS discharge is decreased during and after the period of adaptation. We should note that the anticipatory "steadying" of the arm is the same stiffening action as that discussed with reference to Fig. 6.7, where it was shown to be caused by appropriately timed and scaled long-loop responses. Recall that these properties of long-loop responses fail in humans during cerebellar dysfunction (Figs. 6.4 and 6.9).

The cerebellar cortex functions as a collection of local, isolated patches in which groups of P cells process their inputs, isolated from other patches by the action of inhibitory interneurons. This remarkable self-limiting arrangement is sustained by the excitatory drive of the parallel fibers on the dendrites of the INs (Figs. 13.9 and 13.11). Golgi cell axons make inhibitory connections with granule cells, forming a simple negative-feedback loop that "disfacilitates" P cells by removing their excitatory input. Basket cells inhibit about a half-dozen P cells each by enveloping their cell bodies with a "basket" of inhibitory connections, as seen in the cross section in Fig. 13.9. The distribution of basket cell axons creates a fence of inhibition that surrounds an active efferent zone of P cells aligned along a folium.

The basic circuitry of the cerebellar cortex is schematized in Fig. 13.11, which also shows a third ("stellate") interneuron that inhibits P-cell dendrites. The innervation of the cerebellar output nuclei by collateral branches of MFs and CFs is also indicated. Another type of cerebellar afferent, to the dendrites of P cells, is shown on the left in Fig. 13.11. These fibers, which are "aminergic," arise from the brain stem. There are adrenergic fibers from the locus ceruleus and serotonergic fibers from the raphe nuclei (Fig. 5.8). Both kinds depress nearby P cells, and also MFs and CFs, through release of catecholamines from vesicles along their axons, without necessarily making synaptic contacts with them. They may be more important for long-term regulation of cortical function than for that

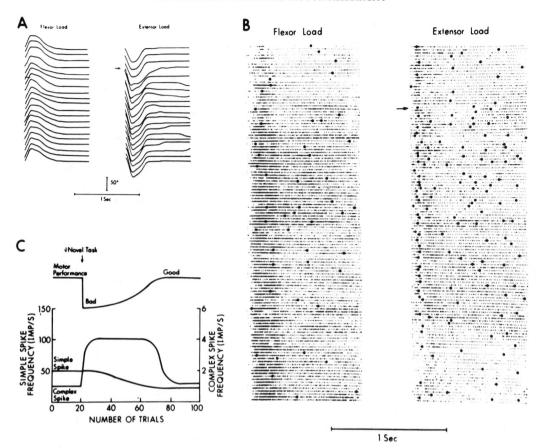

Fig. 13.10. Climbing fibers fire infrequently (i.e., seconds rather than milliseconds) and randomly, except during adaptive changes of movements. Task is to restore a handle to a central target position and to hold it there after it has been displaced in a horizontal arc (for about 0.3 second) by loads that continue to resist flexions or extensions during restoration by monkey's wrist action as in Fig. 13.5. (A) Position traces during successive restoration trials. Note uneven corrections of novel extensor load (right column, below *arrow*). Corrections against unchanged flexor load continue smoothly as before. (B) Task relation and frequencies of complex spikes *(large dots)* change for load-related Purkinje cell in the same trials, with novel extensor load at arrow (simple spikes: *small dots*). Rasters are aligned with time of load switching as in (A). (C) Relationship of motor performance and frequencies of simple and complex spikes (left and right ordinates). [(A) and (B) From Gilbert and Thach, 1977; (C) from Thach, 1980; in Brooks and Thach, 1981; also in Brooks, 1984, Ito, 1984]

of its impulse traffic. The origin of the adrenergic group from the locus ceruleus makes it a candidate for autonomic influences on the cerebellum, but, as pointed out at the end of Chap. 5.1, that small nucleus is likely related to the distribution of states of arousal and vigilance. The serotonergic fibers may be related to neurogenesis, that is, the proper formation of the cerebellum. Glutamate and GABA are the main candidates for excitatory and inhibitory transmitters in the cerebellar cortex, much as in the cerebral cortex (cf. Fig. 12.6).

Finally, note in Fig. 13.11 that the output of P cells is inhibitory, not excitatory like that of cerebral pyramidal cells. The activity of the cerebellar output nuclei, including the vestibular nuclei, is thus shaped by "inhibitory sculpturing," as Eccles put it, in whose laboratory most of the cerebellar circuit was worked out. During postural adjustments, MFs change their tonic firing rates (and that of the P cells

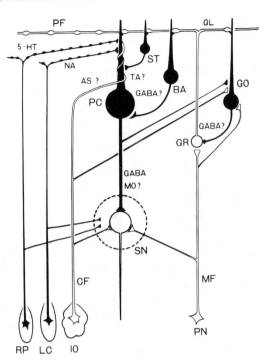

Fig. 13.11. Basic neuronal circuitry of the cerebellum (schematized from Fig. 13.9) and putative neurotransmitters. Abbreviations: PC, Purkinje cell; GO, Golgi cell; BA, basket cell; ST, stellate cell; GR, granule cell; PF, parallel fiber; MF mossy fiber; CF, climbing fiber; SN, vestibular or cerebellar nuclear cell; PN, precerebellar neuron that issues mossy fibers; IO, inferior olive; LC, locus ceruleus; RP, raphe nuclei. Inhibitory neurons and synapses are *filled,* and excitatory ones are *hollow.* Candidates for neurotransmitters are indicated at some synapses: GL, glutamate; AS, aspartate; TA, taurine; MO, motilin; NA, noradrenaline; 5-HT, 5-hydroxytryptamine (Serotonin). (From Ito, 1979, 1984)

they innervate; see Figs. 13.10C and 13.13A). As the rate increases for movement onset, nuclear output is increased by MF collaterals to the output nuclei. Nuclear frequency is then decreased a few milliseconds later by the inhibitory P cells, which impress the outputs of the side loops through the cerebellar cortex on the cerebellar nuclei (see Figs. 13.9 and 13.11). The reverse sequence happens at the end of movements. Inhibitory sculpturing thus shapes the MF frequency step (from one tonic level to another) into a pulse between the initial and final levels. This pulse-step sequence is useful for the prompt starting and stopping of movements (Figs. 13.3 and 13.4). It is fed forward to the motor cortex and to subcortical targets for activation of muscles (e.g., Figs. 7.5 and 7.6).

Many postural changes involve less abrupt alternations between agonists and antagonists than those in sudden movements (as in Figs. 7.5, 12.12, 13.3, and 13.4). For instance, unskilled movements are made with more co-contraction than well-practiced ones whose trajectories have already been learned (Chaps. 5.1 and 7.1). The brain has to steady a limb that it is guiding entirely by means of peripheral feedback. Less steadying is required when the movement (i.e., the reference trajectory) has been learned and is initiated through the descending limb of long-loop paths (Chaps. 6.2 and 7.1). The need for steadying is reduced progressively by strengthening the propelling boost of the initial agonist muscle burst and by weakening the braking opposition offered by opposing muscles. This continues toward optimal control even after the movements have been programmed (i.e., learned). An example of this progression was presented as "tuning" of trajectories in Chap. 5.1. The program for rapid, single elbow flexions, for example, becomes degraded when co-contractions increase owing to loss of premovement inhibition during cerebellar dysfunction (Fig. 13.12). Tanaka has shown that patients with cerebellar disorders co-contract the muscles that move the elbow more than normal subjects while making slow pursuit movements with the forearm to follow a slowly moving target (not illustrated). The cerebellar cortical circuit thus is critically involved in adjusting the degrees of tonic and phasic activity of muscles.

Co-contractions find their greatest use when something is held in the hand (power grip, Fig. 12.16A) or between the fingers (precision grip, Fig. 12.15A), both of which bring all the hand muscles into simultaneous action. The cerebellar cortex plays an important role in our prehensile ability as judged by the activity of P cells. Task-related P cells in the intermediate cortex fire SSs when particular joints are tensed (e.g., Fig. 13.10C). Most stop firing SSs, however, during task-related co-contractions (without necessarily changing the frequency of CSs for a familiar task, as in Fig. 13.10B). Cerebellar function during a precision grip, studied by Smith with the task shown in Fig. 12.15A, is illustrated in Fig. 13.13A. Smith has suggested that the strength of antagonist muscles could be balanced in the cerebellar cortex by a simple anatomical arrangement, drawn in Fig. 13.13B. Co-contraction would be produced if basket cells that receive parallel fiber input from *both* agonists and antagonists inhibit P cells that re-ceive input from only *one* or the other (Fig. 13.13B).

This suggestion opens the question of the functional organization of the cerebellar cortex. Does it contain enough specialized subareas to deal with all the complex body functions, and how could the messages be steered efficiently to the correct one? This is the topic of Chap. 13.6. In the meantime, we conclude from the clinical findings and their experimental counterparts that the cerebellum helps to establish how many muscles function at any one time; that is, *the cerebellum helps to determine the relative timing and intensity of the action of the muscles needed to operate task-related joints.*

How are these determinations made? We know that large movements are programmed for the action of alpha MNs, as are large corrections of intended movements or postures. The activity of gamma MNs is adjusted in subsidiary fashion. It was argued in Chaps. 4.2 and 12.3 that intended motor acts and their adjustments follow commands to alpha MNs conveyed to them through the descending limb of transcortical, long-loop paths, perhaps

Fig. 13.12. Cerebellar dysfunction removes premovement inhibition of antagonist muscles (stippled area), normally acquired as adaptation during motor learning. Elbow flexions of a normal human subject (A) compared to those of a patient with cerebellar deficit (B). EMG of biceps brachii (top) and triceps (bottom). (From Hallett, Shahani, and Young, 1975a,b.; also in Brooks and Thach, 1981)

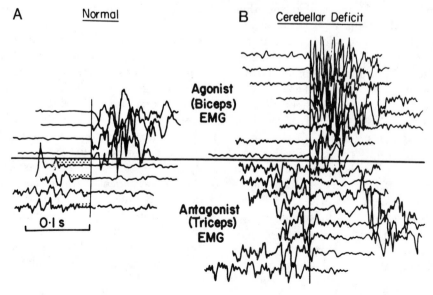

A   Normal   B   Cerebellar Deficit

Agonist
(Biceps)
EMG

0·1 s

Antagonist
(Triceps)
EMG

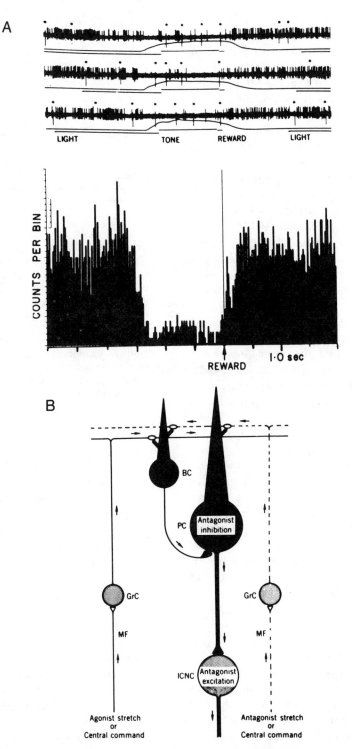

Fig. 13.13 Discharge levels of Purkinje cells (PCs) relate to co-contraction of opposing muscles. (A) Three traces of a PC firing simple (SSs) and complex spikes (CSs, marked by *dots*) when the monkey executes a precision grip; traces of force and of signals appear below (as in Fig. 12.15.). Reduction of SSs, seen at top, is more obvious in histogram summarizing many trials (bottom, same alignment to time of reward). (B) Scheme to show how discharge of P-cell connected to one muscle, could suppress co-contraction of opposing muscles, if basket cell (BC) were to receive input from both the agonist and antagonist. Cerebellar output from intracerebellar nuclear cells (ICNC). Conventions and abbreviations as in histology schema in Fig. 13.11. (From Smith, 1981)

working in conjuction with the reticulo-
tended motor acts and their adjustments
follow commands to alpha MNs conveyed
to them through the descending limb of
transcortical, long-loop paths, perhaps
working in conjuction with the reticulospinal system. (This alpha route is pictured
as the rack-and-pinion control in Fig.
6.10.) In contrast, small, slow movements
and their corrections may also include
programs for gamma MNs if it benefits the
sensitivity of spindles (Fig. 4.12). This may
be particularly useful when the degree of
co-contraction is changed in the shift from
isotonic to isometric actions (i.e., from
movement to posture). This view fits the
modest effects of gamma bias on reflex
gain, and one possible effector path is the
vestibulospinal system.

Granit viewed the cerebellum as the
chief adjustor of alpha–gamma coactivation, because cerebellar dysfunction de-
pressses the bias exerted by static and dynamic gamma MNs on primary spindle
afferents. (Responses of secondary afferents to fast stretches are also depressed.)
Figure 13.14 illustrates his experiment,
made with the decerebrate cat preparation.
Alpha–gamma coactivation was evoked
during contraction of the soleus muscle as
part of a positional reflex elicited by head
ventroflexion (as in Fig. 9.8, bottom row).
Coactivation is made evident by the
greater speeding up of the spindle discharge when the anterior lobe of the cerebellum functions at its normal temperature (top record) than when it is cooled or
ablated (middle and bottom records). During anterior lobe dysfunction, the spindle
becomes more passive as demonstrated by
the slowing of its discharge during contraction and by its acceleration as the muscle relaxes. Yet the reflex contraction is
hardly changed! What has changed is the
degree of alpha–gamma coactivation. It is
reduced by cerebellar dysfunction: that is,
alpha–gamma dissociation occurs, and
gamma drive is replaced by alpha drive.
(Pathways relevant for the decerebrate and
decerebellate animal are illustrated in Fig.
8.3.)

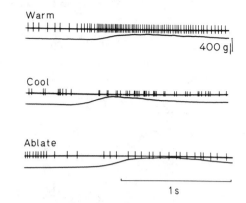

Fig. 13.14. Normal cerebellar function promotes alpha–gamma coactivation, which decreases during cerebellar dysfunction. Spindles
in soleus muscle, activated during positional reflex induced by head ventriflexion (see Fig. 9.8)
of a decerebrate cat, become abnormally passive
during cerebellar cooling (**b**) or ablation (**c**).
Alpha-MN drive continues, as witnessed by the
minimal changes of reflex tension (lower
traces). The descending pathways for alpha and
gamma activation are indicated in Fig. 8.3.
(From Granit, Holmgren and Merton, 1955; in
Brooks, 1983)

The cerebellar Purkinje cells were regarded by Granit as directing excitation
into the alpha or gamma route, with fusimotor drive falling or rising with Purkinje
cell activity. The levels of P-cell discharge
would thus determine muscle tone, among
other things. Loss of muscle tone (hypotonia) is a common consequence of cerebellar lesions (Fig. 8.5), but it often re-
covers after some months while other
symptoms of cerebellar dysfunction per-
sist. The cerebellum is necessary for
gamma support of the tonic stretch reflex,
by which tone is maintained. Since tone is
the resistance offered to imposed stretch
(Chap. 8.1), it depends heavily on the prevailing motor set, which we know is degraded in cerebellar patients. (The conditions in which gamma adjustments are
useful were discussed in Chap. 4.2.) The
cerebellum could influence alpha–gamma
coactivation to accommodate the kinematic conditions for alpha-MN task
groups (cf. Figs. 4.7, 4.11, and 4.12). In this
respect, the cerebellum might be looked at

as the "head ganglion of the proprioceptive system" (Sherrington's term).

Evaluation in behaviorally active animals, without the abnormally high extensor drive of the decerebrate preparation, suggests that the degree of alpha–gamma coactivation may indeed be governed by the cerebellum in some conditions. Thach and associates have shown that during adaptation for learning to make very slow flexions and extensions of the arm (like that in Fig. 4.13), monkeys' P cells discharge *bi*directionally in concert with spindle afferents, which, he suggests, may indicate cerebellar guidance for the assumption of a new relation between the discharge of alpha and gamma MNs. In other words, adaptation and motor learning would be accompanied by the dissociation of the previously existing degree of alpha–gamma linkage, to be replaced by a new, more appropriate one. ("Motor learning" includes the use of various new adaptations on the basis of past experience; that is, it includes further improvements even though the task conditions remain the same; see Chap. 13.7.)

6. Climbing Fibers

All climbing fibers originate in the inferior olive. The olivary nuclei receive spinal, medullary, midbrain inputs, projections from cortical areas 4 and 6, as well as visual and vestibular inputs. The spinal paths project, via the olive, to separate longitudinal zones in the intermediate cerebellar cortex; they are called spino-olivocerebellar paths (SOCPs). The paths arising in the ventral funiculus of the spinal cord (VF-SOCPs) carry direct spino-olivary fibers, while the dorsal paths (DF-SOCPs) ascend to the dorsal column nuclei, which project to the contralateral inferior olive. In addition, there are dorsolateral paths (DLF-SOCPs). The various SOCPs converge onto overlapping groups of olivary neurons. The flexor reflex afferents (FRA; Fig. 5.6) provide the most potent input for spino-

olivary paths, except the DLF-SOCP, which is highly sensitive to cutaneous stimuli. All inputs to the olive are transmuted into CF projections that overlap with the MF projections from the same, or other relevant, parts of the body. This convergence provides the anatomical substrate for olivary corrections of limb movements. Eye movements are corrected by means of the vestibulo-ocular reflex (VOR), which depends on visuo-olivary fibers from pretectal nuclei. They project, via the olive, to the flocculus to participate in the VOR, which maintains the gaze in the intended direction by compensating for unexpected changes in head position (Figs. 9.3 and 13.17).

For all input modalities—somatic, vestibular, or visual—the inferior olive can be thought of as a comparator of the control signals for the intended and actual events. In Fig. 13.15, Oscarsson pictures the comparator as consisting of a cortical sagittal zone, an olivary region, the cerebellar output nucleus, and a lower motor center (in the spinal cord or brain stem). By comparing information from these sources, the olive could detect perturbations of the commands introduced in the lower center by reflex activity and perturbations in the evolving movement due to unexpected changes in load. Information about these perturbations is used by the P cells in the sagittal zone to form corrective signals to be sent to lower and higher centers.

The functional comparator units are much smaller than the whole sagittal zones. Climbing fibers project to narrow strips within the sagittal zones of the cerebellar cortex. These "microzones" (discovered through plotting of convergent inputs by Oscarsson) create multiple "representations" of particular parts of the body in areas as small as 0.1 to 0.2 mm wide and a few millimeters long (Fig. 13.16). Each zone contains a stack of about 500 P cells and is linked reciprocally with a distinct group of neurons distributed in its output nucleus. Microzones receive additional inputs both from CFs innervating other zones and from MFs that carry a va-

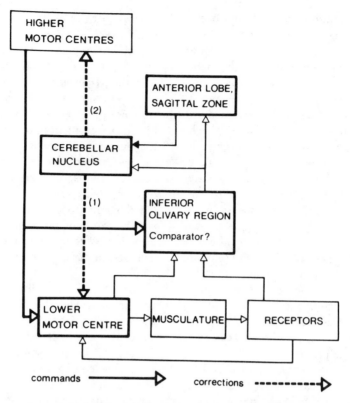

Fig. 13.15. Connections of the inferior olive suggest that it can compare the control signals from higher and lower motor centers. The diagram concentrates on a functional unit *(heavy outlines)* consisting of a sagittal zone of cerebellar cortex with its olivary input region, cerebellar output nucleus, and lower motor center. Note that cerebellum is on a side loop to the efferent line from the higher to lower motor center, as in Fig. 13.1. (From Oscarsson, 1980; in Brooks and Thach, 1981; also in Brooks, 1983, 1984)

riety of related inputs. The question was raised in relation to Fig. 13.13 whether the cerebellar cortex contains an adequate number of subareas that are suitably connected for specialized tasks. Microzones could be the answer because the entire cerebellar cortex may be so organized, although it has been demonstrated so far only in the vermis and flocculus. The important point is that the *microzones constitute the smallest operational units of the cerebellar cortex,* equivalent to the columns of the primary sensory, motor, and visual cortices (cf. Figs. 11.12, 12.4, and 12.8). The sagittal, longitudinal shape of cerebellar microzones is dictated by the histological arrangements of P cells in relation to the parallel fibers (Fig. 13.9).

Since the microzones receive convergent inputs, they are delineated more precisely by their outputs, which can be established, for instance, through electrical microstimulation of floccular zones. Ito showed that this inhibits relay cells of the vestibulo-ocular reflex (VOR) in the vestibular nuclei. The activity in cerebellar cortex and its output nuclei are correlated by their common excitatory inputs from CFs and MFs. The cortical microzone and its nuclear target constitute a corticonuclear "microcomplex" for corrective computations for the control of the functions executed by the represented body parts.

Figure 13.17 illustrates the cerebellar side-loop operation for the VOR. The vestibular reflex (from the vestibular organs to

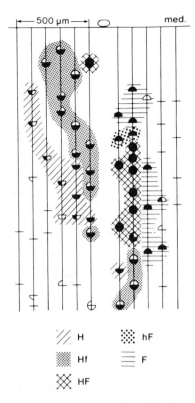

<!-- legend -->
H   hF
Hf   F
HF

Fig. 13.16. Sagittal microzones (in the vermal cortex of the cat), established by stimulation of the appropriate afferent nerves (ulnar and sciatic). Note the small size of microzones compared to the entire sagittal zones in Fig. 13.2. Abbreviations: F, f, short- and long-latency forelimb activation; H, h, similar for hindlimb. Microzones are cerebellar equivalents of input–output assemblies in the cerebral cortex (cf. Figs. 11.2, 12.4, and 12.8). (From Andersson and Oscarsson, 1978; in Ito, 1984)

the external muscles of the eye) traverses the vestibular and oculomotor nuclei. Afferents from the vestibular organs (that signal head movement) also form an MF side loop through the cerebellar cortex, whose output impinges on oculomotor neurons (by way of the vestibular nuclei). The reflex effects (moving the eyes to compensate for head movements to stabilize the retinal image) are not fed back to the vestibular system; they would get there too late to modify quick saccades (see Fig. 9.3). What *is* fed back, by way of the CFs, is visual information from the accessory optic

tract about slip of the retinal field, that is, about imperfections (errors) of the control system that attempts to fixate the gaze.

The climbing fibers *adapt* the responses of P cells to input from MFs, making the cerebellum an adaptive control device. Corrective computations of cerebellar microzones are fed forward to the cerebellar outputs and thus adapt the program. Programs are therefore distributed between the cerebellum and other parts of the brain, such as the premotor and primary motor cortices (as well as other parts of the circuit connected to these structures), and also subcortical targets of the cerebellum such as the components of the VOR. Cerebellar corrections are used in open-loop fashion on the basis of predictive programming. This is one aspect of the model of cerebellum–cerebrum interaction introduced in Fig. 13.1 and elaborated further for limb movements in this chapter. Predictive commands from motor cortex depend on cerebellar triggering (Figs. 13.3–13.5). Movements of the trunk, head, and limbs are slower than those of the eyes, however. Therefore, peripheral feedback is used at all times not just for reflex control but also for updating programs, that is, for adaptive control (Fig. 4.13; and Chap. 13.7).

An example of functional microzone connections with regard to limb movements is drawn in Fig. 13.18, involving alpha- and gamma-MN activation. The figure illustrates a reflex path through a lower motor center, from cutaneous and FRA afferents to alpha and gamma MNs (as in Fig. 5.6; and compare to Fig. 13.15). Ascending collaterals from the lower motor center form a side loop ("reefference") to the cerebellum, with a descending limb through the (rostral, parvicellular) red nucleus back to the lower motor center, passing on the way through the reticular formation of the medullary bulb and ending on spinal INs. This rubrobulbospinal path (RBSP) descends in the dorsolateral reticulospinal tract, which activates spinal segmental INs by releasing them

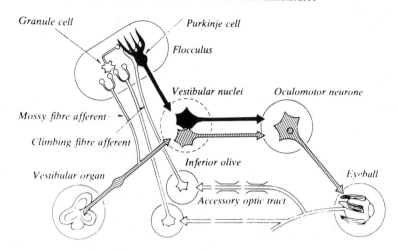

Fig. 13.17. Neural connections in the vestibulo-ocular reflex *(hatched)*, stressing the side-loop connection through the cerebellum, as in Fig. 13.1. Inferior olive receives and forwards error signals about control of eye position ("retinal slip"). Inhibitory neurons are drawn in *black*. (From Ito, 1979)

from segmental reflex functions. (This action was explained in Fig. 5.6B, which is equivalent to the lower part of Fig. 13.18.) The inferior olive receives a collateral branch from the rubrobulbar projection (the "higher motor center" in Fig. 13.18) as well as from the branches of a spinal IN ("lower motor center") ascending in the DLF-SOCP. The curved arrow between the two olivary inputs denotes a *comparator* function of these two independent control signals. Ito stresses that the comparison is made between two central control signals and not between peripheral events. The essence of the scheme is that the control errors of this system are monitored through two independent channels, which do not compare each other.

Recognition by the comparator of a difference between the two controls leads to CF impulses in the dentate and in one of its sagittal microzones (d_1-zone). The comparator function consists of the sequential arrival in the olive of the synaptic potentials generated by the corollary branch from the higher motor center, followed by that from the lower motor center (through the DLF-SOCP). The sequence is analogous to that discussed for VSCT neurons (Fig. 5.5).

The d_1-zone controls a spinal motor center that facilitates dynamic gamma MNs and inhibits, through an inhibitory IN, postsynaptic effects by the FRA on alpha MNs (and also presynaptic effects on primary afferents through depolarization, PAD). The dentate, in turn, projects back to the same part of the inferior olive, besides its main projection to the cerebral cortex via the VL thalamus (see Figs. 13.1 and 13.2). This circuit provides an example of an anatomical basis for cerebellar involvement in movement programming. With regard to dynamic gamma MNs, we know that they emphasize the reports by spindles about changes of length, rather than about its maintenance (Chaps. 4.2 and 5.2; Fig. 13.14). Little is known, however, about the modes of their descending control in behaviorally active animals.

7. Adaptation and Motor Learning

Adaptation

Adaptation is a long-lasting change of task-related responses in a novel task situation. The example in Fig. 6.4 illustrates how human subjects optimize within a few

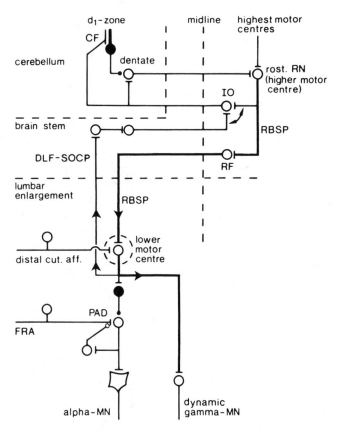

Fig. 13.18. Proposed comparison by the inferior olive (IO) of higher motor commands, from red nucleus (RN), with reefference from a lower motor center. The result is forwarded to a microzone in cerebellar cortex (d_1). Comparator function of IO, indicated by *curved arrow*, is an example of the IO function blocked out in Fig. 13.15. IO is on side loop to the efferent *(heavy)* line from higher to lower motor center. Abbreviations: CF, climbing fiber; DLF-SOCP, dorsolateral funiculus spino-olivocerebellar path; PAD, primary afferent depolarization; RBSP, rubrobulbospinal path; RF, reticular formation. The lower part of this figure, dealing with FRA, flexor reflex afferents, is comparable to Fig. 5.6B. (From Ekerot, Larson, and Oscarsson, 1979; in Oscarsson, 1980; based largely on Jeneskog and Johannson, 1977, in Brooks and Thach, 1981; Brooks, 1983, 1984)

trials the use of their leg muscles to regain their balance on shifting ground. Optimal solutions are arrived at by successive approximations through trial and error that, of course, need not be conscious. Dependence on consciousness distinguishes adaptation from "habituation," which was introduced in Chap. 3.1 as a change in directed attention when a sensory stimulus has lost its significance for the subject, a conscious activity by definition. (The habituated state is lost during light anesthesia, but the adapted state persists during and after periods of unconsciousness, including sleep). A familiar example is how we "get out sea legs" after some days (or weeks!) on board ship. The vestibular system becomes adapted to the heaving deck—that is, to the changing slopes of the surface supporting the stance of the legs (cf. Fig. 9.12). Adaptation leads to (unconscious) expectation of these changes; witness the common illusion of the ground seeming to heave as we step ashore. We also adapt to the visual scene of the rising and falling horizon, which ceases to induce nausea. Nausea is caused by sensory conflict when the two senses do not adapt equally or when we fail to suppress the one that has not yet adapted (Chap. 9.6).

Adaptation is part of motor learning, as noted in relation to Fig. 13.10, but adaptation is less versatile. The same trials and errors are repeated during adaptation in successive exposures to a novel stimulus, whereas the optimum is achieved faster during learning because the explorations are more varied and are improved from one time to the next. An example of poorly remembered adaptation was mentioned in Chap. 5.1, the "loosening up" ("tuning") of joints during practice of a simple motor task. Tuning increases the agonist drive that propels the limb and decreases the co-contraction of opposing muscles, including premovement inhibition. This form of adaptation repeats its sequence of improvement during each trial, with only fair carryover from one work session to the next. In contrast, "learning" uses the experience gained in previous trials. Learning and adaptation are usually mixed together.

Recall the distinction made in Chap. 2.3 between learning by "insight" and by "rote." Insight learning requires intact connections with the hippocampus and the amygdala which relate meaning to memory formation. They are connected to the limbic system and receive input from the higher association cortex, relayed through the entorhinal cortex (Figs. 2.8 and 11.15). Rote learning, in contrast, can still be carried out after disconnecting lesions of the hippocampus and amygdala. The details of how this capability is related to cerebellar function are still unknown. Adaptation has access to some rudimentary form of memory but no access to associative capabilities. Cerebellar function is essential for adaptation, because it is lost in cerebellar patients and in animals during cerebellar dysfunction. Postures and movements are adapted by changes in the timing and intensity of task-related adjustments of joint position and stiffness (e.g., Figs. 6.4, 8.5, and 9.12). This is accomplished by alterations of alpha- or gamma-MN activation, in whatever way is best suited to the task execution (see Fig. 4.12).

Through what mechanism does the cerebellum enable the process of adaptation? The discussion of Fig. 13.10 revealed that a likely mechanism may be the firing of complex spikes (CSs) that accompany adaptations from old to new tasks and change the subsequent firing levels of simple spikes (SSs; e.g., Fig. 13.10B, right, and C). For familiar tasks, in contrast, commands pass from the cerebellar cortex to its output nuclei as SSs without necessarily involving CSs (e.g, Figs. 13.10B, left, and 13.13A). The change of CS firing implicates the participation of the inferior olive in the adaptation and learning of motor performance. This argument is strengthened by the consequences of olivary dysfunctions, which degrade the use of programmed movements in the same way as cerebellar lesions. In other words, the inferior olive is an essential component of the cerebellocerebral circuit for successful task execution.

How is the olivary action exerted? We already know of Oscarsson's proposal that olivary function is based on forwarding, to the cerebellar cortex, comparisons of what is and what should be (Figs. 13.15, 13.17 and 13.18). Ito points out that the inferior olive is the forwarding agent, although it need not be the actual comparator. For instance, the vestibulo-ocular reflex that adjusts the position of the eyes (gaze) in relation to the head (VOR, Chap. 9.1; Fig. 13.17) is based on the comparison of controls for head and eye movements that are made in the retina, not in the olive (retinal slip). Melvill Jones has shown that vestibulo-ocular conflict is resolved when vision adapts, together with the VOR (within a few days) for individuals wearing prisms that reverse the visual scene left to right. The similarity with which the VOR adapts in humans, monkeys, and other animals, presents the opportunity to investigate how the circuit functions (Fig. 13.17). The way was pointed by Marr's proposal that adaptation occurs in the cerebellar cortex, specifically because CFs modify the responses of P cells to MF input.

How the side loop through the cerebellum produces adaptation of "reflex" outputs was shown by Ito for the VOR (of rabbits). The VOR can adapt, as proved by its change when the visual environment moves past the rabbits' eyes instead of standing still. Such optokinetic stimulation is produced by rotating the animals on a turntable inside a drum that presents a visual environment of vertical stripes, rotating at slightly different speeds from that of the animals. Established adaptation of the VOR is lost after lesioning of those parts of the vestibulocerebellum or of the inferior olive involved in the original establishment. The retinal error signals reach particular microzones in the flocculus, whose SSs adapt to the optokinetic stimulation when the VOR adapts. The precise localization of VOR adaptation in the cerebellar cortex enabled Ito, and others, to examine the nature of this plasticity.

Ito's experiments prove Marr's theory that coincident inputs from MFs and CFs to a P cell adapt subsequent responses of that P cell to the particular MF input. Coincident ("conjunctive") electrical stimulation, at natural frequencies, of vestibular afferent (MF) fibers and of the inferior olive or its CFs for some seconds produces adaptations of P-cell responses to input from those MFs lasting about 1 hour. Similar experiments with other animal preparations in various parts of the cerebellum have confirmed the general applicability of this finding. The adaptation consists of a change of postsynaptic responsiveness of P-cell dendrites to the transmitter from parallel fibers, glutamate (cf. Fig. 13.11). Postsynaptic responsiveness is decreased by calcium ion entry into P-cell dendrites during their plateau depolarizations by complex spikes, reducing their response to standard amounts of glutamate. There is no presynaptic change at the MF terminals to the P-cell dendrites. (The postsynaptic desensitization of P-cell responsiveness stands in contrast to the presynaptic mechanism of adaptation in the hippocampus, where calcium ion entry into presynaptic terminals alters the amount of transmitter released by the presynaptic impulses.) Adaptive reduction of P-cell excitability by CFs fits Albus' version of Marr's theory.

Motor Learning

Motor learning is by no means only a cerebellar function. It is accomplished in successive stages of giving selective responses to a stimulus. It is a transition from nonspecific responses to highly selective associations. This "multiple-trace" view, put forward by Thompson, is based on studies of classical Pavlovian conditioning of animals, such as pairing a conditioned and unconditioned stimulus to elicit foot flexion or eyeblink. The *first*, most general responses are usually autonomic, but also include generalized body movements that prepare the subject to respond in some manner. Such conditioned emotional states, or acquired drives, are generated by the limbic system, particularly the amygdala (Chap. 11.1 and 11.2). Once the subject has been well conditioned, however, limbic participation is no longer essential. Classical conditioning leads to short-term changes of the order of one day, and long-term changes lasting a week or more. Short-term changes are produced by alterations of existing synapses, while long-term changes depend on the formation of new synapses made by new branches of neurons that sprout during repeated participation in the conditioning process.

The *second* stage of learning applies to operant conditioning, in which correct performance is rewarded, as well as to classical conditioning. The second stage is exactly what has been described above as the normal cerebellar functions in performing intended movements! Neurons in the cerebellar output nuclei emit predictively timed discharges as much for classically as for instrumentally conditioned responses. These nuclear discharges and conditioned responses fail when the cerebellar nuclei are incapacitated by local application of a GABA antagonist or when the nuclei are lesioned. During the conditioning process the number of effective, preferred synaptic paths increases, which has been demonstrated (by Tsukahara) to result from sprouting of afferent fibers in the active path.

The *third* level of learning involves insight and depends on use of the hippocampus and amygdala, as already discussed in Chaps. 1.3, 2.1, and 11.2. This process presumably is reflected in the upturn of the learning curve near 50% correct behavior of Fig. 1.5C. Successful cerebellar activity presumably is enabled by this circuit through repeated testing, making operative changes, and testing again. In other words, the selective action improves with knowledge of results and execution, knowledge that need not be conscious. The hippocampus and amygdala are engaged by the association and cingulate cortices (Fig. 11.5B). The limbic, cingulate cortex (Fig. 11.15) probably assists motor learning by enabling insight into appropriate behavior to yield optimal increase of motor skill (cf. Fig. 1.5). It may do this through its connections with cortical association areas, the motor loop of the basal ganglia (Fig. 11.8) and the pontine (PN) input to the cerebellum (Fig. 13.7).

8. Summary

The cerebellum is essential for learning and executing motor acts. It optimizes postures and movements by coordinating and adapting their components, including the required muscle synergies. Cerebellar dysfunction decomposes intended movements into sequential constituents and causes errors of direction, force, velocity, and amplitude. Motor programs are thus degraded, because predictive control of trajectories is lost. Similarly, co-contractions of opposing muscles for maintenance of intended limb postures are decomposed,

causing inaccurate corrective movements (intention tremor). Decomposition of postures of the whole body leads to sway and gait disturbances, and decomposition of gaze (posture of the eyeball) leads to nystagmus. However, there is no loss of sensory activity, of intellectual ability and awareness, or of thought processes.

Cerebellar control is based on comparisons of premotor commands and their actual implementation. Moreover, the cerebellum has the special ability to adapt intended postures and movements to changing task conditions, that is, to change task-related motor acts for a long time. Adaptation, which is based on comparisons of commands from the middle and lower levels of the motor hierarchy, operates by means of climbing fiber modulations of mossy fiber inputs to Purkinje cells. Adaptation assists motor learning by enabling the predictive implementation of trajectories, as described below. This level of cerebrocerebellar learning in turn engages the hippocampal circuit, presumably through the association and limbic cortices.

Cerebellar inputs and outputs are organized in three sagittal zones, of which the medial and lateral ones, respectively, receive only peripheral and central information, and the intermediate one both. Cortical input to the lateral (neo) cerebellum comes mostly from area 6, and to the intermediate one from area 4. There is also some input from the visual, auditory, and autonomic systems but only very little input from higher association cortex. In addition, there are inputs from the brain stem and midbrain. Peripheral input reaches the intermediate and medial zones through the spinocerebellar paths. The lateral zone projects, through the dentate nucleus, to areas 6 and 4; the intermediate zone (through the nucleus interpositus anterior) to area 4 and the brain stem; and the medial one (through the fastigial nucleus) to the spinal cord and brain stem. The flocculonodular lobe is connected with the vestibular nuclei.

The output of the lateral cerebellum is related to the intent of movements and precedes their onset, whereas that of the intermediate cerebellum reflects properties of movements during their execution. Dentate discharge can encode the reaction time of intended movements, their direction, intensity, and the patterns of muscles used. Its trigger signals activate the motor cortex (or subcortical targets) to generate optimal movement speeds along the straightest paths possible, that is, the reference trajectories. They are (for compound and simple movements) established by the lateral cerebellum and are updated by the intermediate zone, through its projections to area 4 where they converge with those from the dentate. Discharges of the intermediate cerebellum largely encode the patterns of muscles used. Loss of predictive start signals degrades motor programs or leads to abandonment of their use, and loss of predictive stop signals degrades damping and leads to tremor. Thus, cerebellar dysfunction prevents the use of the smooth matching of move and hold programs, acquired during motor learning of reference trajectories.

The cerebellar cortex receives inputs from all sources as mossy fibers (MFs), except from the inferior olive that gives rise to climbing fibers (CFs). MFs innervate granule cells, whose horizontal axon branches form parallel fibers, of which a large number innervate the dendrites of Purkinje (P) cells within reach, evoking "simple spikes" (SSs). In contrast, only one CF innervates the entire dendritic tree of each cell, evoking "complex spikes" (CSs). P cells are the sole cortical output cells and modify the activity of the cerebellar deep nuclei by inhibitory "sculpturing." The high frequency of SSs can encode the usual tonic and phasic neural commands. In contrast, CSs only fire a few times during a movement and are not driven by the intentional consequences of movements. Instead, they synchronize only with movements during their adaptation to new task conditions. They forward, to the cerebellar cortex, error signals about the central control of movements. CSs alter (adapt) the rates of subsequent SSs by postsynaptic desensitization of P-cell dendrites to the transmitter released by parallel fibers, thus reducing P-cell responses to MF input.

Projections from MFs and CFs overlap in very small, sagittal "microzones" of cerebellar cortex, which combine inputs from relevant parts of the body. The very numerous microzones and their target cells in cerebellar output nuclei constitute the smallest operational units of the cerebellum. These "microcomplexes" are specialists for particular forms of corrective control of particular parts of the body represented in them, by virtue of their selected inputs and outputs.

References

Albus, J. S. 1971. A theory of cerebellar function. *Math. Biosci.* 10:25–61.

Allen, G. I., and Tsukahara, N. 1974. Cerebrocerebellar communication systems. *Physiol. Rev.* 54:957–1006.

Andersson, G., and Oscarsson, O. 1978. Climbing fiber microzones in cerebellar vermis and the projection to different groups of cells in the lateral vestibular nucleus. *Exp. Brain Res.* 32:565–579. [Fig. 13.16]

Arshavsky, Yu. I., Gelfand, I. M., and Orlovsky, G. N. 1983. The cerebellum and control of rhythmical movements. *Trends Neurosci.* 6:417–422.

Beppu, H., Suda, M. and Tanaka, R. 1983. Slow visuomotor tracking in normal man and in patients with cerebellar ataxia. In *Motor control mechanisms in health and disease*, ed. J. E. Desmedt. *Adv. Neurol.* 39:889–895.

Bloedel, J. R., and Courville, J. 1981. Cerebellar afferent systems. In *Motor control*. Sect. 1, vol. 2. *Handbook of physiology*, ed. V. B. Brooks, pp. 735–829. Bethesda, Md.: American Physiological Society.

Brooks, V.B. 1986. How does the limbic system assist motor learning? *Brain, Behav. Evol.* In press.

Brooks, V. B. 1984. Cerebellar functions in motor control. *Human Neurobiol.* 2:251–260. [Figs. 13.1; 13.2; 13.4; 13.10; 13.15; 13.18]

Brooks, V. B. 1983. Study of brain function

by local, reversible cooling. *Rev. Physiol. Biochem. Pharmacol.* 95:1-109. [Figs. 13.14 and 13.15, 13.18]

Brooks, V. B., and Thach, W. T. 1981. Cerebellar control of posture and movement. In *Motor control.* Sect. 1, vol. 2. *Handbook of physiology,* ed. V. B. Brooks, pp. 877-946. Bethesda, Md.: American Physiological Society. [Figs. 13.1, 13.2, 13.4, 13.10, 13.12, 13.14, 13.15, 13.18]

Dichgans, J. 1984. Clinical symptons of cerebellar dysfunction and their topodiagnostical significance. *Hum. Neurobiol.* 2:269-279.

Eccles, J. C. 1969. The dynamic loop hypothesis of movement control. In *Information processing in the nervous system,* ed. K. N. Leibovic, pp. 245-268. Heidelberg: Springer Verlag.

Eccles, J.C. 1967. Circuits in the cerebellar control of movement. *Proc. Natl. Acad. Sci. USA* 58:336-343. [Fig. 13.9]

Eccles, J. C. 1979. Introductory remarks. In *Cerebro-cerebellar interactions,* eds. J. Massion and K. Sasaki, pp. 1-18. Amsterdam: Elsevier/North Holland.

Eccles, J. C. 1973. *The understanding of the brain.* New York: McGraw-Hill Book Co. [Fig. 13.9]

Eccles, J. C., Ito, M., and Szentagothai, J. 1967. *The cerebellum as a neuronal machine.* Berlin: Springer Verlag.

Ekerot, C.-F., Larson, B., and Oscarsson, O. 1979. Information carried by the spinocerebellar paths. In *Reflex control of posture and locomotion,* eds. R. Granit and O. Pompeiano. *Prog. Brain Res.* 50:79-90. [Fig. 13.18]

Fox, C. A. 1962. The structure of the cerebellar cortex. In *Correlative anatomy of the nervous system.* New York: Macmillan. [Fig. 13.9]

Gilbert, P. F. C., and Thach, W. T. 1977. Purkinje cell activity during motor learning. *Brain Res.* 70:1-18. [Fig. 13.10A,B]

Gilman, S. 1970. The nature of cerebellar dyssynergia. In *Modern trends in neurology,* ed. D. Williams. pp. 60-79. Vol. 5. London: Butterworths.

Gilman, S., Bloedel, J. R., and Lechtenberg, R. 1981. *Disorders of the cerebellum.* Philadelphia: F. A. Davis. [Fig. 13.8]

Gonshor, A. and Melvill Jones, G. 1976. Short-term adaptive changes in the human vestibulo-ocular reflex arc. *J. Physiol. (Lond.)* 256:381-414.

Granit, R. 1977. Reconsidering the "alphagamma" switch in cerebellar action. In *Physiological aspects of clinical neurology,* ed. F. R. Rose, pp. 201-213. Oxford: Blackwell Scientific Publications.

Granit, R., Holmgren, R., and Merton, P. A. 1955. The two routes for excitation of muscle and their subservience to the cerebellum. *J. Physiol. (Lond.)* 130:213-224. [Fig. 13.14]

Hallett, M., Shahani, B. T., and Young, R. R. 1975a. EMG analysis of patients with cerebellar deficits. *J. Neurol. Neurosurg. Psychiatry* 38:1163-1169. [Fig. 13.12B]

Hallett, M., Shahani, B. T., and Young, R. R. 1975b. EMG analysis of stereotyped voluntary movements in man. *J. Neurol. Neurosurg. Psychiatry* 38:1154-1162. [Fig. 13.12A]

Holmes, G. 1939. The cerebellum of man (The Hughlings Jackson Memorial Lecture). *Brain* 62:1-30.

Hore, J. and Vilis, T. 1984. A cerebellar-dependent efference copy mechanism for generating appropriate muscle responses to limb perturbations. In *Cerebellar functions,* eds. J. R. Bloedel, J. Dichgans, and W. Precht, pp. 24-35. Berlin: Springer Verlag.

Ito, M. 1984. *The cerebellum and neural control.* New York: Raven Press. [Figs. 13.6, 13.10, 13.11, and 13.16]

Ito, M. 1979. Is the cerebellum really a computer? *Trends Neurosci.* 2:122-126. [Figs. 13.11 and 13.17]

Jeneskog, T., and Johannson, H. 1977. The rubro-bulbospinal path. A descending system known to influence dynamic fusimotor neurones and its interaction with distal cutaneous afferents in the control of flexor reflex afferent pathways. *Exp. Brain Res.* 27:161-179. [Fig. 13.18]

Lamarre, Y., Bioulac, B., and Jacks, B. 1978. Activity of precentral neurones in conscious monkeys: effects of deafferentation and cerebellar ablation. *J. Physiol. (Paris)* 74:253-264.

Lamarre, Y., Spidalieri, G., and Chapman, C. E. 1983. A comparison of neuronal discharge recorded in the sensori-motor cortex, parietal cortex and dentate nucleus of the monkey during arm movements triggered by light, sound or somesthetic stimuli. In *Neural coding of motor performance,* eds. J. Massion, J. Paillard, W. Schultz, and M. Wiesendanger. *Exp. Brain Res.* Suppl. 7, pp. 140-156. [Fig. 13.3]

Llinas, R. R., and Simpson, J. I. 1981. Cerebellar control of movement. In *Motor coordi-*

nation. Vol. 5. *Handbook of behavioral neurology,* eds. A. L. Towe and E. S. Luschel, pp. 231–302. New York: Plenum Press.

Lundberg, A. 1971. Function of the ventral spinocerebellar tract. A new hypothesis. *Exp. Brain Res.* 12:317–330.

MacKay, W. A., and Murphy, J. T. 1979. Cerebellar modulation of reflex gain. *Prog. Neurobiol.* 13:361–417.

Marr, D. 1969. A theory of cerebellar cortex. *J. Physiol. (Lond.)* 202:437–470.

Melvill Jones, G., and Mandl, G. 1983. Neurobionomics of adaptive plasticity: integrating sensorimotor function with environmental demands. In *Motor control mechanisms in health and disease,* ed. J. E. Desmedt. *Adv. Neurol.* 39:1047–1071.

Meyer-Lohmann, J., Hore, J., and Brooks, V. B. 1977. Cerebellar participation in generation of prompt arm movements. *J. Neurophysiol.* 40:1038–1050. [Fig. 13.4]

Oscarsson, O. 1980. Functional organization of olivary projection to the cerebellar anterior lobe. In *The inferior olivary nucleus: anatomy and physiology,* eds. J. Courville, C. de Montigny, and Y. Lamarre, pp. 279–289. New York: Raven Press. [Fig. 13.18]

Oscarsson, O. 1979. Functional units of the cerebellum: sagittal zones and microzones. *Trends Neurosci.* 2:143–145.

Rispal-Padel, L. 1983. Neocerebellar synergies. In *Neural coding of motor performance,* eds. J. Massion, J. Paillard, W. Schultz, and M. Wiesendanger. *Exp. Brain Res.* Suppl. 7, pp. 213–223.

Sasaki, K. 1979. Cerebro-cerebellar interconnections in cats and monkeys. In *Cerebro-cerebellar interactions,* eds. J. Massion and K. Sasaki, pp. 105–124. Amsterdam: Elsevier/North-Holland. [Fig. 13.6]

Sasaki, K., and Gemba, H. 1983. Premovement cortical potentials associated with self-paced and reaction time movements. In *Neural coding of motor performance,* eds. J. Massion, J. Paillard, W. Schultz, and M. Wiesendanger. *Exp. Brain Res.* Suppl. 7, pp. 88–96.

Smith, A. 1981. The coactivation of antagonist muscles. *Can. J. Physiol. Pharmacol.* 59:733–747. [Fig. 13.13]

Strick, P. L. 1983. The influence of motor preparation on the response of cerebellar neurons to limb displacements. *J. Neurosci.* 3:2007–2020. [Fig. 13.5]

Thach, W. T., Schieber, M. H., and Elble, R. H. 1985. Motor programs: trajectory versus stability. In *Cerebellar functions,* eds. J. R. Bloedel, J. Dichgans, and W. Precht, pp. 36–51. Berlin: Springer Verlag.

Thach, W. T. 1980. Complex spikes, the inferior olive, and natural behavior. In *The inferior olivary nucleus: anatomy and physiology,* eds. J. Courville, C. de Montigny, and Y. Lamarre, pp. 349–360. New York: Raven Press. [Fig. 13.10C]

Thach, W. T. 1980. The cerebellum. In *Medical physiology,* ed. V. B. Mountcastle, pp. 837–858. 14th ed. St. Louis: C. V. Mosby Co. [Fig. 13.2]

Thach, W. T. 1978. Correlation of neural discharge with pattern and force of muscular activity, joint position, and direction of the intended movement in motor cortex and cerebellum. *J. Neurophysiol.* 41:654–676.

Thompson, R. F., Clark, G. A., Donegan, N. H., Lavond, D. G., Lincoln, J. S., Madden, J., Mamounas, L. A., Mauk, M. D., McCormick, D. A., and Thompson, J. K. 1984. Neuronal substrates of learning and memory: a "multiple trace" view. In *Neurobiology of learning and memory,* eds. G. Lynch, J. L. McGaugh, and N. M. Weinberger, pp. 137–164. New York: Guilford Press.

Tsukahara, M. 1984. Classical conditioning mediated by the red nucleus: an approach beginning at the cellular level. In *Neurobiology of learning and memory,* eds. G. Lynch, J. L. McGaugh, and N. M. Weinberger, pp. 165–180. New York: Guilford Press.

Tsukahara, N. 1981. Sprouting and the neuronal basis of learning. *Trends Neurosci.* 4:234–237.

Wiesendanger, M. 1983. Cortico-cerebellar loops. In *Neuronal coding of motor performance,* eds. J. Massion, J. Paillard, W. Schultz, and M. Wiesendanger, *Exp. Brain Res.* Suppl. 7, pp. 41–53. [Fig. 13.7]

14

The Basal Ganglia

In this chapter we gain an overview of the anatomy of the basal ganglia circuits (14.1), examine their functional properties (14.2), and integrate these properties into an understanding of the diseases of the basal ganglia (14.3).

The basal ganglia are important for carrying out motor plans. They were introduced as three subcortical forebrain systems that are connected to the sensorimotor system and the limbic system (Fig. 2.4; Chaps. 2.1, 2.2, 11.2, and 11.3). Figure 2.7 shows the two types of circuits of the dorsal basal ganglia: the caudate one is linked to the higher level of the motor hierarchy, and the putamen circuit is linked to the middle level. The loop through the higher level is thought to control the assembly of overall motor plans, while the loop through the middle level is thought to scale the intensity of execution of motor patterns in the context of the task requirements. The third circuit, through the ventral basal ganglia (not shown in Fig. 2.7), contains the ventral striatum, which has limbic innervations. The ventral basal ganglia contribute to the conversion of need-directed intentions (created by the limbic system and the higher level association cortex) into specific, goal-directed motor acts. The ventral basal ganglia project through the nucleus accumbens to the midbrain locomotor centers, and can, but

need not, be accessed by the cerebral cortex to induce locomotion (Chaps. 2.1 and 11.2). In the cortical bypass mode, this oldest circuit presumably enables the organism to move about in order to fill biological or sublimated needs. The nucleus accumbens also projects to the rostral cingulate cortex by way of the dorsomedial nucleus of the thalamus (MD, Fig. 11.15).

1. Anatomical Orientation

Constituent Parts

The basal ganglia are structures in the basal forebrain and midbrain. They consist of the most basal, ventral "old" system (not shown in Fig. 14.1) and of a dorsal "new" system. The *ventral system* contains the limbically innervated nucleus accumbens. The inputs to the dorsal basal ganglia derive from all areas of the cerebral neocortex, and the outputs are directed to the frontal association cortex and to motor regions of the cortex (Fig. 14.1A,B). The *dorsal system* has three anatomical parts. The first includes the putamen, globus pallidus, and caudate nucleus (which is separated from the other two by the internal capsule). The putamen and the caudate nucleus (the most rostral components, called the new, or "neostriatum") are the main receptive areas for extrinsic inputs to the basal ganglia. The second part consists of the substantia nigra, which is a sheet of tissue overlying the cerebral peduncle in the midbrain, and the third is the subthalamic nucleus. Figure 14.1A indicates three inputs to the basal ganglia: the major one descends from the cerebral cortex, and others ascend from the thalamus and the raphe nuclei in the reticular formation (see Fig. 5.8; the limbic inputs are not shown). The largest thalamostriate projection is from the centromedian nucleus to the putamen. Figure 14.1B shows two sets of outputs from the system: one from the globus pallidus to the thalamus and the pons, and the other from the substantia nigra to the thalamus, superior colliculus, and reticular formation. [Recall that the "enhancement" of task-related activity in the superior colliculus (Fig. 11.2) depends on the influence of the substantia nigra, pars reticulata (SNpr, Fig. 14.2).]

The *interconnections* of the dorsal basal ganglia are highlighted in Fig. 14.1C. The SN projects to the caudate and to the putamen, which, together with the external segment of the globus pallidus (GP), use the internal palladial segment as their collective output. All efferents from the striatum go to the GP and the SN. The subthalamic nucleus receives from the external pallidum (GPe) and projects topographically to the internal pallidum (GPi) as well as to the SN. The GPi is also reciprocally connected in topographic manner with the SNpr. The subthalamic nucleus is under the influence of the premotor and motor cortex (Fig. 14.2), which enables the middle level of the motor hierarchy to modulate the output of the basal ganglia.

The connections of the basal ganglia described above are schematized in Fig. 14.2, which shows the nucleus accumbens (ACC) as a part of the ventral, old ("paleo") striatum, which was omitted from Fig. 14.1A–C. The SN is split into the densely pigmented pars compacta (SNpc) and the less dense pars reticulata (SNpr).

The densely pigmented structures, including those in the ventral tegmentum (VTA), give rise to ascending paths transmitting by release of dopamine. The *dopaminergic* (DA) paths are organized in three systems of which the first is the "nigrostriatal" DA system from the SNpc to the striatum. The two others, the "mesolimbic" and "mesocortical" systems, arise from the VTA with projections to the ventral striatum (nucleus accumbens) on the one hand, and on the other to the frontal and cingulate cortex, the olfactory tubercle, and the central nucleus of the amygdala. The DA paths provide tonic support for the neural traffic in their target centers. The intensity of tonic control is probably governed by cortical and thalamic fibers reaching the SNpc. When DA paths fail, as in parkinsonism, some previously controlled functions go awry in the basal ganglia, not unlike the diverse failures in electronic devices when a section of the power supply has burned out. The dorsal raphe (DR) nuclei transmit by means of *serotonin*.

We can now summarize the *inputs to the striatum* as arising from the cerebral cortex and the intralaminar nuclei of the thalamus (e.g., CM, see Fig. 11.14) and, as DA paths from the SNpc, the VTA, and the DR. The most intense corticostriatal projections are organized on a simple basis: cortical regions connect with those striate structures that are nearest to them. In addition, there are longitudinally arranged projections to caudate regions from diverse cortical areas (not illustrated). The same sort of convergent–divergent sorting is at work here as was encountered for thalamocortical connections in Chap. 11.3. The *outputs from the striatum* are organized topographically; those from the caudate nucleus and the putamen are segregated in the pallidum and the SNpr as well as in their thalamic projections: VL and VA (Figs. 11.7, 11.9, and 11.14). This important separation of the two functional circuit types is considered in greater detail in relation to Figs. 14.3–14.5. The connections, histological features, and cellular

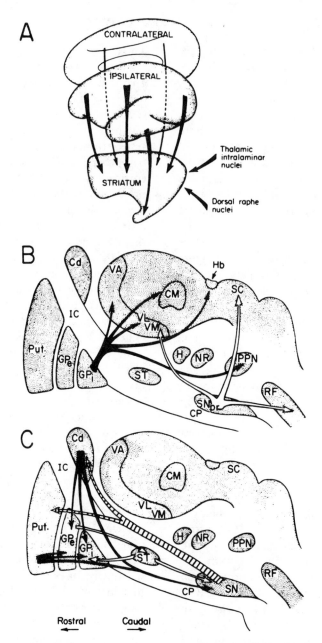

Fig. 14.1 The main afferent, efferent, and connecting paths of the basal ganglia. (A) Afferents originate from ipsilateral and contralateral cerebral cortex and from ipsilateral thalamic intralaminar nuclei and dorsal raphe n. (B) Efferent axons leave from the internal globus pallidus (GPi) and substantia nigra, pars reticulata (SNpr) to the ventroanterior (VA) and ventrolateral (VL) and centromedian (CM) thalamic nuclei, the habenula (Hb), and the pedunculopontine n. of the mesencephalic-pontine tegmentum (PPN). Nigral axons terminate more medially in the thalamic ventromedial n. (VM), in the superior colliculus (SC), and in the pontomedullary reticular formation (RF). Abbreviations: Put., putamen; GPe, external globus pallidus; Cd, caudate n.; IC, internal capsule; ST, subthalamic n.; H, Forel's field; NR, red n.; CP, cerebral peduncle. Compare to thalamic nuclei shown in Fig. 11.14. (C) Both striatal nuclei (putamen and caudate n.) send axons to the substantia nigra and both pallidal segments *(filled arrows)*. Axons of GPe terminate in ST, which sends axons to GPi and SN *(hollow arrows)*. Nigrostriatal axons from pars compacta of SN go to the putamen and caudate *(hatched arrows)*. (From Anderson and Crill, 1979; in Anderson, 1981)

properties of GPi and SNpr suggest that they are the medial and lateral parts of a single functional entity.

The scheme of Fig. 14.2 indicates that the main business of the dorsal basal ganglia is to refine the information transferred to the association and motor areas of the cerebral cortex. An important develop-

ment in primates has been the control of the basal ganglia by the sensorimotor cortex, through progressive enlargement and differentiation of the globus pallidus, especially GPi, and its control by the subthalamic nucleus (STN). It would be well to review some of the structures mentioned above.

Fig. 14.2. Diagram of the main intrinsic and extrinsic connections of the basal ganglia. Abbreviations as in Fig. 14.1, except for ACC, nucleus accumbens; SNpc, substantia nigra, pars compacta; STN, subthalamic n.; VTA, ventral tegmental area. *Hollow lines and arrows,* excitatory; *filled lines and arrows,* inhibitory; *dashed lines,* paths transmitting with dopamine (DA) from VTA, SNpc, and with serotonin from dorsal raphe nuclei (DR). Compare to cerebellum in Fig. 13.1. (Adapted from DeLong and Georgopoulos, 1981; Spann and Grofova, 1984)

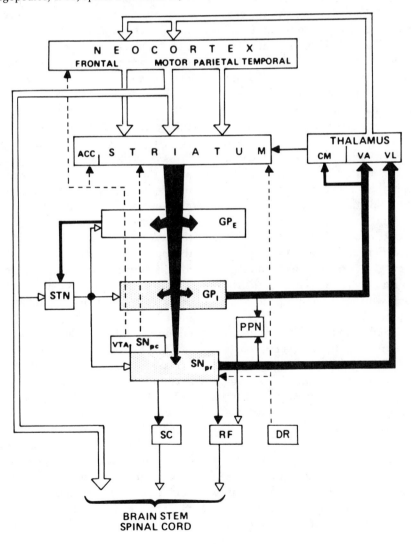

Review of Related Structures

The cingulate areas 23 and 24 receive hypothalamic input ascending through the amygdala, as well as input from the hippocampus, by way of the subiculum, mammillary body, and anteroventral (AV) and mediodorsal (MD) nuclei of the thalamus (Fig. 11.15). We saw in Chaps. 2.1 and 11.12 that the ventral tegmentum (VTA, Fig. 2.3B), another "limbic" structure, consists of the preoptic area, the lateral hypothalamus, and the ventral striatum (the most ventral, "basal" part of the basal ganglia). The ventral striatum, that is, the nucleus accumbens and the striatal part of the olfactory tubercle, projects to the ventral pallidum, which contains the limbically oriented substantia innominata. The latter projects to the rostral cingulate gyrus (area 24) and the prefrontal cortex after relay in the mediodorsal (MD) nucleus of the thalamus. The rostral cingulate, in turn, projects back to MD, while the caudal cingulate (area 23) projects back to the anteroventral nucleus (AV) (Chap. 11, Figs. 11.8 and 11.15). The nucleus accumbens, in the ventral striatum, also projects to the SNpc that, in turn, may modulate activity in the dorsal striatum.

The raphe nuclei were introduced in Chap. 5.2 with regard to one of their properties: they give rise to monoaminergic (serotonergic) fibers descending to the spinal cord, which can inhibit pain-transmitting spinothalamic neurons (Figs. 5.8 and 5.11). The VA and VL thalamic nuclei are also familiar from Chap. 11.3, where they were characterized as having movement-related functions (Fig. 11.14B, **a,b**), and CM as transmitting arousal from the ascending reticular formation. The frontal association cortex (marked as areas 8, 9, and 10 in Fig. 11.1 and as PrCo in Fig. 11.5B) is connected with its rostral neighbor, the orbitofrontal cortex (e.g., area 46). The latter projects to the limbic system, in fact to the hypothalamus and midbrain tegmentum, which project back up to the basal ganglia and down to the spinal cord, respectively, The tegmentum receives input from the prefrontal cortex as well as from the cingulate gyrus. The ventral (paleo) circuit has already been described adequately in Chap. 14.1 above and in Chaps. 2.1 and 11.2.

Functions of the Basal Ganglia in Relation to Their Connections

The general course of the two separate circuits through the dorsal basal ganglia is blocked out in Fig. 14.3A. This diagram makes it plain that the two nuclei, the caudate and the putamen, are located in side loops that parallel corticocortical projections. This suggests to us that the basal ganglia are parts of control circuits that may operate somewhat like those of the cerebellum, that is, by comparing intended outputs with their actual execution. For the cerebellum, this applies as much to central "control" outputs as to those addressed to the lower level for muscle use. Since the basal ganglia have only central inputs, it appears likely that *the basal ganglia control the nature and quality of corticocortical processing* in the context of the task requirements. They might achieve this by comparison of the original cortical messages (monitored as efference copies) with the final messages emerging from the corticocortical chain, and by also adding ingredients provided by their subcortical circuit components, the thalamus, GP and the SNpr. This idea was summarized in Fig. 2.10, discussed in Chap. 11.3, and is examined further below.

The "motor" and "complex" loops are shown in more detail in Fig. 14.3B. The caudate loop receives its cerebral inputs from the "higher" association areas. This loop runs through the magnocellular and parvicellular parts of the ventral anterior nucleus of the thalamus (VAmc, VApc), and projects to frontal association areas (e.g., prefrontal cortex). Note that the caudate loop actually also includes a part of the anterior putamen. The putamen loop receives its cerebral input somatotopically from the sensorimotor areas, including the middle-level premotor areas 6 and 5. The loop runs through the oral and medial parts of the ventral lateral nucleus (VLo, VLm) of the thalamus, and projects to the supplemental motor area (SMA, medial area 6, Figs. 11.2 and 11.7).

Both circuits relay in the internal segment of the globus pallidus (GPi) and the SNpr, but they remain separated in each case rostrocaudally and mediolaterally (rostrodorsal vs. caudoventral GPi, and rostromedial vs. caudolateral SNpr). The SMA serves as primary gateway for the circuit through the putamen (Figs. 11.2, 11.7, 11.11 and 11.14), a parallel arrangement to that through the premotor area of the cortex, which serves as primary gateway to the sensorimotor system from corticocortical (transcortical) fiber loops and the circuit through the lateral cerebellum. Recall from the discussion of Fig. 11.7 that the cortical fiber connections between area 4 and the lateral and medial areas 6 provide routes for mutual influences between the cerebellum and the basal ganglia.

The scheme of Fig. 14.3B differs from the well-known diagram of Kemp and Powell that pictures the cerebellum and the basal ganglia as "funneling" inputs to the sensorimotor cortex. In the current view presented here, loops through the basal ganglia refine cortical processing of inputs provided through other routes. Inputs to one of the loops consist of limbic signals dealing with biological or sublimated "needs" and cortical signals dealing with attention, recognition of significant inputs, and selection of responses. Ascending limbic inputs reach the SMA, the ventral putamen, and the caudate, for instance, from the hypothalamus via the amygdala, and descending limbic influences from the cingulate cortex. These connections are important for motor learning (Chap. 13.7).

Comparison of the Circuits through Basal Ganglia and the Cerebellum

The cerebellum and the basal ganglia each contain "complex" and "motor" loops. Each loop ends at different targets from its origin. (This is obscured in Fig. 2.7–2.10 but is apparent in Figs. 13.1, 13.2, and 14.1–14.3). Information from both the complex and the motor loops of the dorsal basal ganglia reaches the premotor cortex by means of transcortical connections, one from prefrontal to premotor cortex (Figs. 2.7 and 11.7), and the other through connections between the lateral and medial aspects of area 6 (PM and SMA, Fig. 11.7). The complex loop of the basal ganglia is the only one in Fig. 14.3 that operates above the middle level.

The primary motor area (MI) influences the putamen by direct projection, and it influences the cerebellar side loop indirectly through the pontine nuclei (Fig. 13.6). The putamen loop projects back to the supplementary motor cortex (SMA, Fig. 14.3), while the intermediate cerebellar loop projects to the primary motor cortex and to subcortical targets (Figs. 11.2 and 13.2). The "complex" and "motor" circuits of the dorsal basal ganglia are entirely separate, while the circuits through the lateral and intermediate cerebellum converge in the primary motor cortex. The cerebellar and basal ganglia loops are separated from each other until they finally pool their influences through indirect paths on output neurons of the primary motor cortex. The two systems converge after transcortical links from the prefrontal cortex and the premotor cortex, and shorter links between the supplementary, premotor, and primary motor areas (Fig. 11.7), as well as from the SMA to the pontine nuclei (Fig. 13.7). In the end, of course, all supraspinal influences merge in the final common path by virtue of the multiple descending supraspinal paths (Chap. 5.2; Fig. 13.1). Finally, we note that the cerebellum and the basal ganglia both influence their targets by inhibitory modulations. Figure 14.2 indicates that the outputs of the striatum are inhibitory, as are the projections from GPi and SNpr to the thalamus, and those to the superior colliculus, that is, the midbrain tectum (from SNpr, and to the subthalamic nucleus (STN, from GPe).

A reminder is worthwhile that major lesions of the basal ganglia reveal particularly the remaining capabilities of the cerebrocerebellar circuit at the middle level (e.g., Fig. 13.1). These are to execute movements according to intact motor plans but to fail in their prompt execution because of degraded sequencing of the constituent motor acts and because of inadequate scaling of their detailed programs. Major lesions of the cerebellum reveal particularly

the remaining capabilities of the cerebrum in concert with the basal ganglia and the higher and middle levels. Again, motor plans can be carried out, but their execution fails because of degraded triggering of their detailed, constituent programs.

Integration in the middle level depends on the recombinations of multiple somatotopic inputs into topographically organized outputs (Chap. 11.3). Topographic "representations" of middle-level components are each provided with multiple afferent, somatotopic codes such as for body parts, adequate stimuli, and types of response (Chaps. 11.3, 12.3, and 13.6). This rule also applies to the motor loop of the basal ganglia. Figure 14.4 presents a scheme to show how the arm, for instance,

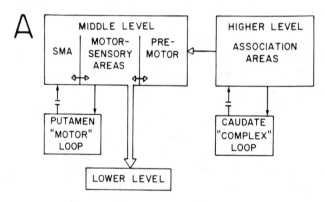

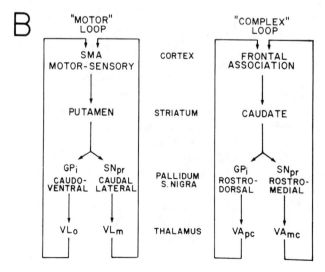

Fig. 14.3. The two parts of the striatum, the caudate and putamen, are parts of segregated pathways, respectively, from the higher association cortex ("complex" loop) and the sensorimotor areas ("motor" loop) through the pallidum, substantia nigra, and thalamus. (A) Simplified scheme to show the relations of the main parts. Compare to Figs. 2.7 and 11.7. (B) More detailed diagram that names the components. [(B) From DeLong, Georgopoulos, and Crutcher, 1983; also in DeLong, Alexander, Georgopoulos, and Mitchell, 1984]

is represented in sequential stages of the putamen motor loop. Cortical areas project to the nearest parts of the striatum, together with convergent projections from related and neighboring areas.

The essence of this scheme is familiar by now from similar ones in the motor cortex and the cerebellum (cf. Figs. 11.7, 11.11, 12.4, and 13.16). "Patchy" projections dealing with equivalent somatotopic subjects are focused on one stage of the sequence (in this case the putamen), bringing together all information that has a bearing on the projection topic, in this case the "arm." (It is no surprise to learn that striatal neurons, like those in other projection systems, surround their dendritic fields with a fence of inhibition powered by the message traffic in their axon collaterals.) The integration of striatal outputs is completed in its passage through the pallidum and the thalamus, from which it leaves for the final coordinating unit, the SMA. From there it enters the chain of commands to enable movements, starting in the motor cortex. Patchy projections have become familiar clues for tracing a distributed system, ever since Eccles first drew attention to their existence in the cerebellum, and Phillips and Mountcastle pointed out equivalents for mapping in motor and sensory association cortex (e.g., Figs. 12.3 and 12.4). We last encountered them in this text as corticothalamic modules (proposed by Strick, Fig. 11.7), Oscarsson's cerebellar cortical microzones (Fig. 13.16), and Ito's corticonuclear microcomplexes (cf. Fig. 13.17).

Corticostriate Connections

Convergence of corticostriate projections, shown for the motor loop in Fig. 14.4, is pictured as a general scheme in Fig. 14.5. Progressive overlap of projections from three cortical areas is drawn through the striatum, pallidum and substantia nigra, and finally the thalamus. The point of this

Fig. 14.4. Diagram of paths for integration of cortical inputs concerning the arm within a long anteroposterior cylinder in the putamen. This cylindrical representation is maintained by topographic projections to the pallidum and ventrolateral n. of the thalamus. Area 6 refers to SMA. Main connections shown as *heavy lines;* projections from reciprocally interconnected cortical areas (cf. Figs. 11.9 and 11.11), *continuous light lines;* those from nonreciprocally connected areas, *broken lines*. These convergent and divergent recombinations are equivalents to those described for the cerebral cortex (Figs. 11.12 and 12.4) and the cerebellar cortex (Fig. 13.16). (From DeLong and Georgopoulos, 1981; also in DeLong, Alexander, Georgopoulos, and Mitchell, 1984)

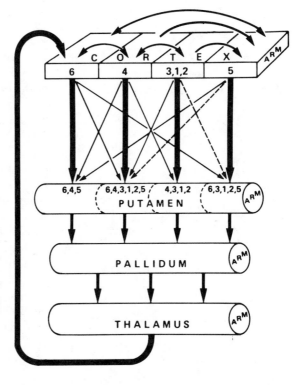

drawing is that such overlap does not extend, however, beyond particular functional loops, which are the motor loop, the caudate loop, and the loop through the anterior cingulate cortex. Their direct projections are essentially separate, as deduced from anatomical data by Alexander, DeLong, and Strick. Separate projections in the return paths from thalamus to cortex

Fig. 14.5. Generalized diagram of a basal ganglia-thalamo-cortical loop (like that in Fig. 14.4). There are at least five such self-contained loops in the dorsal and ventral basal ganglia. Each receives inputs from several, functionally related, cortical areas (A,B,C) that send partially overlapping projections to a restricted, specific portion of the striatum. The striatal regions send further converging projections to the globus pallidus and substantia nigra, which in turn project to a specific region of the thalamus. Each thalamic region projects back to one of the cortical areas that provides input into the circuit (see Fig. 11.14), thus closing the loop. (From Alexander, DeLong, and Strick, 1986)

GENERALIZED
BASAL GANGLIA-THALAMOCORTICAL
CIRCUIT

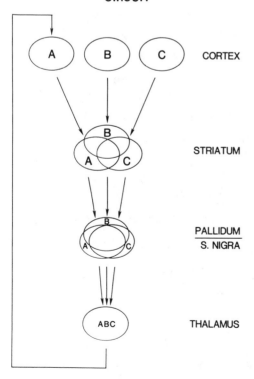

(the long upward-going arrow on the left in Figs. 14.4 and 14.5) are familiar from our consideration of the thalamic nuclei (Fig. 11.14). The proposed strong separation between the loops leaves the unsolved puzzle how integration of functions between the loops might occur. One loop could presumably influence others through cortico-cortical fiber projections and through subsidiary overlaps at synaptic relays.

Subsidiary overlaps might arise among the numerous projections from cortical association areas to the caudate nucleus. These projections fall into two overlapping geometric patterns. The *first* pattern shows separate terminal fields that are ordered rostrocaudally, going from frontal projections to the head, through parietal and occipital cortex, to temporal projections to the tail of the caudate. This is based on degeneration methods that reveal the densest connections, corresponding to observable defects following lesions. For instance, bilateral damage to the dorsolateral aspect of the prefrontal cortex, or to their projections to the anterodorsal portion of the heads of the caudate nuclei, interferes with spatial aspects of *where* to respond (e.g., in delayed alternation tasks). Damage to the orbitotemporal cortex, or of its projection to the ventrolateral aspect of the head of the caudate, interferes with the timing aspects or *when* to respond (e.g., in tasks involving object reversal and "go" or "no go" decisions). Lesions of the inferotemporal association cortex, or its projection to the tail of the caudate, disrupt visual discrimination based on recognition of previously experienced scenes, such as choosing to press one of two differently marked buttons.

The *second* pattern is obtained with stains based on axonal transport, which reveal an additional separation along the sagittal plane. Goldman-Rakic points out that her result resembles an equivalent sagittal thalamocortical organization, found by Kuypers with the same methods, an organization that can be superimposed on the conventional nuclear anatomy illustrated in Fig. 11.14. The two patterns presumably supplement each other and represent perhaps a convergent–divergent sorting of inputs.

There are three separate "complex" loops through the caudate nucleus, according to Alexander, DeLong, and Strick. These loops each have separate main inputs from the oculomotor, prefrontal, and orbitofrontal cortex respectively, and traverse separate parts of the caudate nucleus, pallidum and substantia nigra, and thalamus. Moreover, the cingulate input to the ventral striatum may constitute yet another separate loop, leaving the puzzle of limbic/non-limbic integration (see Fig. 11.8). Oculomotor functions are served by convergent inputs from the anterior cingulate, frontal eyefields, the dorsolateral prefrontal cortex, and the posterior parietal cortex (see Figs. 11.1 and 11.4). Higher functions are served primarily by the dorsolateral prefrontal cortex, the posterior parietal cortex, and the arcuate premotor area (APA, Fig. 11.8). Integration of species-preserving actions is served by the lateral orbitofrontal cortex, the superior and inferior temporal gyri, and the anterior cingulate area. This new scheme, which probably is still incomplete, does not provide for closure between the limbic and non-limbic systems. Yet, recall the convergence from non-limbic higher cortical areas on the limbic system (Fig. 11.5). At this time we can only guess that limbic influences are brought to bear through yet unspecified sites of convergence, perhaps still including the basal ganglia.

The most important *neurotransmitters* in the basal ganglia are dopamine (DA), acetylcholine (ACh), and gamma-amino butyric acid (GABA). The cell bodies in the substantia nigra, pars compacta (SNpc) and their axon terminals in the striatum have the greatest DA concentrations in the nervous system. DA is the transmitter both in the nigrostriatal branch to the caudate and putamen (i.e., from the ventral tegmentum to the dorsal striatum; region

"A9," not illustrated), and in the mesolimbic branch to the nucleus accumbens (i.e., from the ventral tegmentum to the ventral striatum; region "A10" located along the medial forebrain bundle in Fig. 2.3, not marked). These projections are inhibitory, probably because DA inhibits excitatory interneurons, although it excites striatal cells directly. The striatal interneurons are cholinergic but their action is very slow, not unlike that of ACh in the neocortex (in the order of seconds, not milliseconds). The transmitter in the inhibitory return path from the striatum to the SNpr is GABA, as well as in the inhibitory output paths from the dorsal striatum to the GPi (dorsal pallidum) and from the ventral striatum to the ventral pallidum. (Neurotransmitters of the middle level were last discussed at the end of Chap. 11.3, Chap. 12.2, and 13.5.)

2. Overview of Functions

The basal ganglia have three main functions: they enable the brain to implement high-level motor plans, to do so in relation to emotional and motivational drives (in our view), and to scale the amplitudes of the motor efforts in the execution of these tasks. The first two functions largely concern the higher level of the motor hierarchy, while the third belongs to the middle level. The complex loops of the dorsal basal ganglia help shape the motor plans being made in the higher association cortex, and the motor loop scales the execution of the programs that implement overall plans. The basal ganglia might presumably help to *enable* the conversion of need-directed, general aims and the memory of significant events into goal-directed, specific motor action. The term "enabling" denotes facilitation by provision of access rather than triggerlike actions of the sort illustrated for the cerebro-cerebellar circuit for movement initiation (Figs. 12.10A, 13.3, and 13.4). The complex loop automates the execution of overall behavioral motor patterns, which multiplies the number of actions we can undertake simultaneously and in sequence.

The scaling by the motor loop is applied to entire *patterns* of action like the handwriting examples in Figs. 2.6 and 7.1, or complex movements like those in Figs. 7.3 and 7.4, or use of muscle synergies like those in Figs. 9.9 and 9.10. This has been inferred from the retention of normal patterns, but with abnormal amplitudes, for complex motor acts during pallidal dysfunction (Fig. 14.8). The ventral basal ganglia can enable locomotor actions without having to "consult" the cortex, although it is open to cortical access for voluntary motion. These specifications of function are still guesses at the current stage of knowledge.

We begin this overview with some deductions about the caudate circuit, and continue with consideration of the putamen circuit. We follow the reasoning in recent reviews by Marsden, by Anderson, and by DeLong and his associates, based on studies of normal as well as of abnormal functions. What information is processed in the basal ganglia can be glimpsed from the correlates of their neural discharges and from the consequences of local lesions.

Evidence from Neural Discharge Properties

Discharge of neurons in the *striatum* reflects calls for action signaled by their cerebral inputs (Fig. 14.1A). The cerebral cortex, like some other parts of the CNS, emits output signals when they are required for "error" corrections of the controlled system (Figs. 1.4 and 4.11). Neural discharge in the basal ganglia loops seem to reflect the need for corrections of *cortical processing*, based presumably on comparisons of what is intended with what actually occurs at the cortical level. For the complex and motor loops these are the formations, respectively, of higher and middle-level commands. The low rates of

"spontaneous" activity of striatal (input) neurons indicates that these commands concern actions that occur only once or twice a second, that is, that they likely concern whole movements rather than their ongoing corrections. This contrasts with the high-frequency message traffic in the cortex, which deals with the details. In this respect, striatal neurons resemble those of the olivary input to the cerebellum. Unlike the climbing fibers, however, striatal neurons can fire bursts in relation to intended movements that have already been learned rather than firing only during correction when they are being learned (cf. Fig. 13.10). What aspect of the nature and quality of corticocortical processing might be adjusted by the basal ganglia in response to cortical "error" messages?

The most likely parameter adjusted by the dorsal basal ganglia is the *intensity* of selected cortical outputs. These are intensities of complex higher functions for the caudate loop, and intensities of simpler motor functions for the putamen loop. Chapter 2.2 pointed out the difference between "insightful" learning (which can occur in very few trials, based on experience and emotional connotations) and "rote" learning, which accrues by mere repetition. Insightful learning depends on active involvement of the hippocampus and the amygdala, whereas rote learning does not. The higher level has these limbic connections, whereas the sensorimotor cortex obtains them mostly indirectly (Fig. 11.8). Mishkin has proposed that the basal ganglia can support rote learning, which might be implemented by relay of corollary discharges of higher cortical functions through the basal ganglia. It is not known if this depends on interaction with the cerebellum through nonprimary motor cortex (cf. Fig. 11.7).

Our formulation is not far from Marsden's proposal that the basal ganglia enable the "automatic" performance of practiced motor acts, by facilitating the use of motor plans that reside elsewhere in the CNS. The cerebrocerebellar circuit, particularly the dentatorubro-olivary loop and the dentate connections with the premotor cortex, might qualify as suitable generators and distributed residences for such motor memories (see Chap. 13). At the same time, limbic connections might create set-points that indicate when "enough is enough" in terms of limbic drive reduction, which, among other things, could also switch off Ito's proposed internal "attention" mechanism necessary for cerebrocerebellar learning (Fig. 2.8). These ideas are still speculative.

Neural discharges in the *caudate* circuit (including the rostrodorsomedial pallidum, Fig. 14.3) are not uniform because of the preferred projections of association areas to different parts of the caudate nucleus (Fig. 14.5). Some relate to the significance of cues for intended motor acts (e.g., previously experienced visual signals) and thus precede movement preparations, let alone onset. Others relate to the general direction of intended motor acts but are not linked as closely to the movements of individual parts of the body as neurons in the putamen. These properties are appropriate in a neural loop originating from and projecting to high-level association cortex that deals with selective aspects of complex motor acts (Chap. 11.1). Caudate lesions destroy the animals' ability to select cues of previously established significance.

In contrast, the cells in the *putamen* circuit reflect the topographic input from the motor cortex. Studies by DeLong and associates have revealed that most neuronal responses in the putamen of behaviorally trained monkeys relate to simple motor acts. Nearly half of all neurons related to arm movements respond to somatosensory input from the arm, mostly to rotation of joints, singly or in synergic combinations. Passively imposed loads can evoke short-latency static or dynamic responses of graded amplitudes that are directionally selective, that is, the familiar kind for many neurons in motor cortex and cerebellum. This indicates that the putamen re-

ceives a place- and modality-specific somatosensory inputs that may be used to enable and modify ongoing movements. Half of the putamen neurons are related exclusively to the direction of movement and the other half to the force, that is, the level of load that is being maintained. One-quarter combine the two properties. The same two factors also help to determine the discharge of neurons in the motor cortex (Figs. 12.10, and 12.12–12.14), in the ventrolateral (VL) nucleus of the thalamus, and in the lateral cerebellum (Figs. 13.5 and 13.10). Thus coding of these movement properties is distributed in the three main components of the middle level of the motor hierarchy. Coding for muscle patterns, however, occurs only in the cerebrocerebellar circuit and *not* in the basal ganglia.

The basal ganglia are not initiators of motor acts; instead they prepare for them and adjust them. Rather few neurons in the putamen discharge before, and most discharge after, first EMG onset, in contrast to the cerebellocerebral sequence. This has been studied with an arrangement like that in Fig. 7.7D, which combines the capability of testing responses to perturbations (as in Fig. 12.12) with that of dissociating the relations between neural discharge to movement direction and to muscle patterns (as in Fig. 12.13). Figure 14.6 shows the result: neurons in monkeys' putamen discharge in relation to step-tracking movements made with the arm, but most fire later than task-related neurons in cerebellum or motor cortex. A glance back at Fig. 14.3 recalls that the putamen receives its input from the SMA and motorsensory cortex, whose neurons mostly discharge before intended movements. This timing implies that the output from the putamen, and generally of the motor loop of the basal ganglia, is used for adjustments of the next, following movement. This form of updating cortical programs was already suggested in relation to Fig. 2.7.

Neurons in the *globus pallidus* and in

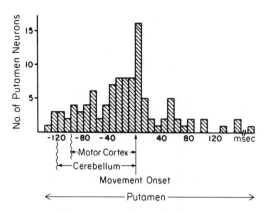

Fig. 14.6. The basal ganglia modify but do not initiate movements. Most putamen neurons discharge *after* the cerebellum and motor cortex have fired (shown in relation to onset of simple, continuous movements made by a monkey in a step-tracking task similar to that in Fig. 12.12A). Compare to Figs. 13.3 and 13.4. (From Crutcher and DeLong, 1984)

the *substantia nigra, pars reticulata* (SNpr) have similar somatotopic, patchy distributions and input–output properties as those of the striatum from which they receive their inputs. Thus, output neurons near one another in the pallidal "patches" relate to active movements of the limb from which sensory (passive) inputs are obtained, which are usually from deep structures. This arrangement resembles that of "efferent zones" in the caudal motor cortex (Fig. 12.4). (Many neurons in SNpr are related to orofacial movements.) Neurons in the pallidum and STN discharge later than those in the motor cortex and the striatum from which they receive their input. Whereas half of the precentral neurons discharge at least 80 msec prior to movement onset, the proportions for GPe and STN are about one-quarter, and for GPi one-tenth. The discharges of most of these neurons during intended movements are modulated in relation to two movement properties: amplitude and direction, particularly the latter. Examples in Fig. 14.7 show that pallidal neurons tend to fire in relation to the direction (and amplitude) of simple step-tracking movements (**M**) rather than to the instructive stimulus (**S**) given to create preparatory motor set for them. As in the putamen, muscle patterns are not a controlled variable. How the controls of amplitude and direction can sum together is depicted in the summary diagram of Fig. 14.8.

Figure 14.2 indicates the projections from the *Substantia Nigra, Pars Compacta* (SNpc) to the neostriatum and from the ventral tegmentum (VTA) to the paleostriatum (nucleus accumbens). Both nigrostriatal lines originate from a relatively small number of neurons with low spontaneous activity that conduct slowly along divergent projections that transmit by means of the inhibitory transmitter DA. These systems are essential for the normal operation of the basal ganglia because their degeneration leads to profound hypokinesia, but they do not transmit specific information of the sort found in the striatopallidal circuit described above. (Chapter 14.1 used the analogy of a power supply in describing the DA support of striatal function.) When tested in behaviorally active monkeys, cellular activity in SNpc relates most to the general level of motor activation rather than to sensory inputs, task cues, or individual muscular acts. Discharge increases during (not before) movements, and may outlast them. Some cells can be activated by appropriate cues for motor action if the waiting period between the cue and the required motor action is less than one second. If the delay in such a task is several seconds, neurons in SNpc can discharge in appropriate as well as in inappropriately made movements. Overall, it appears that *neurons in the SNpc modulate the level of tonic DA release in the striatum.*

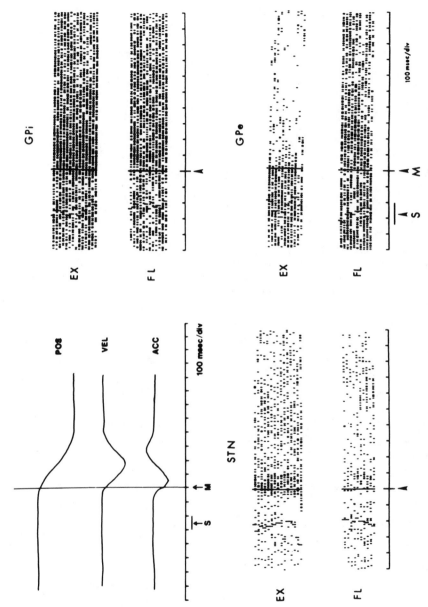

Fig. 14.7. Neurons in the pallidal circuit discharge mostly in relation to the direction of movements (when tested as described in Fig. 14.6). (top left) traces of position (POS), acceleration (ACC), and velocity (VEL), averaged for 10 successive movements that begin at **M**. Appearance of target stimulus, **S**. Horizontal bar = ± 1 SD. Rasters of the activity in single cells in GPe, GPi, and STN during flexions (FL) and extensions (EX) of the elbow. Cell activity differs between the two directions of movement. (From Georgopoulos, DeLong, and Crutcher, 1983; also in DeLong, Alexander, Georgopoulos, and Mitchell, 1984)

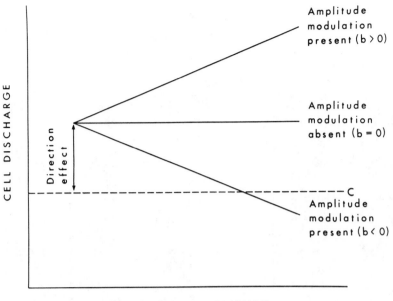

Fig. 14.8. Schematic diagram to illustrate the idea that single-cell discharge levels in the globus pallidus and the subthalamic n. may reflect a movement direction-related step change (indicated by the *vertical arrow*) in addition to movement amplitude-related modulations (*b*). C represents a control baseline. (From Georgopoulos, DeLong, and Crutcher, 1983; also in DeLong, Alexander, Georgopoulos, and Mitchell, 1984)

Evidence from Lesions

Striatal projections inhibit their target neurons in the GP. Since the thalamic nuclei are in turn inhibited by the projections from the GPi and SNpr (VA and VL, Fig. 14.2), the successive inhibitory links disinhibit (i.e., in effect facilitate) the thalamic projections, which excite the ipsilateral motor cortex. The conclusion from unit records is that the globus pallidus facilitates the motor cortex. This fits the cortical disfacilitation produced by pallidal lesions.

Pallidal lesions prolong movement durations of contralateral limbs. Examples are illustrated in Fig. 14.9 for small pallidal lesions made in monkeys trained to depress a lever and then to reach up and press an illuminated button. There is no change in the personal, idiosyncratic habits that each animal uses for its task execution, that is, no change in the order of the sequential, multi-joint movements. Figure 14.9 illustrates how two monkeys each preserved their postural habits and sequences in making reaching movements. Retention of habits implies that the basal ganglia control neither the selection of the object of greatest attention for the central nervous system nor that of its preferred, continuous trajectory (Figs. 7.3 and 7.4). These selections are presumably made as functions of the higher association cortex and are implemented by the cerebrocerebellar circuit. The globus pallidus is, however, involved in the achievement of the chosen reference trajectory by enabling the appropriate supraspinal commands for recruitment of spinal motoneurons. Furthermore, the monkeys take about 50 msec longer to complete the movement patterns during GP dysfunction. This is indicated by the numbers of the movie frames in Fig. 14.9 and by the time courses of EMG buildup for these movements in Fig. 14.10. Reaction time, however, remains essentially normal.

The consequences of pallidal lesions described above can be related to the slowness of movements made by patients with Parkinson's disease. Figure 14.11 shows an example for a patient whose elbow flexions are slowed and of poorly sustained amplitudes. The slow buildup is caused by recruitment of spinal motoneurons that is about 10 times slower than normal. However, there is no change of recruitment order or change of the detailed pattern or timing of alternate use of opposing muscles. Prolonged occurrence of small steps resembles co-contraction. When patients try very hard to speed up, they tend to emit almost synchronous bursts that lead to rapid, brief contractions resembling bursts for ballistic movements of normal subjects (cf. Fig. 1.3). Something akin to the clinical picture, including flexor drift of the affected limb, has been observed in monkeys during reversible dysfunction of the GP produced by local cooling (Fig. 14.12). As in the clinical case, "simple" (no choice) reaction time remains unchanged. (Fig. 14.10).

The *subthalamic nucleus* (STN) controls the output of the entire globus pallidus (GPe and GPi), as well as of SNpr. This control is under the influence of somatotopic projections from motor and premotor cortices and a massive inhibitory feedback from GPe. Neurons in STN have input–output properties comparable to those in the middle-level cortical areas (cf. Fig. 14.7). As might be expected from their connections (Fig. 14.2), they discharge after cortical neurons but before the pallidal ones. The control of GP by STN is a moderating one, because lesions of STN release large involuntary movements in humans and monkeys (hemiballismus, see below in Chap. 14.3). Monkeys also exhibit writhing (choreoid) motions. All forms of these dyskinesias are abolished by subsequent lesions of GP or of its output projections through the motor cortex and the pyramidal tract. It thus appears that *dyskinesias are caused by release of uncontrolled, abnormal output from GPi.* In-

cidentally, note that such GP lesions do not abolish normal, voluntary movements, presumably because the projection from SNpr acts as an adequate backup. The balance between the two components, GPi and SNpr, is signaled to the reticular formation and the thalamus through the nucleus tegmenti pedunculopontinus (PPN, Fig. 14.2).

3. Diseases of the Basal Ganglia

The function of the basal ganglia is degraded by two kinds of diseases, one kind of which produces excessive activity and abnormal involuntary movements. These *dyskinesias* include chorea, hemiballismus, and torsion dystonia. Pallidal lesions produce subtle effects that are visible in be-

Fig. 14.9. Patterns of complex movements are preserved after lesioning the globus pallidus (GP) using the neurotoxin kainic acid. Monkeys were trained to start test sequence by depressing a lever (*hatched*) and then to reach toward, and push, an illuminated button. We see preservation of personal habits in the mode of task execution (A) before and (B) after GP lesions of two monkeys (upper and lower rows) by means of numbered frames from high-speed movies, taken at 10 msec/frame. (From Horak and Anderson, 1984)

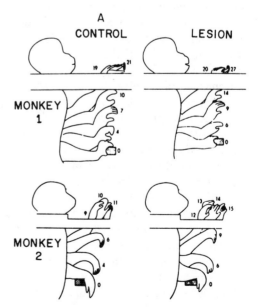

A
CONTROL   LESION

MONKEY 1

MONKEY 2

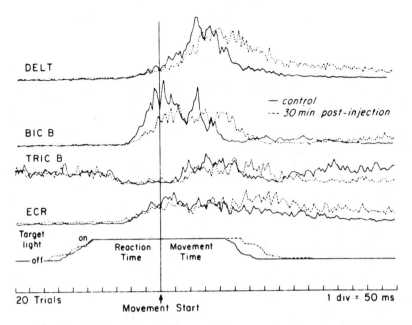

Fig. 14.10. Dysfunction of the globus pallidus prolongs movement time by slowing the buildup of EMG activity. Tests made with a monkey that points at a target light, using shoulder, elbow, and wrist movements as in Fig. 14.9. Reaction time to appearance of target light (bottom line) is not prolonged. Comparison of control EMGs *(solid lines)* and those from trials 30 minutes after microinjection of kainic acid into the globus pallidus *(dotted lines)*. Abbreviations: DELT, anterior deltoid muscle; BIC B, biceps brachii; TRIC C, triceps brachii, ECR, extensor carpi radialis. Averages of 20 traces synchronized on movement start. (From Horak and Anderson, 1984)

haviorally trained animals, but pallidal atrophy in humans produces akinesia, rigidity, and dystonia (abnormal involuntary postures). Involuntary movements are produced not only by striatal lesions, however. Destruction of the STN, which regulates the output of the pallidum (see above), leads to involuntary, often violent, movements of contralateral, proximal limbs (hemiballismus). Destruction of the SN produces irregular (choreiform), or even writhing, distal movements. These imbalanced movements resemble those seen in clinical situations (but not in parkinsonism), thus *dyskinesias are caused by abnormalities of the STN and/or the SN.*

The best known disease is *parkinsonism,* which is characterized primarily by poverty of movement (hypokinesia) and resistance to stretch (rigidity), and secondarily by tremor at rest. The most consistent lesion is degeneration of dopaminergic (DA) neurons in the SNpc and where its axons terminate in the striatum, more so in the putamen than in the caudate. The effects of this deficiency can be counteracted by L-dopa, which passes through the blood–brain barrier. Despite this clinical result, not all the signs of parkinsonism can be explained by dysfunction of the SNpc. For instance, the parkinsonian syndrome can be reproduced by combined destruction of the main outputs of the basal ganglia to the thalamus (i.e., the globus pallidus together with the SNpr), but not either one alone (see Fig. 14.2). The combined destruction (which follows poisoning with carbon disulfide) leads to hypokinesia, incoordinated walking, exaggerated flexor position of the trunk and limbs, and plastic rigidity, cogwheeling, and tremor. The pathological changes in parkinsonism are not restricted to DA paths in the dorsal basal ganglia; DA is

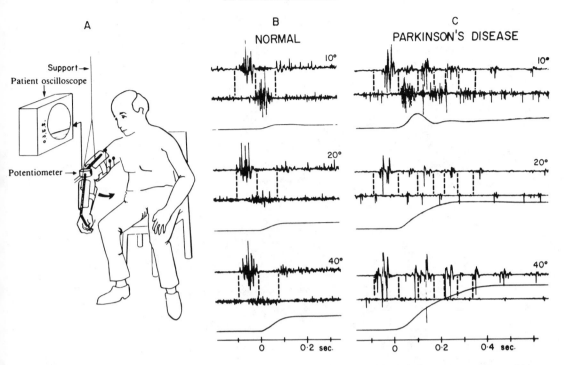

Fig. 14.11 Bradykinesia in Parkinson's disease is caused by the patient's inability to generate agonist EMG bursts of adequate amplitude. In their place there is an excessive number of small bursts that still produce slow movement rise times. (A) Subject grasps a handle to make self-paced horizontal elbow flexions *(horizontal arrow)* as "rapidly and accurately" as possible toward target positions indicated on the "patient oscilloscope." (B) Position and EMG traces of a normal 83-year-old person. Note the usual triphasic EMG pattern of the agonist and antagonist (separated by *vertical broken lines*), as in Fig. 7.5C with a similar task. (C) Traces of a 68-year-old man with Parkinson's disease, showing repeated, weak bursts of both muscles with consequent slow rise time of movements. (From Hallett and Khoshbin, 1980)

also deficient in mesolimbic and mesocortical projections. Damage extends to the nucleus basalis, which projects cholinergically from the basal forebrain to the neocortex, and to the locus ceruleus, which projects noradrenergically to the neocortex and other structures. Loss of these projections causes cerebral atrophy of the kind seen in Alzheimer's disease (cf. Fig. 11.2).

Marsden has pointed out that patients with Parkinson's disease (like patients with cerebellar lesions) suffer no general loss of perceptual intellectual or thought processes. Despite extreme motor difficulties, there often is little or no difficulty in perception, understanding, learning, imagination, thinking, and speech. The senses can be acute, and the memory for special skills need not be impaired. Chapter 2.2 showed that poverty of movement includes degradation of automatic coordination of high-level motor plans, such as loss of the ability to perform two motor tasks simultaneously or to concentrate adequately for stringing together successive acts of a motor performance. In the example of a person standing up and extending the hand to greet a friend, the friend was recognized (a function of "insightful memory" involving the inferotemporal cortex and its caudate projection). The complex function could not be completed, however, because continuity was lost from one phase of the task to the next (e.g., when the patient concentrated on standing

EXTENSIONS

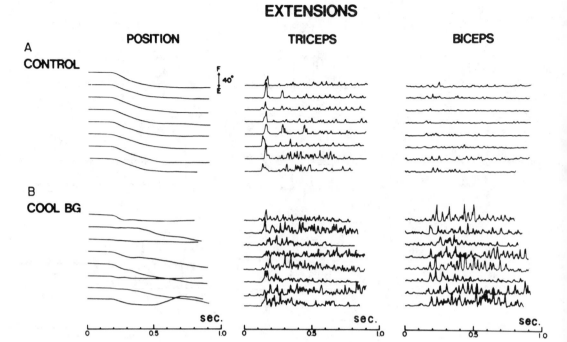

Fig. 14.12. Dysfunction of the globus pallidus can produce co-contraction of opposing muscles. Tests made with a monkey in the step-tracking task situation of Fig. 12.12A. Individual control records (A) are contrasted with records obtained during local cooling of the globus pallidus (B). Note abnormal, prolonged movements in position traces (left), and also that EMGs of triceps and biceps are linked with respect to movement onset. (From Hore and Vilis, 1980)

up, at which point he could not connect to the follow-up, to extending the arm). This is a failure of the prefrontal cortex, because similar defects are caused by lesions of this part of the cortex or of its projection targets in the caudate nucleus (in monkeys). In addition, smooth function of serial motor acts is also interrupted by lesions of the SMA (that receives prefrontal input; Chap. 11.1).

The failure to devote sufficient attention to the management of two simultaneous learned motor tasks (because they cannot be run automatically as before) in practice disrupts the swift continuity of successive components of a complex act. To succeed, they have to be performed very slowly, one after the other. Many, but not all patients with Parkinson's disease, have prolonged ("complex") reaction times in tasks that involve choices such as visual discriminations. They make errors when criteria

change in tasks with alternate possibilities, and inappropriate responses are not corrected well. For instance, patients perform poorly at pursuit- and/or step-tracking, evincing signs of defects in predictive control, which leads to more errors and poorer corrections than with age-matched normal subjects. Patients do not recognize the predictable nature of a pattern that they are following, and even when told they fail to institute predictive tracking patterns. The defect appears to be between the highest level and the motor cortex, that is, in the caudate circuit. As we saw before, it takes the cooperation of all parts of the higher level to establish appropriate motor plans, and all parts of the middle level to convert them into usable motor set (Chap. 11.1 and 11.2). Patients with Parkinson's disease and those with cerebellar problems suffer the consequences of related problems. Parkinsonian patients experience the decomposition of high-level motor plans, and cerebellar patients experience the decomposition of their planned, constituent motor acts (Chap. 13.3 and 13.5).

Normally, efference copies remind appropriate parts of the brain what they should expect. This, for instance, protects the execution of intended movements from undue interference by reflex mechanisms (Chap. 7.4). Conversely, encountering consistent, unexpected sensorimotor consequences requires our brains to recalibrate, for example when the support surfaces for postural support are shifted (Chap. 9.6), or when vision is inverted by prisms (Chap. 13.6), or when we hear the sound of our own speech delayed like an echo. Unlike normal subjects, patients with Parkinson's disease, for instance, do not recalibrate their posture with correctly sized long-loop responses, although they can emit their components, albeit with wrong amplitudes, that is, wrong postural strategies are used (Fig. 9.13). The excessively large M2 responses (Fig. 8.4) bespeak the main abnormality of these patients: alpha MNs are overdriven when long-loop responses are released from the normal, restraining influence of the basal ganglia. There is no distinctive disorder of the fusimotor system; patients' elevated tonic stretch reflexes resemble those of tense, normal subjects who cannot relax (Chap. 8.2).

The preparation for motor acts of parkinsonian patients appears near normal, as judged by the regular occurrence of "readiness" potentials (Fig. 6.1), although they have abnormally long rise times, which would be expected because of lost automatic call-up routines. Patients preserve the use of complex muscle synergies. They can, for instance, co-contract triceps when biceps is used to steady the elbow joint of the supinated forearm, or relax triceps when biceps is used to flex the elbow (cf. Figs. 5.3 and 9.11). They err, however, in the details of their execution. As mentioned above, long-loop responses to per-

turbations are too large, while self-initiated programmed movements are too small (Fig. 14.11). In this connection we recall that the major consequences of nigrostriatal DA loss are in the putamen (i.e., in the "motor" loop).

Altogether, patients fail to make movements automatically, as if something is awry with their programming. Simple motor programs, the components of motor plans, are intact but are used inappropriately. Purdon Martin has shown, for example, that akinetic patients can be assisted to start walking by tilting them sufficiently to initiate the postural support and attitude responses (Chaps. 9.3 and 9.4). Furthermore, they can be made to continue walking by giving them successive visual or auditory cues for each step, as illustrated in Fig. 14.13A,B. The normal walking cycle is not restored by such aids, however, as shown by Forssberg. The steps are larger but they retain their shuffling character (Fig. 14.13C). Normal programs are restored only when the basal ganglia can be made functional again, for instance by reenergizing them with L-dopa therapy, which restores stance and swing phases with an initial knee flexion in early stance (Fig. 14.13C; cf. Fig. 10.2). Forssberg suggests that basal ganglia dysfunction prevents use of adult walking programs, causing patients to return to immature walking patterns (cf. Fig. 10.1). When patients cannot perform motor tasks "automatically," they behave as if the guidance usually provided by internal corollary discharges (Chap. 7.4) cannot be adapted to the abnormally slow and small recruitment of spinal motoneurons.

In summary, patients with Parkinson's disease cannot execute simultaneous or sequential motor programs, indicating a defect in the use of motor plans for complex motor acts, and they cannot emit programs for rapid movements. These dysfunctions suggest that the basal ganglia normally contribute to the automatic use of motor plans. One aspect of this use would be the selective inhibition of mus-

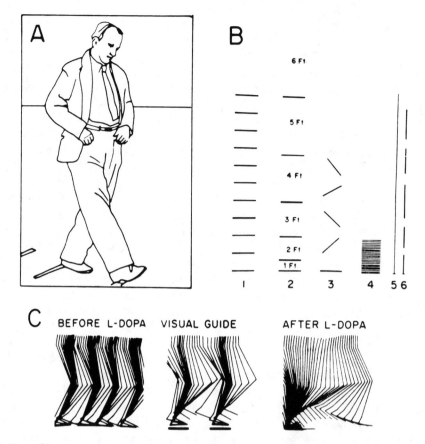

Fig. 14.13. Akinetic patients with Parkinson's disease can walk with visual cues for stepping, although the normal walking cycle is often not restored. (A) An akinetic patient stepping over white stripes on the ground. (B) Cue lines are most effective if spaced at about normal stepping distance (**1**), but can serve up to two to three steps' distance (**2**). Ineffective spacings and orientations in **3** to **6**. (C) Diagrams of parkinsonian shuffling gait before medication (left) with white stripes on the ground (middle), and (right) after medication, which restores use of normal swing phase. [(A, B) Adapted from J. Purdon Martin, 1967; (C) from Forssberg, Johnels, and Steg, 1984]

cles that are called up to form synergies (Fig. 9.9). Since the basal ganglia project to the cortex rather than to the spinal cord, they can be thought of as dealing with, and providing, corollary discharges. Marsden has suggested that this constitutes "a 'write-out' of motor instructions ... for the automatic execution of learned motor plans," and "that as motor skill is learned, the basal ganglia increasingly take over the role of automatically and accurately running the motor plan.... When the basal ganglia are damaged, the patient must revert to employing cortical mechanisms for

motor behavior, but these are more ponderous."

The disruption of continuity in performing learned motor tasks is often first detected on the contralateral side in the early stage of Parkinson's disease. Dependence of task performance on visual cues after unilateral disruption of the pallidum has been reproduced by temporary, experimental dysfunction of GPi. Figure 14.14 shows this disruption of an arm step-tracking task when carried out during cooling of the contralateral GPi (with the experimental arrangements shown in Figs. 1.5,

12.12A and 13.4). The first of two monkeys (Fig. 14.14A) exhibits hypometric movements, prolonged holding periods, and drift toward the flexion position during cooling. The beginnings of the "cool" trace in Fig. 14.14B shows that the second monkey cannot perform the task at all without the visual cues for movements (that is, seeing the positions of the handle cursor on the oscilloscope screen). The animal knows, however, what it is expected to do, as witnessed by repeated hypometric attempts that are occasionally successful. When visual cues are restored (at the arrow: "handle cursor displayed"), motor performance returns to near normal during pallidal dysfunction. This result, which resembles assisted walking of patients in Fig. 14.13, at first glance seems to run counter to the continued performance of a complex reaching task such as that illustrated in Fig. 14.9. The difference may be due to the rapid timing required in the task of Fig. 14.14, which calls for the succession of large movements made at relatively high speeds, followed quickly by maintained muscular efforts for holding in the target. The two components of the

task cannot be put together in normal single-step actions without visual aid because of degraded automatic sequencing at the middle level.

There are still sufficient contradictory laboratory results to preclude coherent statements about reproducing parts of the parkinsonian syndrome reliably by restricted, local lesions. At any rate, no single lesion will suffice. We know that human basal ganglia disease is due to disruption of more than one pathway. Akinesia, rigidity, and tremor each have independent pathological bases. Moreover, the symptoms could be due to abnormal functioning of diseased neurons (rather than to cell loss) that give pathological outputs in response to having lost one (or more) of their several inputs.

Hypokinesia of parkinsonian patients is manifested in various ways. They initiate voluntary movements slowly (bradykinesia; Figs. 14.10 and 14.11) and maintain fixed postures for long periods of time (akinesia). The face presents fixed facial expressions (masked faces), and the arms do not swing during walking. Erect postures are assumed on command, but appro-

Fig. 14.14. Dysfunction of the globus pallidus can destroy the ability to perform a previously learned step-tracking task in the absence of visual guidance. (A) and (B) Tests with two monkeys (in the task situation of Fig. 12.12A, X, Extend; F, flex) moving the elbow to place the forearm into target position indicated on the right in Fig. 14.14, before (left) and during cooling of the globus pallidus (right). The visual display was withdrawn during cooling in (B) and restored at the *arrow* with concurrent, immediate restoration of the ability to carry out the sequential pattern of flexion, holding, extension, and holding of the elbow. (From Hore, Meyer-Lohmann, and Brooks, 1977)

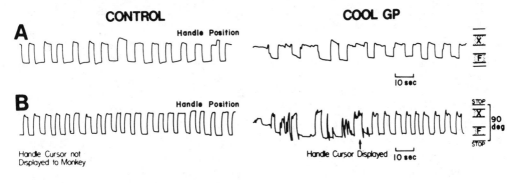

priate postures are not maintained. Reactions to tilt are also abnormal, recalling the role of long-loop responses in both functions, and their abnormally large amplitudes in such patients (Fig. 8.4).

Unilateral lesions of the SN in animals do not produce major changes, but bilateral lesions produce permanent akinesia. More specifically, destruction of the nigrostriatal dopaminergic path (by 6-hydroxydopamine) produces hypokinesia, contralateral neglect, postural asymmetries, and circling toward the lesioned side in experimental animals. [Circling is also produced by lesions of the caudate, but not of the putamen, which leads only to some contralateral neglect that may be due to interference with other ascending dopaminergic (DA) paths.] The conclusion is that *akinesia is produced by destruction, or blockage, of the mesolimbic DA path ascending from the VTA* (Fig. 14.2). Motor activity can be restored, at least partially, by injection of drugs that release DA, such as amphetamine. Injection of DA into the striatum abolishes rigidity, as described above, but not akinesia. The major recipient of the mesolimbic DA projection is the nucleus accumbens, whose injection with DA relieves akinesia but not rigidity.

Also limiting motor activity of parkinsonian patients is *rigidity,* the presence of motor unit activity that would be absent in equivalent normal subjects, even when they try to relax completely (Chap. 8.2). Resistance to stretch is present throughout the full range of movements, irrespective of speed. We saw earlier that such patients have unduly large, saturated long-loop responses. Rigidity can be produced by interfering with the DA metabolism of the striatum, for example by blocking DA receptors or by depleting DA from synaptic endings with reserpine. Since injections of DA into the striatum relieve reserpine-induced rigidity, we conclude that *rigidity is caused by insufficiency of the nigrostriatal DA system, which leads to dysfunction of the putamen, in turn, resulting in abnor-*

mal pallidal output. Not surprisingly, lesions of the pallidum or of its efferent paths abolish this rigidity. A promising new development is the compensation of behavioral disturbances following lesions in the nigrostriatal path by implantation of embryonic SN neurons (which are not rejected by the body).

A highly visible motor defect in Parkinson's disease is *tremor* at rest (static tremor, at 3 to 6 beats/second), which usually first appears between the thumb and forefinger ("pill-rolling") and which disappears when voluntary movements begin. Not all patients exhibit this tremor, however, or its faster, equivalent during maintained postures (6–7 Hz). *Tremor follows the loss of cells in the SN, with consequent depletion of DA in the striatum.* It is exacerbated, for instance, by amine oxidase inhibitors such as harmaline. The tremor reflects some imbalance in the thalamus, since neurons in the posterior part of the nucleus ventralis oralis (posterior part of VL) fire in rhythm with the tremor, and since tremor is abolished by lesions of this part of the thalamus.

This type of tremor can be mimicked in the animal model by combined manipulation of the basal ganglia and the cerebellum. Poirier has produced tremor, associated with hypotonia and/or hypokinesia, by lesions of the rubro-olivocerebellorubral loop in the midbrain tegmentum and pons. This tremor, at 3 to 6 Hz, requires an intact VL nucleus and motor cortex, but it is not abolished by pyramidal lesions (unlike the dyskinesias following damage of the STN). Neurons in the pallidum and its efferent paths, such as VL and motor cortex, discharge in rhythm with the experimental tremor, and do so in self-sustaining oscillations without the need for peripheral input. Tremor and rigidity produced by experimental bilateral tegmental lesions can be abolished by pallidectomy, and the pallidal neurons can be silenced by administration of L-dopa. Tremor thus is not necessarily a consequence of basal ganglia lesions, but instead indicates the additional involvement of the cerebrocerebellar circuit.

4. Summary

The basal ganglia are important for fulfilling intended motor plans. Three *general functions* are proposed: (1) the dorsal basal ganglia are essential for the execution of learned motor acts by scaling the results of corticocortical processing to fit in the context of the task requirements, (2) the ventral basal ganglia provide essential access to midbrain locomotor centers, and (3) the basal ganglia are involved in the conversion of general motor activity into specific, goal-directed motor actions. This conversion is thought to involve both the higher and middle levels of the motor hierarchy, whose transcortical processing is enhanced ("enabled") by the actions of the side-loop circuits through the caudate and putamen, respectively. The extensive cortical connections of these "complex" and "motor" circuits involve the basal ganglia in a wide range of functions. How these circuits interact in integrative function, however, is still unknown. Control by the basal ganglia might involve comparisons of efference copies from successively linked areas of higher association cortex. Similarly, comparisons for the middle level might be made by means of the conveyance of prefrontal outputs to the supplemental motor area (SMA) through transcortical connections and the additional projection to the "motor" side loop of the basal ganglia. In addition, the basal ganglia might compare limbic drives from the hypothalamus and messages ascending through the amygdala with their processed cortical forms that descend from the cingulate gyrus.

Specifically, the basal ganglia are needed (1) for the simultaneous or successive behavioral use of learned motor acts that are usually chained together by cues interpreted at the higher level, and (2) for the smooth integration of programmed movements and postures that make up the learned motor acts. Dysfunction of the basal ganglia decomposes (1) behavior into isolated motor acts, and (2) intended motor acts into movements of inappropriate amplitudes and into postures of inappropriate durations. (In Parkinson's disease, movements are too short and postures too long, while the reverse is true in the dyskinesias that are release phenomena, such as hemiballismus.) Overall motor plans are thus degraded because of the loss of predictive use of high-level cues and of middle-level programs. Yet, there is no loss of sensory acuities, intellectual abilities and awareness, or thought processes.

Inputs to the dorsal basal ganglia arise from all areas of the neocortex, and impinge on the neostriatum (caudate and putamen for the higher and middle-level loops, respectively). Inputs and outputs of the dorsal basal ganglia are organized in two types of parallel, closed loops, one through the association cortex of the higher level and the other through the SMA of the middle level. These loops are separate anatomically, and contain separate component loops.

The basal ganglia modify but do not initiate muscular efforts. Striatal (input) neurons discharge after those in the cerebral cortex from which they receive their inputs. Correspondingly, (output) neurons in the globus pallidus and in the reticulated part of the substantia nigra (SNpr) discharge even later. The outputs close a loop through the VL and VA thalamic nuclei to the cerebral cortex, and through the CM nucleus to the striatum. The cerebral cortex exerts a feedback control on the pallidum through the subthalamic nucleus, whose dysfunction releases uncontrolled pallidal activity (e.g., hemiballismus). Neurons in the putamen and in the connected part of the globus pallidus reflect the properties of the sensorimotor cortex, in that they deal with the intensities and directions of movements. Muscle patterns, however, are only dealt with in the cerebrocerebellar circuit, as are the adaptations of neural connections of the middle level. Neurons in the caudate nucleus mostly reflect the selective actions of the high-level association cortex to highlight significant cues for motor actions. Caudate lesions abolish the ability to make such selections. Activity of the striatum is maintained by dopaminergic (DA) projections from the dense, compact part of the substantia nigra (SNpc) and the ventral tegmentum. Degeneration of this DA path is the most obvious (but not the only) pathology in Parkinson's disease, which is characterized primarily by hypokinesia and rigidity, and secondarily by tremor at rest.

A third loop, through the ventral basal ganglia, traverses the nucleus accumbens of the (paleo) striatum, which receives strong limbic inputs and connects with the midbrain locomotor centers, without looping through the cerebral cortex. The nucleus accumbens is accessible, however, to signals from the middle level and projects to the cingulate gyrus through the dorsomedial nucleus of the thalamus. Lesions of the nucleus accumbens produce akinesia.

References

Alexander, G. E., DeLong, M. R., and Strick, P. L. 1986. Parallel organization of functionally segregated circuits linking basal ganglia and cortex. *Ann. Rev. Neurosci.* 9 (In press). [Fig. 14.5]

Anderson, M. E. 1981. The basal ganglia and movement. In *Motor coordination.* Vol. 5. *Handbook of behavioral neurobiology,* ed. A. L. Towe and E. S. Luschei, pp. 367–399. New York: Plenum Press. [Fig. 14.1]

Anderson, M. E., and Crill, W. E. 1979. The basal ganglia and cerebellum. In *Physiology and biophysics,* eds. T. C. Ruch and H. D. Patton, Vol. 1, pp. 123–156. 20th ed. Philadelphia: W. B. Saunders. [Fig. 14.1]

Carpenter, M. B. 1981. Anatomy of the corpus striatum and brain stem integrating systems. In *Motor control.* Sect. 1, vol. 2. *Handbook of physiology,* ed. V. B. Brooks, pp. 946–995. Bethesda, Md.: American Physiological Society.

Crutcher, M. D., and DeLong, M. R. 1984. Single cell studies of the primate putamen. II. Relations to direction of movement and pattern of muscular activity. *Exp. Brain Res.* 53:244–258. [Fig. 14.6]

DeLong, M. R., Alexander, G. E., Georgopoulos, M. D., Mitchell, S. J., and Richardson, R. T. 1984. Role of basal ganglia in limb movements. *Hum. Neurobiol.* 2:235–244.

DeLong, M. R., and Georgopoulos, A. P. 1981. Motor functions of the basal ganglia. In *Motor control.* Sect. 1, vol. 2. *Handbook of physiology,* ed. V. B. Brooks, pp. 1017–1061. Bethesda, Md.: American Physiological Society. [Figs. 14.2 and 14.4]

DeLong, M. R., Georgopoulos, A. P., and Crutcher, M. D. 1983. Cortico-basal ganglia relations and coding of motor performance. In *Neural coding of motor performance,* eds. J. Massion, J. Paillard, W. Schultz, and M. Wiesendanger. *Exp. Brain Res.* Suppl. 7, pp. 30–40. [Figs. 14.3 and 14.7]

Forssberg, H., Johnels, B., and Steg, G. 1984. Is parkinsonian gait caused by a regression to an immature walking pattern? In *Parkinson-specific motor and mental disorders. Role of the pallidum: pathophysiological, biochemical, and therapeutic aspects.* eds. R. G. Hassler and J. F. Christ, *Adv. Neurol.* 40:375–379. [Fig. 14.13C]

Fuster, J. M. 1981. Prefrontal cortex in motor control. In *Motor control,* Sect. 1, vol. 2. *Handbook of physiology,* ed. V. B. Brooks, pp. 1149–1178. Bethesda, Md.: American Physiological Society.

Georgopoulos, A. P., DeLong, M. R., and Crutcher, M. D. 1983. Relations between parameters of step-tracking movements and single cell discharge in the globus pallidus and subthalamic nucleus of the behaving monkey. *J. Neurosci.* 3:1586–1598. [Figs. 14.7 and 14.8]

Graybiel, A. M., and Ragsdale, C. W., Jr. 1979. Fiber connections of the basal ganglia. In *Development and chemical specificity of neurons,* eds. M. Cuenod, G. W., Kreutzberg, and F. E. Bloom. *Prog. Brain Res.* 51:239–283.

Hallett, M., and Khoshbin, S. 1980. A physiological mechanism of bradykinesia. *Brain* 103:301–314. [Fig. 14.11]

Heimer, L., Switzer, R. D., and Van Hoesen, G. W. 1982. Ventral striatum and ventral pallidum. Components of the motor system? *Trends Neurosci.* 5:83–87.

Horak, F. B., and Anderson, M. E. 1984. Influence of globus pallidus on arm movement in monkeys. I. Effects of kainic acid-induced lesions. *J. Neurophysiol.* 52:290–304. [Figs. 14.9 and 14.10]

Hore, J., Meyer-Lohmann, J., and Brooks, V. B. 1977. Basal ganglia cooling disables learned arm movements of monkeys in the absence of visual guidance. *Science* 195:584–586. [Fig. 14.14]

Hore, J., and Vilis, T. 1980. Arm movement performance during reversible basal ganglia lesions in the monkey. *Exp. Brain Res.* 39:217–228. [Fig. 14.12]

Ito, M. 1984. *The cerebellum and neural control.* New York: Raven Press.

Kemp, J. M., and Powell, T. P. S. 1971. The connexions of the striatum and globus pallidus: synthesis and speculation. *Phil. Trans. R. Soc. London Ser. B.* 262:441–457.

Kitai, S. T. 1981. Electrophysiology of the corpus striatum and brain stem integrating systems. In *Motor control.* Sect. 1, vol. 2. *Handbook of physiology,* ed. V. B. Brooks, pp. 997–1015. Bethesda, Md.: American Physiological Society.

Marsden, C. D. 1984. Motor disorders in basal ganglia disease. *Hum. Neurobiol.* 2:245–250.

Marsden, C. D. 1983. Neurotransmitters and CNS disease: basal ganglia disease. *Lancet* 2:1141–1147.

Martin, J. Purdon. 1967. *The basal ganglia and posture.* London: Pitman. [Fig. 14.13A,B]

Mishkin, M., Malamut, B., and Bachevalier, J. 1984. Memories and habits: two neural systems. In *The neurobiology of learning and memory,* eds. J. L. McGaugh, G. Lynch, and N. M. Weinberger, pp. 65–77. New York: Guilford Press.

Morgenson, G. J., Jones, D. L., and Yim, C. Y. 1980. From motivation to action; functional interface between the limbic system and the motor system. *Prog. Neurobiol.* 14:69–97.

Poirier, L. J., Pechadre, J. C., Larochelle, L., Dankova, J, and Boucher, R. 1975. Stereotaxic lesions and movement disorders in monkeys. In *Primate models of neurological disorders,* eds. B. S. Meldrum and D. C. Marsden. *Adv. Neurol.* 10:5–22.

Rolls, E. T. 1983. The initiation of movements. In *Neural coding of motor performance,* eds. J. Massion, J. Palliard, W. Schultz, and M. Wiesendanger. *Exp. Brain Res.* Suppl. 7, pp. 97–113.

Rolls, E. T. 1981. Processing beyond the inferior temporal visual cortex related to feeding, memory, and striatal function. In *Brain mechanisms of sensation,* eds. Y. Katsuki, R. Norgren, and M. Sato. pp. 241–269. New York: John Wiley & Sons.

Schultz, W., Ruffieux, A., and Aebischer, P. 1983. The activity of pars compacta neurons of the monkey substantia nigra in relation to motor activation. *Exp. Brain Res.* 51:377–387.

Schwab, R. S., and Zieper, I. 1965. Effects of mood, motivation, stress and alertness on the performance in Parkinson's disease. *Psychiatr. Neurol. (Basel)* 150:345–357.

Selemon, L. D., and Goldman-Rakic, P. S. 1985. Longitudinal topography and interdigitation of cortico-striatal projections in the rhesus monkey. *J. Neurosci.* 5:776–794.

Spann, B., and Grofova, I. 1984. Ascending and descending projections of the nucleus tegmenti peduncolopontinus in the rat. *Abstr. Soc. Neurosci.* 10:657. [Fig. 14.2]

Stein, R. B., and Lee, R. G. 1981. Tremor and clonus. In *Motor control.* Sect. 1, vol. 2. *Handbook of physiology,* ed. V. B. Brooks, pp. 325–343. Bethesda, Md.: American Physiological Society.

Author Index

Subject Index